SUCCESS!
for the Critical Care Paramedic

Bryan E. Bledsoe, DO, FACEP, EMT-P
Clinical Professor of Emergency Medicine
University of Nevada School of Medicine
Department of Emergency Medicine
University Medical Center of Southern Nevada
Las Vegas, Nevada

Steven "Kelly" Grayson, NREMT-P, CCEMT-P
Critical Care Transport Paramedic
Acadian Ambulance
Kinder, Louisiana

Katharine P. Rickey, NREMT-P, NH EMS I/C
EMS Educational Consultant – Becker Training Associates, LLC
Barnstead Fire-Rescue / Penacook Rescue
Barnstead, New Hampshire

Brady
is an imprint of
Pearson

Boston   Columbus   Indianapolis   New York   San Francisco   Upper Saddle River
Amsterdam   Cape Town   Dubai   London   Madrid   Milan   Munich   Paris   Montreal   Toronto
Delhi   Mexico City   Sao Paulo   Sydney   Hong Kong   Seoul   Singapore   Taipei   Tokyo

Library of Congress Cataloging-in-Publication Data

Bledsoe, Bryan E.
　Success! for the critical care paramedic / Bryan E. Bledsoe, Steven "Kelly" Grayson, Katharine P. Rickey. — 1st ed.
　　p. ; cm.
　Includes index.
　ISBN-13: 978-0-13-240509-6
　ISBN-10: 0-13-240509-1
　1. Emergency medical technicians—Examinations—Study guides. 2. Critical care medicine—Examinations—Study guides. I. Grayson, Steven Kelly. II. Rickey, Katharine P. III. Title.
　[DNLM: 1. Critical Care—methods—Examination Questions. 2. Emergency Treatment—methods—Examination Questions. 3. Allied Health Personnel—education—Examination Questions. 4. Emergency Medical Services—methods—Examination Questions. WX 18.2 B646s 2010]
　RC86.9.B545 2010
　616.02'5076—dc22

2009023741

Publisher: Julie Levin Alexander
Publisher's Assistant: Regina Bruno
Editor-in-Chief: Marlene McHugh Pratt
Senior Managing Editor for Development: Lois Berlowitz
Editorial Assistant: Jonathan Cheung
Director of Marketing: Karen Allman
Executive Marketing Manager: Katrin Beacom
Marketing Specialist: Michael Sirinides
Marketing Assistant: Judy Noh
Managing Editor for Production: Patrick Walsh

Production Liaison: Faye Gemmellaro
Production Editor: Erika Jordan, Laserwords Maine
Manufacturing Manager: Ilene Sanford
Manufacturing Buyer: Pat Brown
Creative Director: Jayne Conte
Cover Design: Solid State Graphics
Interior Design: Janice Bielawa
Composition: Laserwords, Inc.
Printer/Binder: Hamilton Printing Company
Cover Printer: Lehigh-Phoenix Color Corp.

Many of the designations by manufacturers and sellers to distinguish their products are claimed as trademarks. Where those designations appear in this book, and the publisher was aware of a trademark claim, the designations have been printed in initial caps or all caps.

Notice: The author and the publisher of this book have taken care to make certain that the information given is correct and compatible with the standards generally accepted at the time of publication. Nevertheless, as new information becomes available, changes in treatment and in the use of equipment and procedures become necessary. The reader is advised to carefully consult the instruction and information material included with each piece of equipment or device before administration. Students are warned that the use of any techniques must be authorized by their medical adviser, where appropriate, in accord with local laws and regulations. The publisher disclaims any liability, loss, injury, or damage incurred as a consequence, directly or indirectly, of the use and application of any of the contents of this book.

Copyright © 2010 by Pearson Education, Inc., Upper Saddle River, New Jersey 07458. All rights reserved. Printed in the United States of America. This publication is protected by Copyright, and permission should be obtained from the publisher prior to any prohibited reproduction, storage in a retrieval system, or transmission in any form or by any means, electronic, mechanical, photocopying, recording, or likewise. For information regarding permission(s), write to: Rights and Permissions Department.

Brady
is an imprint of

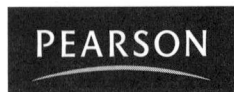

www.bradybooks.com

10 9 8 7 6 5 4 3 2 1
ISBN 13: 978-0-13-240509-6
ISBN 10: 　　0-13-240509-1

Dedication

Thanks to Larry Johnson, Rickey Reed, Donnie Beeson, DO, and the others who stuck their necks out when we started our Critical Care Paramedic program in North Texas. We all took some risks—but it worked!

—BEB

This book is dedicated to my partners, both present and past, who have watched my back, corrected my mistakes, completed my sentences, and occasionally bought me lunch for the past fifteen years. Many thanks.

To my students, who have provided me with inspiration.

And to Richard Pace and Randal Howard, my original EMT instructors—you two set me on this path, and I am forever grateful for it.

To Bryan Bledsoe, friend and mentor and untiring advocate for excellence in EMS—your example is one I strive to emulate.

—SKG

Dedicated to Bryan for all his years of inspiration and guidance, with sincere thanks. My love to my husband and my children for their support, and my gratitude to all the students who have allowed me access to their minds and hearts over these many years

—KPR

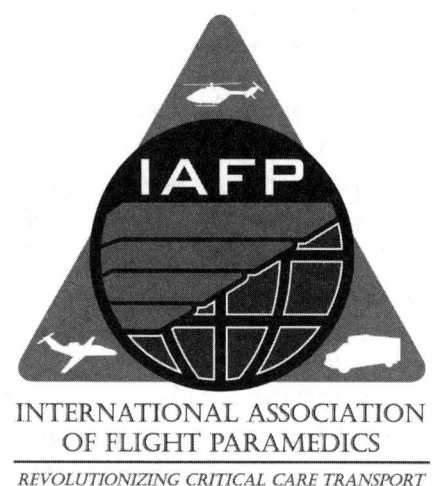

The International Association of Flight Paramedics (IAFP) endorses this review as an adjunct to Brady Publishing's critical care textbook, *Critical Care Paramedic*, by Bryan E. Bledsoe and Randall W. Benner. The International Association of Flight Paramedics supports, through education and EMS professionalism, critical care paramedics practicing in expanded scopes world wide.

Contents

Reviewers / vii
Introduction / ix

1. Introduction to Critical Care Transport / 1
2. Critical Care Ground Transport / 5
3. Critical Care Air Transport / 8
4. Altitude Physiology / 12
5. Flight Safety and Survival / 19
6. Patient Assessment and Preparation for Transport / 27
7. Airway Management and Ventilation / 34
8. The Shock Patient: Assessment and Management / 42
9. Cardiac and Hemodynamic Monitoring / 46
10. ECG Monitoring and Critical Care / 52
11. Critical Care Pharmacology / 64
12. Interpretation of Lab and Basic Diagnostic Tests / 80
13. Introduction to Trauma / 86
14. Neurologic Trauma / 91
15. Thoracic Trauma: Assessment and Management / 100
16. Abdominal and Genitourinary Trauma / 108
17. Face/Ear/Ocular/Neck Trauma / 116
18. Burns and Electrical Injuries / 124
19. Principles of Orthopedic Care / 135
20. Special Patients: Pediatric, Geriatric, and Obstetrical Trauma / 141
21. Pulmonary Emergencies / 150
22. Cardiovascular Emergencies / 162
23. Neurologic Emergencies / 175
24. Gastrointestinal Emergencies / 191
25. Renal and Acid-Base Emergencies / 200
26. Infectious Disease Emergencies / 206
27. Pediatric Medical Emergencies / 219
28. High-Risk Obstetrical/Gynecological Emergencies / 227

29 Neonatal Emergencies / 234
30 Environmental Emergencies / 243
31 Diving Emergencies / 249
32 Toxicological Emergencies / 255
33 Weapons of Mass Destruction / 267
34 Organ Donation and Retrieval / 275
35 Quality Improvement in Critical Care Transport / 279
36 Communications and Documentation / 282
37 The Critical Care Paramedic in the Hospital Environment / 286

Answer Key / 289
Final Review: Practice Examination / 315
Answers for Final Review / 339
Index / 342

Reviewers

We would like to thank the following reviewers for their comments and suggestions, which have been helpful in ensuring the accuracy and clarity of questions.

Randall Benner, MEd, MICP, NREMT-P
Director, Emergency Medical Technology
Youngstown State University
Youngstown, OH

Harvey Conner, AS, NREMT-P
Professor of EMS
Oklahoma City Community College
Oklahoma City, OK

Michael Fisher, NREMT-P, CCP
Program Director, Emergency Medical Technology
Greenville Technical College
Greenville, SC

Russell Griffin
Critical Care Flight Paramedic
CareFlight
Dallas/Fort Worth, TX

James S. Lion, Jr.
Williamsville Fire Department EMS Lt., AEMT-I
Erie County EMS Instructor
Decatur, IL

Brian Petrone, PA-C, EMT-P
Emergency Department
Newton-Wellesley Hospital
Newton, MA

Bobby R. Thomas, NREMT-P
Integrity EMS of Oklahoma
Cassville, MO

Matt Zavarella, MS, RN, NREMT-P, CFRN, CCRN, CEN
LifeFlight
St. Vincent's/Medical University of Ohio
Toledo, OH

Introduction

ABOUT THE SUCCESS! SERIES

SUCCESS! is a complete review system that combines relevant exam-style questions with a self-assessment format to provide you with the best preparation for your exam.

- Build your experience and exam confidence!
- Practice with realistic exam-style questions.

The SUCCESS! program is a complete method for increasing pass rates in many health professions from EMS to Nursing Assisting. We invite you to use our exam preparation system and HAVE SUCCESS!

Prentice Hall's complete SUCCESS! system includes review for the following areas:

Clinical Laboratory Science/ Medical Technology	Massage Therapy
	Medical Assisting
Dental Assisting	Nursing Assisting
Dental Hygiene	Pharmacy Technician
Emergency Medical Services	Phlebotomy
Health Information Management	Surgical Technology

ABOUT SUCCESS! FOR THE CRITICAL CARE PARAMEDIC

Prentice Hall is pleased to present ***SUCCESS! for the Critical Care Paramedic*** as part of a review series on the various EMS education levels. The authoritative text gives you expert help in preparing for certifying examinations.

ABOUT THE BOOK

- **Multiple-choice questions:** This manual has been designed to help you prepare for the written course and certification exams. It can also be used as a review for currently certified EMT-Paramedics. The multiple-choice items are similar to those found on teacher-made exams and certifying exams. Working through these items will help you assess your strengths and weaknesses in each section.
- **Answers:** Correct answers are provided, along with page references from *Critical Care Paramedic* (CCP), *Paramedic Care: Principles and Practice* (PCPP), *Prehospital Emergency Pharmacology* (PEP), and *Anatomy and Physiology for Emergency Care* (AP). These citations offer a more detailed explanation of the answers.

STUDY TIPS

So, you're getting ready for an exam. Congratulations for making it to this point; now let's help you make the next step—doing your best on this exam. Some people find test taking unsettling, while many consider tests unnerving and even scary! Use this book as an opportunity to practice preparation, information review, and exam techniques.

PHYSICAL PREPARATION

The key to maximizing your potential on a test is to be at your personal best. Along with mental preparation, physical preparation should be included in a good study strategy. Physical preparation includes getting adequate rest and exercising. It also includes eating a balanced meal the night before and the morning of the exam. Your brain works best when it has access to a supply of glucose, so fruits, grains, vegetables, and pasta are important foods. Try to avoid caffeine and foods with high sugar content on the morning of the exam. These foods provide a short burst of energy, but when they are used up, the slump will significantly reduce your ability to function.

Try some physical exercise the days before the exam but not to the point of exhaustion. Increasing cardiovascular perfusion will also increase perfusion to the brain. More oxygen circulating in the brain can only be good, right? Exercise is also an outlet for stress, making it easier to get a good night's sleep.

INFORMATION REVIEW

Against popular belief, preparing for the exam should not include extensive studying. You've been studying for months, you know the material, and cramming now will probably cause an intellectual shutdown. Review the material for short periods of time, and take frequent breaks. Try study groups of three to five people for review; the active discussion will be an excellent way to reinforce the material and retain the information.

While knowing the material is essential, physical preparation is equally important. Remember: Review only in brief intervals, use a study group, and don't cram.

TAKING THE EXAMINATION

An exam is not written by happenstance; it's an art and a science. Each time you take an exam it's a chance to evaluate your knowledge, as well as to master the test-taking process. It might seem hard, but exams are generally built to measure *minimum* competency. Certification or recertification exams are usually not designed to test total knowledge, ability to expertly function in the field, or even your level of professionalism. They are an attempt to evaluate your reading comprehension and judgment.

There are three basic kinds of questions found on most certification exams: multiple-choice, true/false, and matching. Each of these question types is built in a specific way to test your ability and your knowledge. Knowing how the questions are constructed may help you during the exam.

Multiple-choice questions consist of two parts: stems and answers. A stem is the actual question part, and the list of answers that follow are called distracters. Distracters are designed to—what else—distract you from the correct response. Multiple-choice questions require you to use knowledge, judgment, and expertise in order to answer the question. *Hint:* Use the process of elimination.

When answering a multiple-choice question, read the question and all of the answers first. Then begin the process of elimination, starting with the most incorrect and sorting your way through until you're left with one or two possible answers. Got a problem picking from those? Then reread the stem. If it would make it easier, rephrase the question, looking for key words that give you a hint about the answer. Don't forget to look at the grammar; is the stem in plural form or singular? Whatever process you use, try not to spend more than 2 minutes on any one question.

You may find a topic is covered in several consecutive questions. In this case, be sure all your answers are similar and seem to fit together. It might be helpful to use the previous answers to validate each new set of choices. Another option is to check the next question because sometimes the answer, or a strong hint to one question, is the stem of the following questions. Remember, when reading multiple-choice responses, the correct answer may be the most comprehensive choice—the one that combines several of the other answers or includes more details.

If the exam contains true/false questions, remember that statements containing absolute terms like *never, always,* and *only* will usually be false. Very little of medicine, or life itself, is absolute. Statements that contain words like *maybe* or *sometimes* tend to be true. These are some hints that may help you when reading true/false questions.

The scientific part of test-building is putting information into questions. The way the questions are put together to evaluate you is an art form. The key is to read each question carefully—try not to scan because you may miss important key words like *incorrect* or *not* that would cause you to waste time or, more important, miss the answer. Be prudent, pace yourself, and use patience, your all-important three "P's."

WRAPPING UP

You've often heard people say to go with your first hunch; well, they're right. Your brain makes immediate connections based on stored information and your experience. Don't be afraid that the answer is wrong just because you didn't go through all the usual steps of logic. Research shows that first impressions tend to be correct.

It's okay to choose the same letter answer two or three times in a row. The answers are put into a question at random so it could be that the same letter shows up as being correct up to five times. Don't change your answer if you have chosen the same letter more than once.

Well, you have done the most you can by participating in class, practicing your skills, and reading your material. You know it all by now so trying to teach yourself the curriculum just won't work and ultimately your patients will suffer. Trust yourself and your abilities. Practice some of the tips in this section as you proceed through this book. In the days before the exam remember to eat well, exercise, and get sleep. Good luck.

Please visit http://www.prenhall.com/success for additional tips on studying, test taking, and other keys to success.

CHAPTER 1

Introduction to Critical Care Transport

DIRECTIONS Each of the questions or incomplete statements below is followed by suggested answers or completions. Select the **one answer** that is best in each case.

1. Critical care paramedics must:
   A. maintain a caring perspective.
   B. preserve human dignity.
   C. provide sophisticated out-of-hospital care.
   D. provide emotional support for the patient.
   E. all of the above.

2. The first report of wounded soldiers being transported from battlefield to surgical care occurred during which of the following wars?
   A. Crimean War
   B. Napoleonic Wars
   C. Spanish-American War
   D. Battle of Vera Cruz
   E. Korean War

3. What year did the Geneva Convention meet and ratify the Geneva Treaty?
   A. 1864
   B. 1901
   C. 1899
   D. 1906
   E. 1900

4. The first use of an ambulance in the United States occurred during which of the following wars?
   A. Revolutionary War
   B. War of 1812
   C. Civil War
   D. World War I
   E. World War II

5. Prehospital advanced life support was first introduced in the late 1950s by which prominent physician?
   A. Dr. Eugene Nagel
   B. Dr. Mickey Eisenberg
   C. Dr. Nancy Caroline
   D. Dr. Peter Baskett
   E. Dr. J. Frank Pantridge

6. Prehospital advanced life support was first introduced in the United States in which city?
   A. Philadelphia
   B. Pittsburgh
   C. Miami
   D. Cincinnati
   E. Seattle

7. Which helicopter operation was the first dedicated exclusively to medical care in the United States?
   A. Maryland State Police (Baltimore)
   B. Ben Taub Hospital (Houston)
   C. Los Angeles Fire Department (Los Angeles)
   D. Parkland Hospital (Dallas)
   E. Saint Anthony's Hospital (Denver)

8. The first reported Intensive Care Unit in the United States was at which of the following hospitals?
   A. Johns Hopkins (Baltimore)
   B. Bellevue Hospital (New York City)
   C. Mayo Clinic (Rochester)
   D. Rampart Hospital (Inglewood)
   E. Charity Hospital (New Orleans)

9. Critical care medicine became a recognized specialty by the American Board of Medical Specialties in what year?
   A. 1996
   B. 1993
   C. 1986
   D. 1983
   E. 1976

10. Critical care paramedics may be employed in which of the following settings?
    A. air ambulance
    B. ground ambulance
    C. hospital intensive care unit
    D. children's hospital pediatric transport
    E. all of the above

11. Critical care paramedics function under whose authority?
    A. Registered Nurse
    B. State Board of Nursing
    C. Licensed Physician
    D. State Board of EMS
    E. State Board of Medical Examiners

12. Which of the following is NOT a professional trait of a critical care paramedic?
    A. sets low goals
    B. earns respect and confidence of colleagues
    C. masters essential skills
    D. critically reviews own performance
    E. checks equipment regularly

13. Rules or standards that govern the conduct of a particular group are referred to as?
    A. Magna Carta
    B. Bill of Rights
    C. Oath of Geneva
    D. Hippocratic Oath
    E. Ethics

14. Which of the following formats can provide continuing education for critical care paramedics?
    A. MTV
    B. "Emergency!" television series reruns
    C. Grand Rounds
    D. A & B
    E. A & C

15. What is the best method for prevention of skills degradation?
    A. periodic refresher training
    B. clinical rotations
    C. periodic skills retesting
    D. frequent use of skills in practice
    E. none of the above

16. The level of ambulance service established by Medicare that calls for ongoing care by one or more health care professionals in an appropriate specialty area is:
    A. paramedic intercept.
    B. specialty care transport.
    C. advanced life support 2.
    D. advanced life support 1.
    E. none of the above.

17. Which of the following board-certified specialists CANNOT be certified in critical care medicine?
    A. internist
    B. anesthesiologist
    C. pediatrician
    D. emergency physician
    E. surgeon

18. The term MASH stands for:
    A. Military Ambulatory Surgical Hospital.
    B. Medical Ambulatory Surgical Hospital.
    C. Military Authorized Surgical Hospital.
    D. Medical Army Surgical Hospital.
    E. Mobile Army Surgical Hospital.

19. The first motorized ambulance was introduced in which United States city?
    A. New York
    B. Cincinnati
    C. Cleveland
    D. Denver
    E. Chicago

20. Which of the following is **NOT** considered a typical critical care paramedic skill?
    A. gastrostomy tube replacement
    B. escharotomy
    C. intraosseous needle placement
    D. continuous waveform capnography
    E. none of the above

CHAPTER 2
Critical Care Ground Transport

DIRECTIONS Each of the questions or incomplete statements below is followed by suggested answers or completions. Select the **one answer** that is best in each case.

1. Which of the following is typically NOT a factor considered in choosing ground-based versus helicopter critical care transport?
   A. weather conditions
   B. patient accessibility
   C. patient acuity
   D. total transfer time, including arrival, departure, and out-of-hospital intervals
   E. none of the above

2. Advantages of helicopter over critical care ground transport include:
   A. speed.
   B. larger patient compartment.
   C. lower cost.
   D. ability to operate in adverse weather conditions.
   E. all of the above.

3. The most common providers of critical care ground transportation are:
   A. for-profit private EMS providers.
   B. third service 911 EMS agencies.
   C. public and private hospitals.
   D. fire department–based EMS.
   E. none of the above.

4. Interfacility critical care ground transport is reimbursed by Medicare as:
   A. specialty care transport.
   B. BLS nonemergency transport.
   C. ALS nonemergency transport.
   D. ALS emergency transport.
   E. none of the above.

5. An interfacility transfer qualifies as specialty care transport when:
   A. the patient requires a level of specialty care beyond the scope of the typical paramedic, such as critical care nursing or respiratory therapy.
   B. more than one crew member is needed to attend the patient.
   C. the patient requires a level of care provided by a specially trained critical care paramedic.
   D. the patient is on a ventilator.
   E. A and C.

6. Medical direction for the critical care paramedic is most commonly provided through:
   A. physician consultation via voice and video satellite links.
   B. on-line medical control via cellular phone or radio communications.
   C. off-line standing orders and protocols.
   D. a physician accompanying the patient during transport.
   E. none of the above.

7. Which of the following is a critical care paramedic skill that is typically beyond the scope of education and training of the paramedic?
   A. transvenous pacing
   B. central venous catheter maintenance and interpretation
   C. invasive hemodynamic monitoring
   D. monitoring and troubleshooting of intra-aortic balloon pumps
   E. all of the above

8. Due to the extra equipment and space needed for most critical care transports, the most common type of ambulance chassis configuration is the:
   A. Type I ambulance.
   B. Type II ambulance.
   C. Type III ambulance.
   D. A and C.
   E. B and C.

9. The critical care paramedic is expected to perform with more autonomy than the typical paramedic due to which of the following factors?
   A. The other members of the critical care transport team usually make patient care decisions and delegate procedures to the critical care paramedic.
   B. The critical care paramedic has a broader knowledge base and skill set and often has to make critical treatment decisions where on-line medical control may not be readily available.
   C. Critical care paramedics are more decisive than typical paramedics.
   D. all of the above
   E. none of the above

10. Specialized equipment found on critical care ground transport units NOT typically carried on paramedic-level ambulances may include:
    A. EKG monitoring equipment.
    B. arterial and central venous catheters and invasive hemodynamic monitors.
    C. airway maintenance equipment such as laryngoscopes and endotracheal tubes.
    D. advanced life support medications.
    E. all of the above.

CHAPTER 3
Critical Care Air Transport

DIRECTIONS: Each of the questions or incomplete statements below is followed by suggested answers or completions. Select the **one answer** that is best in each case.

1. The _____ coordinates the daily operations and plans the strategy and growth of the flight program.
   A. lead medic
   B. medical director
   C. shift supervisor
   D. program director
   E. none of the above

2. The _____ creates and implements medical protocols, coordinates and conducts crew training, and conducts the quality assurance program.
   A. lead medic
   B. medical director
   C. shift supervisor
   D. program director
   E. none of the above

3. Which of the following is NOT typically a responsibility of the program director of the critical care aerial transport program?
   A. planning and implementing the program operating budget
   B. directing marketing and growth strategies
   C. training the flight crews in advanced emergency medical procedures
   D. serving as the representative of the program to hospitals and public entities
   E. none of the above

4. An essential job requirement of the program director of a critical care aerial transport program is:
   A. the ability to pilot any of the aircraft in the fleet.
   B. competence to perform the job duties of any medical crew member.
   C. a degree in business or a high level of business acumen.
   D. a medical degree.
   E. all of the above.

5. The typical duties of the medical director of a critical care aerial transport program include:
   A. creation and implementation of administrative policy.
   B. initial and continuing crew training and education.
   C. conducting disciplinary action toward crew members.
   D. providing on-line consultation and guidance to flight crews in situations not covered under standing orders or protocols.
   E. B and D.

6. The medical director may train the flight crews to perform such procedures as:
   A. surgical airways.
   B. amputations.
   C. opening burr holes to evacuate subdural hematomas.
   D. thoracic escharotomies.
   E. A and D.

7. The most common flight crew configuration for both helicopter and fixed-wing critical care transport is:
   A. two paramedics.
   B. one RN, one paramedic.
   C. one RN, one physician.
   D. one physician, one paramedic.
   E. none of the above.

8. Advantages of the RN/paramedic crew configuration include:
   A. lower cost.
   B. a team with a very broad skill set and knowledge of both in-hospital and prehospital emergency care.
   C. the RN's ability to serve as an intermediary for on-line medical direction and consultation with the medical director.
   D. the RN's ability to perform procedures that are beyond the paramedic's scope of training and education.
   E. none of the above.

9. Which of the following is NOT typically a duty of the flight program communications center?
   A. fielding 911 calls and providing pre-arrival emergency care instructions to callers
   B. gathering and coordinating essential information such as LZ coordinates, ground contact radio frequencies, and other logistical information
   C. coordinating and relaying communication to the receiving facility
   D. following the flight of the aircraft and keeping the flight crew updated with current information such as patient condition, weather, and LZ conditions
   E. none of the above

10. Fixed-wing air transport is most commonly used:
    A. in IFR flight conditions.
    B. when transport distances are well over 100 miles.
    C. for more critically ill patients requiring a large team of caregivers.
    D. when greater speed is needed.
    E. none of the above.

11. Factors to be considered in international fixed-wing transports include:
    A. crew safety in foreign and often unfriendly countries.
    B. obtaining clearance to enter foreign airspace.
    C. ground transport and refueling.
    D. crew rest.
    E. all of the above.

12. The most common mode of air medical transportation in the United States is:
    A. fixed-wing transport.
    B. dirigible transport.
    C. rotor-winged (helicopter) transport.
    D. hovercraft.
    E. none of the above.

13. Scene flights with helicopter air medical transport usually involve:
    A. cardiac arrest victims.
    B. high-acuity cardiac patients.
    C. high-acuity interfacility transports.
    D. trauma victims.
    E. none of the above.

14. Small-airframe rotorcraft are best suited for:
    A. remote geographic locations where long flights require the need to carry a large fuel load.
    B. short, frequent interfacility transports.
    C. remote scene flights that may require transport of two patients in one helicopter.
    D. higher cruising speed.
    E. none of the above.

15. Which of the following is NOT an FAA requirement for rotorcraft operation under visual flight rules (VFR)?
    A. minimum standards for cloud ceiling and horizontal visibility
    B. minimum cruising altitudes
    C. two pilots
    D. minimum surface reference (landmark) recognition requirements
    E. minimum fuel supply requirements

16. FAA regulations setting minimum standards for use of VFR in conjunction with the use of specialized navigation instruments during times of poor visibility or bad weather are known as:
    A. instrument landing system (ILS).
    B. microwave landing system (MLS).
    C. wide area augmentation system (WAAS).
    D. global positioning satellite (GPS) system.
    E. instrument flight rules (IFR).

17. Factors that always favor the choice of rotor-wing air medical transport include:
    A. patients with time-critical illness or injury that require high-level care and minimization of time spent outside the hospital environment.
    B. long transport distances (over 100 miles).
    C. poor weather.
    D. patients with head or chest trauma.
    E. none of the above.

18. Your air-medical transport program is called to do an interfacility transport of a 19-year-old pregnant female from a small community hospital 35 minutes (flight time) away. The tertiary care center (also your flight base) is 90 miles from the community hospital. Your patient is an obese (350-pound) woman who is Gravida 3, Para 1. The woman is in preterm labor at 26 weeks gestational age. Delivery is not imminent. Knowing that your aircraft allows only limited access to the patient's pelvis and lower extremities, and that the tertiary care center has a dedicated NICU ground transport team, your best option would be to:
    A. instruct the physician at the referring hospital to deliver the baby and begin ALS ground transport to the tertiary care center.
    B. coordinate dispatch of the NICU ground transport team to the community hospital.
    C. dispatch your flight crew, with instructions to load the patient into the aircraft backward.
    D. send your flight crew, with instructions to accompany the patient to the tertiary care center in a ground transport unit from the local EMS service.
    E. none of the above.

19. Which of the following might be considered an indication for air medical transport?
    A. patient with isolated closed femur fracture without hemodynamic compromise
    B. patient with multiple penetrating trauma to the chest and abdomen, accompanied by hypotension. The trauma center is 30 minutes away by ground transport, and your flight time to the scene is 25 minutes
    C. patient with Lefort III fracture and airway compromise, and the ground ALS crew does not have the capability to perform RSI or surgical cricothyrotomy
    D. patient with ischemic stroke, 3 hours after symptom onset
    E. none of the above

20. You are flying a patient from the scene of a motor vehicle accident. Ground EMS crews have administered oxygen to the patient, established bilateral large-bore IVs, and packaged the patient on a spine board. The patient has multiple rib fractures over the left anterior chest, slightly diminished breath sounds on the left side, facial fractures, and an open femur fracture. You have secured the airway with an endotracheal tube and begun to package the patient for loading into the aircraft. Which of the following equipment should be readily accessible during the flight?
    A. PASG
    B. Hare traction splint
    C. thoracostomy tray and chest drainage equipment
    D. burn sheets
    E. none of the above

CHAPTER 4

Altitude Physiology

DIRECTIONS: Each of the questions or incomplete statements below is followed by suggested answers or completions. Select the **one answer** that is best in each case.

1. Which of the following layers of the earth's atmosphere is closest to the earth's surface?
   A. stratosphere
   B. mesosphere
   C. terrasphere
   D. thermosphere
   E. troposphere

2. Weather primarily occurs in which layer of the earth's atmosphere?
   A. troposphere
   B. stratosphere
   C. meterosphere
   D. mesosphere
   E. thermosphere

3. Which of the three atmospheric zones CANNOT support life even with 100% oxygen?
   A. physiological zone
   B. pathological zone
   C. pathophysiological zone
   D. physiologically deficient zone
   E. space-equivalent zone

4. Helicopters primarily operate in which of the three atmospheric zones?
   A. pathological zone
   B. physiological zone
   C. space-equivalent zone
   D. physiologically deficient zone
   E. none of the above

5. Armstrong's line can be defined as which of the following?
   A. a line of demarcation between the physiological zone and the space equivalent zone
   B. altitude where the vapor pressure of water is less than the barometric pressure
   C. approximately 63,500 feet
   D. altitude where useful consciousness is lost
   E. point at which gas molecules are converted to plasma

6. The pressure of a gas is measured in which of the following units?
   A. joules
   B. newtons/meter^2
   C. torr
   D. kelvins
   E. kiloPascals

7. Which of the following gases does NOT routinely impact aviation medicine?
   A. nitrogen
   B. carbon dioxide
   C. water vapor
   D. oxygen
   E. hydrogen

8. A gas sample contains four different gases. The partial pressures of these gases are:

   water vapor = 125 mmHg
   nitrogen = 225 mmHg
   xenon = 10 mmHg
   oxygen = "X" mmHg

   The total pressure of the gas sample is 550 mmHg. What is the partial pressure of oxygen in this mixture?
   A. 225 mmHg
   B. 125 mmHg
   C. 350 mmHg
   D. 190 mmHg
   E. 360 mmHg

9. In regard to question 8, what is the percentage of water vapor present in the gas sample?
   A. 39%
   B. 41%
   C. 23%
   D. 2%
   E. 64%

10. The gas law that states that a volume of gas is inversely proportional to the pressure, assuming the temperature remains constant, is:
    A. Dalton's Law.
    B. Charles' Law.
    C. Ideal Gas Law.
    D. Graham's Law.
    E. Boyle's Law.

11. What gas constitutes the majority of the earth's atmosphere?
    A. oxygen
    B. argon
    C. carbon dioxide
    D. nitrogen
    E. hydrogen

12. A gas has a pressure of 76 kPa and a volume of 220 cm^3. If the pressure is increased to 167 kPa, what would the volume be?
    A. 100 cm^3
    B. 78 cm^3
    C. 34 cm^3
    D. 120 cm^3
    E. 26 cm^3

13. A gas at a temperature of 220 K has a volume of 500 cm^3. If the temperature is increased to 300 K, what would the volume be?
    A. 500 cm^3
    B. 650 cm^3
    C. 681 cm^3
    D. 24 cm^3
    E. 381 cm^3

14. In a gas, molecular motion results in which of the following?
    A. plasma
    B. vapor
    C. brownian movement
    D. heat
    E. cold

15. Which gas law states "At equilibrium, the amount of gas dissolved in a given volume of liquid is directly proportional to the partial pressure of that gas above the liquid"?
    A. Graham's Law
    B. Henry's law
    C. Gay-Lussac's Law
    D. Boyle's Law
    E. Dalton's Law

16. The net diffusion rate of a gas across a fluid membrane is proportional to the difference in partial pressure, proportional to the area of the membrane, and inversely proportional to the thickness of the membrane. This is known as:
    A. Avogadro's Law.
    B. Boyle's Law.
    C. Fick's Law.
    D. Charles' Law.
    E. Gay-Lussac's Law.

17. A gas that exactly obeys Charles' Law, Boyle's Law, and Avogadro's Law is referred to as what type of gas?
    A. noble gas
    B. ideal gas
    C. partial gas
    D. theoretical gas
    E. plasma

18. Which of the following is NOT a type of hypoxia?
    A. stagnant hypoxia
    B. anemic hypoxia
    C. chemotoxic hypoxia

D. histotoxic hypoxia

E. hypoxic hypoxia

19. When breathing atmospheric air, compensatory hypoxia begins at approximately which of the following altitudes?
    A. 10,000–15,000 feet
    B. 15,000–20,000 feet
    C. 5,000–10,000 feet
    D. 20,000–23,000 feet
    E. 25,000–30,000 feet

20. Altitude hypoxia is a form of which of the following hypoxia types?
    A. anemic hypoxia
    B. histotoxic hypoxia
    C. hypoxic hypoxia
    D. stagnant hypoxia
    E. none of the above

21. Carbon monoxide poisoning would result in which of the following hypoxia types?
    A. anemic hypoxia
    B. histotoxic hypoxia
    C. hypoxic hypoxia
    D. stagnant hypoxia
    E. none of the above

22. Which of the following is one of the stages of hypoxia?
    A. indifferent stage
    B. compensatory stage
    C. disturbance stage
    D. critical stage
    E. all of the above

23. The amount of time a person is able to perform flight duties in an environment with inadequate oxygen levels is referred to as:
    A. time to functional impairment.
    B. period of useful usefulness.
    C. hypoxic interval.
    D. effective performance time.
    E. effective time to functional impairment.

24. An endotracheal tube cuff holds 4.5 cm^3 of air at sea level with a cuff pressure of 15 cm/H$_2$O. At 18,000 feet the barometric pressure is 380 mmHg. What is the volume of air in the cuff at this altitude?
    A. 13.5 cm^3
    B. 9.0 cm^3
    C. 10.0 cm^3
    D. 4.8 cm^3
    E. 6.75 cm^3

25. Failure of the inner ear space to ventilate upon ascent to altitude is referred to as:
    A. barotitis media.
    B. derous otitis.
    C. otitis media.
    D. myringitis.
    E. labrynthitis.

26. As you descend from altitude, the ambient air has:
    A. less water.
    B. less oxygen.
    C. more water.
    D. less atmospheric pressure.
    E. none of the above.

27. The percentage of air saturated with water is called which of the following?
    A. barometric pressure
    B. dew point
    C. relative humidity
    D. heat index
    E. wind chill index

28. Which of the following factors can adversely impact patient care during flight?
    A. noise
    B. vibration
    C. gravitational forces
    D. all of the above
    E. none of the above

29. The law that states that a body in motion will remain in motion unless acted on by an outside force is:
    A. Sagan's First Law.
    B. Gay-Lussac's Law.
    C. Newton's First Law.
    D. Third Law of Thermodynamics.
    E. Newton's Second Law.

30. A change in speed without a change in direction is referred to as:
    A. centripetal acceleration.
    B. radial acceleration.
    C. angular acceleration.
    D. linear acceleration.
    E. centrifugal acceleration.

31. When a person is accelerated in a foot-first (caudad) manner, in the result is what form gravitational (G) forces?
    A. negative G
    B. positive G
    C. forward G
    D. lateral G
    E. backward G

32. Which of the following effects of acceleration affects humans in flight?
    A. duration
    B. intensity
    C. body area and size
    D. impact direction
    E. all of the above

33. You are transporting a patient with increased intracranial pressure from a closed head injury. As you place the patient into your Cessna Citation jet, which is the best positioning for the patient?
    A. head toward the front
    B. head toward the back
    C. Trendelenburg position
    D. any of the above
    E. none of the above

34. An individual's inability to determine his or her position, altitude, or motion relative to the surface of the earth (or other fixed objects) is called:
    A. pilot vertigo.
    B. labrynthitis.
    C. atmospheric disorientation.
    D. spatial disorientation.
    E. combat fatigue.

35. A helicopter pilot is flying in marginal weather conditions. He believes that his instruments are not functioning properly. This is referred to as:
    A. Type I spatial disorientation.
    B. Type II spatial disorientation.
    C. Type III spatial disorientation.
    D. Type IV spatial disorientation.
    E. none of the above.

36. A helicopter in south Texas experienced a controlled flight into terrain (CFIT), resulting in loss of the aircraft and death of the crew. The NTSB found the following to be factors in the accident:
    - Smoke from fires in Mexico had blown north into Texas.
    - Pilot had minimal IFR time.
    - There were few lights in the area.
    - The pilot was uncomfortable flying at night.

    Which of the following most likely caused the accident?
    A. mechanical failure
    B. instrument failure
    C. spatial disorientation
    D. tail rotor failure
    E. none of the above

37. A disturbance in inner ear equilibrium that causes a person to feel as if he is spinning is called:
    A. déjà vu.
    B. myosotis.

C. labrynthitis.
D. ataxia.
E. vertigo.

38. A flight paramedic develops nausea and dizziness on several occasions when landing at an accident scene where multiple strobe lights are operating. He might be suffering from:
    A. flicker vertigo.
    B. occupational vertigo.
    C. spatial disorientation.
    D. altitude vertigo.
    E. none of the above.

39. A mountain climber ascends Mount Harvard in Colorado. Upon reaching the summit he develops worsening tachycardia, fever, difficulty breathing, orthopnea, and cough. He is most likely suffering which of the following conditions?
    A. acute pulmonary embolism
    B. high-altitude pulmonary edema (HAPE)
    C. pyogenic granuloma
    D. bacterial pneumonia
    E. mediastinitis

40. For the patient presented in question 39, which of the following would NOT be an appropriate treatment?
    A. high-concentration oxygen
    B. removal to a lower altitude
    C. BiPAP
    D. PEEP
    E. empiric antibiotics

41. You are part of a mountain rescue team and have begun treatment of a 23-year-old female with headache, altered mental status, nausea, and dizziness. You suspected high-altitude cerebral edema (HACE). Which of the following is the most important treatment for her condition?
    A. acetazolamide (Diamox)
    B. dexamethasone (Decadron)
    C. BiPAP
    D. CPAP
    E. move to lowest possible altitude

42. High-altitude pulmonary edema, high-altitude cerebral edema, and high-altitude headache (HAPE, HACE, and HAH) are all features of what illness?
    A. Caisson's disease
    B. acute mountain sickness
    C. nitrogen narcosis
    D. hypoxic hypoxia
    E. lateralizing substantia nigra syndrome

43. What is the role of carbonic anhydrase?
    A. enhances the conversion of water and carbon dioxide to carbonic acid
    B. blocks the conversion of pyruvate to lactic acid
    C. enhances the conversion of alcohol to acetic acid
    D. promotes gluconeogenesis
    E. none of the above

44. Which of the following factors affects the rate of accidental cabin decompression?
    A. the volume of the cabin
    B. the size of the opening
    C. the pressure differential
    D. A and C only
    E. all of the above

45. Which of the following does NOT indicate loss of cabin pressurization?
    A. frost on the exterior of windows
    B. fogging
    C. noise
    D. temperature change
    E. presence of flying debris

46. In October 1999, golfer Payne Stewart's Learjet Model 35 crashed in rural South Dakota during a flight from Orlando to Dallas. After the plane failed to make a turn, U.S. Air Force F-16s were dispatched. They found the plane cruising at 45,000 feet with the windows obscured by fog or frost. What was the likely cause of death for the occupants of the plane?
   A. blunt trauma from rapid decompression
   B. hypothermia
   C. blunt trauma from collision with terrain
   D. high-altitude cerebral edema
   E. hypoxia

47. Which of the following does NOT usually result from expansion of a trapped gas?
   A. abdominal pain
   B. ear pain
   C. sinus pain
   D. priapism
   E. toothache

48. Which of the following statements about barodontalgia is FALSE?
   A. Altitude of onset varies between 5,000 and 15,000 feet.
   B. Pain may or may not become more severe as altitude increases.
   C. Pain is usually relieved on descent.
   D. Expansion of gas under dental restorations is the most common cause.
   E. It is invariably associated with some degree of preexisting dental pathology.

49. Which of the following measures will NOT minimize the risks of altitude for flight crews?
   A. being well-rested
   B. avoiding gas-producing foods
   C. avoiding smoking at altitude
   D. using beta agonists routinely on ascent
   E. avoiding flying with an ear infection or "head cold."

50. What is the volume of 1.0 mol of an ideal gas at 2.5 atm of pressure at 0° C (273.15 K)?
   A. 9.0 L
   B. 22.4 L
   C. 11.2 L
   D. 5.3 L
   E. 8.0 L

CHAPTER 5
Flight Safety and Survival

DIRECTIONS Each of the questions or incomplete statements below is followed by suggested answers or completions. Select the **one answer** that is best in each case.

1. The tasks of a flight program safety committee include:
   A. maintaining an open forum.
   B. identifying workplace hazards.
   C. implementing risk reduction programs.
   D. reviewing safety program components.
   E. all of the above.

2. The _____ is an independent federal agency with a mandate to investigate civil aviation accidents in the United States as well as significant accidents involving other modes of transportation.
   A. National Highway Traffic Safety Administration (NHTSA)
   B. National Transportation Safety Board (NTSB)
   C. United States Department of Transportation (USDOT)
   D. Federal Aviation Administration (FAA)
   E. Federal Communications Commission (FCC)

3. The main mission/objective of the Federal Aviation Administration (FAA) includes:
   A. regulation of the aerospace industry.
   B. communications between aircraft.
   C. safety of the aerospace community.
   D. numbering aircraft according to size.
   E. A and C.

4. The term "acceptable risk" is normally considered to be:
   A. an informal group concept.
   B. an employer concept.
   C. an individual concept.
   D. a "risk/benefit" ratio promulgated by insurance carriers.
   E. a qualitative number assigned to a particular mission by the pilot.

5. Safety consciousness includes:
   A. recognizing risk.
   B. understanding risk.
   C. decreasing or eliminating risk.
   D. all of the above.
   E. A and C only.

6. The critical care paramedic should have a good understanding of how flight safety is affected by which four factors?
   A. flight dynamics, weather, mechanical issues, workplace controls
   B. meteorology, aerodynamics, fuel type, in-flight movement
   C. mechanical failures, flight dynamics, weather issues, in-flight movement
   D. acceptable risk, aerodynamics, meteorology, aircraft type
   E. none of the above

7. Which of the following would NOT be required personal protective equipment for medical helicopter work?
   A. eye protection
   B. hearing protection
   C. fire-resistant clothing
   D. helmet
   E. athletic cup

8. The most common rotor-wing aircraft currently used in critical care transport is/are:
   A. the BK-117, Sikorsky S76, and Bell 407.
   B. the Sikorsky D76, Bell 477, and AK-117.
   C. the Bell Jet Ranger.
   D. all of the above.
   E. none of the above.

9. The term "airframe" is normally used to describe the:
   A. size of a fixed-wing aircraft.
   B. length-to-width ratio of an aircraft.
   C. general description of an aircraft type.
   D. height of the aircraft.
   E. none of the above.

10. Concerns about the use of single engine aircraft for medical flight programs are:
    A. catastrophic engine failure will not allow a controlled emergency landing.
    B. smaller payload capability than dual-engine aircraft.
    C. additional fuel tanks limit patient compartment space.
    D. A and B.
    E. A and C.

11. Examples of fixed-wing aircraft used in the transport of critical patients include:
    A. the Learjet 35A and the Sky King 600.
    B. the Learjet 65 and the Sky King 267.
    C. the Beech King 250 and the Learjet 55.
    D. the Beech King Air 200 and the Learjet 35A.
    E. none of the above.

12. A safety issue that occurs more commonly in fixed-wing than in rotor-wing aircraft may be:
    A. loss of balance while standing up in the cabin.
    B. rapid cabin depressurization at altitude.
    C. engine or hydraulic system failure.
    D. gyro systems failure.
    E. all of the above.

13. The _____ is the external body of the aircraft that surrounds the airframe and all its components.
    A. aileron
    B. skin
    C. fuselage
    D. skeleton
    E. none of the above

14. The "tail boom" is the structure extending aft of the airframe that houses the _____, and provides points of fixation for the _____ and _____ stabilizers.
    A. tail rotor, lateral, vertical
    B. tail rotor, forward, aft
    C. blade rotor, horizontal, lateral
    D. tail rotor, horizontal, vertical
    E. top rotor, aft, vertical

15. The smaller vertical rotor blade at the end of the tail boom is called the _____ and compensates for the _____ induced by the turning of the main rotor system.
    A. aft rotor, torque
    B. tail rotor, spin
    C. tail rotor, torque
    D. aft rotor, spin
    E. none of the above

16. The "main rotor system" located above the fuselage produces the _____ and _____ for the aircraft.
    A. lift, thrust
    B. thrust, lateral motion
    C. lift, lateral motion
    D. thrust, lateral motion
    E. none of the above

17. The _____ converts the power from the engines into rotational power.
    A. rotor system
    B. transmission
    C. drive shaft
    D. all of the above
    E. none of the above

18. The act of an airworthy aircraft being inadvertently flown into the ground, water, or some other stationary object without attempt to avert the problem is called a:
    A. mistake.
    B. crash.
    C. controlled flight into terrain.
    D. controlled flight into terra firma.
    E. none of the above.

19. The lever that changes the angle of the main rotor blades, thereby controlling altitude, is called the:
    A. rotor torque control.
    B. cyclic pitch control.
    C. collective pitch control.
    D. rotor attitude control.
    E. cyclic altitude control.

20. The stick that controls the direction and airspeed of the helicopter is called the:
    A. rotor torque control.
    B. collective pitch control.
    C. cyclic altitude control.
    D. rotor attitude control.
    E. cyclic pitch control.

21. The _____ control is the rpm control of the rotor systems. As the rpms increase, causing the rotors to turn quicker, it provides more thrust for flight.
    A. throttle
    B. pitch
    C. altitude
    D. attitude
    E. airspeed

22. The foot pedal system allows the pilot to control the _____ angle of the tail rotor, counteracting the _____ effect of the main rotor and allowing for the _____ of the aircraft.
    A. rotor, pitch, turning
    B. height, lateral, landing
    C. pitch, torque, turning
    D. pitch, torque, landing
    E. pitch, lateral, turning

23. The four kinds of weight that MUST be considered in the loading of the helicopter include the:
    A. empty weight, useful load, gross weight, and maximum gross weight.
    B. gross weight, minimum gross weight, equipment weight, and fuel load.
    C. empty weight, equipment weight, fuel load, and maximum gross weight.
    D. A and C.
    E. none of the above.

24. The term that refers to the weight of the helicopter, including the airframe structure, all fixed equipment, engine fuel, transmission oil, and total hydraulic fluid is:
    A. dead load.
    B. useful load (payload).
    C. empty weight.
    D. gross weight.
    E. maximum gross weight.

25. _____ is the term used to describe the specific weight of the pilot, passengers, and portable medical equipment taken aboard the aircraft for flight.
    A. Dead load
    B. Useful load (payload)
    C. Empty weight
    D. Gross weight
    E. Maximum gross weight

26. It is within the aeromedical provider's control to ensure that each mission is completed as safely as possible. The commonly accepted components of this control area include the pilot safety brief, crew comfort with flights, annual safety training, safe operations, personal safety (fitness standards), personal protective equipment (PPE), and assigned crew member responsibilities. The totality of this concept is also known as:
    A. job description/performance review.
    B. crew resource management.

C. quality assurance.
D. quality improvement.
E. personnel policy and procedures.

27. The _____ not only serves the purpose of maintaining a safe working environment but also facilitates an understanding of normal flight operations and reinforces the constant need for communication between pilot and crew members.
    A. crew preflight meeting
    B. crew safety meeting
    C. employee safety meeting
    D. pilot safety briefing
    E. crew safety briefing

28. Factors that can adversely affect crew comfort level include:
    A. inclement weather conditions.
    B. poor visibility.
    C. unfamiliar or potentially dangerous landing zones.
    D. real or perceived aircraft mechanical issues.
    E. all of the above.

29. An in-depth understanding of helicopter operations, including the use of transponder codes, proper arming and use of the emergency locator transmitter (ELT), and aircraft-specific emergency shutdown procedures, should be included in:
    A. annual safety training.
    B. preflight checks.
    C. postflight checks.
    D. employment interviews.
    E. none of the above.

30. The main rotor system of a helicopter generally consists of:
    A. two to five blades that turn at a range of 290–400 rpm
    B. blades moving as fast as 500 mph
    C. blades that can flex as low as 4 feet from the ground at low rpms
    D. all of the above
    E. none of the above

31. _____ is the airflow produced around the helicopter while the rotor systems are spinning.
    A. Back wash
    B. Rotor wash
    C. Down draft
    D. Up draft
    E. Rotor draft

32. In securing a landing zone (LZ), ground EMS/fire personnel can assist by ensuring that the _____ remains outside of the main rotor system, usually no less than _____ feet from the aircraft, and in direct view of the pilot.
    A. perimeter guard, 100
    B. LZ coordinator, 50
    C. LZ commander, 100
    D. perimeter guard, 50
    E. none of the above

33. Personal safety and fitness standards are the responsibility of the flight crew members. The three main areas the aeromedical community considers critical are:
    A. rest, nutrition, and standardized fitness testing.
    B. rest, physical capability, and nutrition.
    C. rest, physical fitness, and weight.
    D. rest, nutrition, and weight.
    E. rest, weight, and standardized fitness testing.

34. Personal protective equipment (PPE) for flight crews should include, at the least:
    A. helmets and hearing protection.
    B. fire-resistant clothing.
    C. protective footwear and eye protection.
    D. A and B.
    E. all of the above.

35. Preflight procedures are the tasks that should be completed prior to each mission that will ensure the highest degree of safety for flight is being maintained. These procedures should include looking for debris on the ground as well as:
    A. checking "cords, covers, and cowlings."
    B. securing interior portable equipment for flight.
    C. donning protective equipment and checking communications headset.
    D. all of the above.
    E. B and C.

36. The "sterile cockpit" is an FAA regulation that necessitates all nonessential communication be ceased during critical phases of flight. Critical phases include:
    A. lift off, taxiing, and landing.
    B. preflight, take off, and landing.
    C. preflight, landing, and postflight.
    D. lift off, landing, and hanger storage.
    E. preflight, lift off, and landing.

37. The only time the FAA permits violation of the "sterile cockpit" regulation is when:
    A. the crew needs to talk to the pilot about an equipment failure.
    B. the patient takes a turn for the worse.
    C. the crew identifies a safety concern to themselves or the aircraft.
    D. all of the above.
    E. A and C.

38. The use of seatbelts and shoulder harnesses, plugging in to the internal communication system, and scanning airspace are examples of:
    A. preflight duties.
    B. in-flight duties.
    C. postflight duties.
    D. maintenance duties.
    E. none of the above.

39. The "clock method" assumes that the nose of the aircraft is oriented to the _____ position, _____ is the left side, _____ is the right side, and _____ is the rear of the aircraft.
    A. 12 o'clock, 3 o'clock, 6 o'clock, 9 o'clock
    B. 6 o'clock, 9 o'clock, 3 o'clock, 12 o'clock
    C. 12 o'clock, 9 o'clock, 6 o'clock, 3 o'clock
    D. 12 o'clock, 9 o'clock, 3 o'clock, 6 o'clock
    E. 6 o'clock, 3 o'clock, 9 o'clock, 12 o'clock

40. You indicate to the pilot that an aircraft is approaching from the "7 o'clock high position." This description tells your pilot the encroaching aircraft is physically located:
    A. directly to the right of your aircraft.
    B. directly to the left of your aircraft.
    C. to the left rear and below your aircraft.
    D. to the right rear and above your aircraft.
    E. to the left rear and above your aircraft.

41. Ensuring that the patient and portable equipment are well secured, that the flight crew is secure in their safety harnesses, and that the crew is plugged in are all considered part of the:
    A. preflight duties.
    B. in-flight duties.
    C. postflight duties.
    D. general patient care procedures.
    E. employee safety policies and procedures.

42. On final approach, the rotor-wing pilot will do a "fly around" and ask the crew to assist in identifying _____ prior to final approach.
    A. uneven terrain, trees, and ground vehicles
    B. radio/electrical towers, wires, and ground personnel

C. loose articles on the ground
D. all of the above
E. A and B

43. If time is pressing and their assistance at the scene is needed immediately, the crew may have to exit the rotor-wing craft:
   A. before the aircraft has fully touched down.
   B. while the aircraft is still running.
   C. before the doors have been fully opened.
   D. without bringing portable equipment along.
   E. none of the above.

44. An in-flight emergency involves an emergency with the _____, rather than the _____.
   A. electrical system, engine
   B. patient, aircraft
   C. aircraft, patient
   D. crew, patient
   E. patient, crew

45. Controlled flight into terrain (CFIT) most often happens during take-off or landing and may involve:
   A. pilot fatigue.
   B. loss of situational awareness.
   C. loss of visual landmarks.
   D. sudden meteorological changes.
   E. all of the above.

46. A rotor-wing pilot may perform an "autorotation" procedure in order to safely land an aircraft experiencing:
   A. complete engine/turbine failure.
   B. mechanical failure of the stick.
   C. electrical failure of the instrument panel.
   D. failure of one or more stabilizers.
   E. failure of the instrument landing computer.

47. A problem may occur to the heating/cooling systems of the aircraft, allowing smoke or fumes to accumulate in the patient compartment. After notifying the pilot of the problem, the attending crew should:
   A. vent the cabin by opening the sliding windows.
   B. unplug all electrical monitoring devices and use battery packs.
   C. make plans for an emergency landing.
   D. all of the above.
   E. A and C.

48. Familiarity with emergency procedures and exit routes from the aircraft, as well as the use of fire extinguishers, the _____ device, and emergency communications such as the _____ should be included in annual safety training programs.
   A. emergency locator transmitter (ELT), CALFON Codes
   B. emergency transmitter locator (ETL), FALCON Codes
   C. emergency locator transmitter (ELT), FALCON Codes
   D. emergency transmitter locator (ETL), NAFCON Codes
   E. none of the above

49. In the event of a crash wherein the pilot is incapacitated, the critical care paramedic should know how to shut off the _____ to reduce the chance for a fire following impact.
   A. rotors, fuel supply, and electrical system
   B. engines, fuel supply, and main batteries
   C. rotors, engines, and main batteries
   D. fuel supply, electrical system, and engines
   E. engines, rotors, and fuel system

50. A device mounted to the aircraft that will automatically emit a distress radio signal upon impact of the aircraft is known as a/an _____ and is designed to automatically activate in an impact exceeding 4 G.
    A. emergency locator transmitter (ELT)
    B. emergency transmitter locator (ETL)
    C. emergency locator (EL)
    D. emergency transmitter (ET)
    E. black box

51. Post-accident emergency duties include:
    A. meeting with surviving crew members at the designated location.
    B. attempting rescue of anyone still trapped in the aircraft.
    C. assessing each other's injuries and performing initial stabilization.
    D. salvaging medical supplies that are still usable from the aircraft.
    E. all of the above.

52. _____, _____, and uncertainty can combine to undermine attempts at crew survival should an aircraft accident occur in a remote location.
    A. Fear, anger
    B. Fear, isolation
    C. Isolation, anger
    D. Anger, exposure
    E. Exposure, fear

53. Most survival kits include basic medical supplies, high-energy foods, tablets for potable water, waterproof matches, space blankets, and signaling devices (e.g., flare gun, signaling mirror). Of the following, which could also aid in survival?
    1. fuselage, wings, and stabilizers (wind break, shelter, signal panels)
    2. fuselage, cowlings, and doors (signal panels, collect water, fire pit)
    3. upholstered seats (insulation, cushions for sleeping, fire material)
    4. intact engine batteries (illumination, signaling, communication)
    5. fuel and insulation (fire, warmth, signaling)
    A. 1, 2, 3, and 5
    B. 1, 2, 4, and 5
    C. 1, 2, and 3
    D. 1, 2, and 5
    E. all of the above

54. _____ states that a person can survive 3 minutes without oxygen, 3 hours in extreme weather without shelter, 3 days without water, and 3 weeks without food.
    A. The NTSB
    B. The FAA
    C. The Wilderness Medical Guide
    D. The "rule of threes"
    E. The Wilderness Survival Guide

55. Geographical location influences specific training regarding crew survival. Crews should take flight paths into consideration when considering the immediate need for:
    A. personal flotation devices and water collection techniques.
    B. protective equipment/shelters for heat and cold weather environments.
    C. sunscreen, gloves, and personal electronic devices.
    D. all of the above.
    E. A and B.

56. Safety:
    A. is the employer's responsibility.
    B. is a minor part of flight crew training.
    C. begins before the flight and precedes all actions.
    D. A and B.
    E. A and C.

CHAPTER 6

Patient Assessment and Preparation for Transport

DIRECTIONS Each of the questions or incomplete statements below is followed by suggested answers or completions. Select the **one answer** that is best in each case.

1. Assessment criteria utilized by the critical care paramedic that are NOT typically used in the prehospital environment may be based on information obtained from:
   A. other prehospital providers.
   B. the patient.
   C. the patient's family.
   D. laboratory diagnostic tests.
   E. a physical examination of the patient.

2. Prearrival information that may assist the critical care paramedic in formulating an assessment and management plan may include:
   A. transport destination.
   B. history of present illness.
   C. insurance information.
   D. patient demographic information.
   E. names of referring and accepting physicians.

3. Which of the following is NOT a reason for selecting critical care transport?
   A. The patient has a central venous catheter and a tracheostomy, is not ventilator-dependent, and is being transferred from an intensive care unit to a long-term skilled nursing facility.
   B. The patient is at a remote location or still entrapped, and the speed of rotor-wing air medical transport would benefit the patient.
   C. The patient is at one medical facility and requires transport to a tertiary care center for more extensive/advanced care.
   D. The patient is being transferred to another facility for economic or insurance reasons and requires specialty care during transport.
   E. none of the above

4. You are called to a rural hospital to transport a patient to a tertiary care center 50 miles away for emergency angioplasty. You arrive to find the patient intubated, being manually ventilated with a BVM device, and with intravenous infusions of both nitroglycerin and heparin in place. The patient is bradycardic and hypotensive with a blood pressure of 64/20, and further examination reveals jugular venous distension and bibasilar rales evident upon auscultation of lung sounds. The Emergency Department (ED) physician seems anxious for you to leave with the patient and finally orders you to package the patient and transport him without providing further intervention. Which of the following is the best course of action for you to take?
   A. Ignore the physician and continue your assessment and treatment plan.
   B. Discontinue the nitroglycerin infusion and attempt to stabilize the patient's blood pressure.
   C. Transport the patient as directed and report the referring physician for an EMTALA violation.
   D. Attempt to explain to the ED physician that the patient needs further stabilization prior to transport, and that you will initiate transport as soon as he takes appropriate interventions to stabilize the patient's heart rate and blood pressure.
   E. Refuse the transport, citing EMTALA regulations that require the referring hospital to stabilize the patient for transport.

5. Of the following, which is most likely to give the critical care paramedic clues as to what further interventions may be required during transport?
   A. history of present illness
   B. reason for transport

C. current interventions and response to treatment
   D. patient allergies
   E. none of the above

6. Your flight team is called to a community hospital to transport a critical burn patient to the regional burn center. Your patient has second- and third-degree burns over 40% of his body surface, including burns to the face and throat. Physical examination reveals sooty nasal passages and stridorous respirations. Current interventions are high-flow humidified oxygen via mask, bilateral large-bore IVs on rapid infusers, and IV analgesia. Concerned with the patient's airway status and potential for deterioration during the expected transport time, you elect to perform rapid sequence induction (RSI) and intubate the patient prior to packaging for transport. This is an example of:
   A. overly aggressive treatment on your part.
   B. exceeding your scope of practice as a critical care paramedic.
   C. preplanning and anticipating needed interventions.
   D. something the community hospital should have done prior to your arrival.
   E. none of the above.

7. Stability for transport is best determined by:
   A. history of present illness.
   B. reason for transport.
   C. current interventions and response to treatment.
   D. current physiological status of the patient.
   E. all of the above.

8. The scene size-up for the critical care paramedic is much like that used in the prehospital setting and includes:
   A. the initial assessment.
   B. evaluating the need for additional resources.
   C. forming a general impression.
   D. initiating life-saving interventions.
   E. all of the above.

9. You arrive at a community hospital to transport an 8-year-old boy to a pediatric tertiary care center. The child fell through the ice while skating on a local lake and was resuscitated in the Emergency Department after a prolonged (30-minute) submersion. Upon your arrival, you find the room crowded with three members of the boy's family, the physician, two nurses, a respiratory therapist, a radiology technician, the hospital pharmacist, and the unit clerk. You quietly ask the physician to ask nonessential team members and all but one family member to leave the room while you assess the patient. This is an example of:
   A. controlling the scene.
   B. overstepping your bounds as a critical care paramedic.
   C. an initial assessment.
   D. determining mechanism of injury.
   E. none of the above.

10. A brief physical examination designed to rapidly detect and manage immediate threats to airway, breathing, and circulatory function is:
    A. the rapid trauma assessment.
    B. the ongoing assessment.
    C. the detailed physical examination.
    D. the initial assessment.
    E. none of the above.

11. The first step of an initial assessment that includes a report of mechanism of injury/nature of illness (MOI/NOI) from EMS personnel on the scene and a visual assessment of the patient is known as a/an:
    A. "sick or not sick" determination.
    B. ongoing assessment.
    C. priority determination.
    D. general impression.
    E. none of the above.

12. One of the first clues that may indicate a high-priority patient in need of rapid intervention and support of airway, breathing, and circulation is:
    A. absent breath sounds.
    B. hypotension.
    C. acute alteration in mental status.
    D. metabolic acidosis as indicated on the arterial blood gas (ABG) report.
    E. none of the above.

13. The general sequence of airway intervention is:
    A. general impression of mental status and airway patency, manual positioning, suctioning, BLS adjuncts, endotracheal intubation or Combitube, surgical or needle cricothyrotomy.
    B. lung auscultation, review of diagnostic imaging, suctioning, BLS adjuncts, Combitube, endotracheal intubation, surgical or needle cricothyrotomy.
    C. review of arterial blood gas values, pulse oximetry, manual positioning, endotracheal intubation, Combitube, surgical or needle cricothyrotomy.
    D. general impression of mental status and airway patency, manual positioning, BLS adjuncts, suctioning, endotracheal intubation or Combitube, surgical or needle cricothyrotomy.
    E. none of the above.

14. The most important parameter to assess in initially determining adequacy of ventilation is:
    A. respiratory rate.
    B. tidal volume and alveolar ventilation.
    C. pulse oximetry.
    D. capnography waveform interpretation.
    E. none of the above.

15. The goal in reviewing circulatory and cardiovascular status prior to transport is:
    A. to determine if the patient is actually sick enough to require critical care transport.
    B. to assure the critical care paramedic that the patient has normal vital signs.
    C. to allow the critical care paramedic the opportunity to minimize potential complications during transport.
    D. to make sure that the referring physician hasn't missed anything.
    E. none of the above.

16. Cardiovascular findings that indicate the need for further stabilizing interventions prior to transport include:
    A. internal bleeding.
    B. lethal prearrest or arrest arrhythmia.
    C. airway stridor.
    D. significantly altered perfusion status.
    E. B and D.

17. For the purposes of critical care transport, high-priority patients can simply be defined as those with:
    A. loss of, or significant deficits in, mental status, airway, breathing, and circulation.
    B. multiple long bone fractures.
    C. critical burns.
    D. injuries from motor vehicle accidents in which one or more vehicle occupants were killed.
    E. internal injuries.

18. The purpose of the rapid physical examination is:
    A. to identify all injuries.
    B. to discover the injuries and physiological conditions that may have contributed to the deficits in airway, breathing, or circulation that were discovered and treated in the initial assessment.

C. to find and treat external hemorrhage.
D. basically the same as the detailed physical examination.
E. none of the above.

19. The purpose of the _____ assessment is to discover if threats to airway, breathing, and circulation are present, and the purpose of the _____ physical examination is to discover why there are deficits to airway, breathing, and circulation.
    A. initial, rapid
    B. rapid, ongoing
    C. rapid, initial
    D. initial, detailed
    E. detailed, ongoing

20. While the critical care paramedic is conducting the rapid physical examination, the other members of the transport team should be:
    A. standing on the other side of the bed, doing the same thing.
    B. copying the patient's medical chart.
    C. making the patient ready for transport by, for example, preparing the cot and replacing the hospital's equipment with the critical care team's portable equipment.
    D. getting consent forms signed by the patient's family.
    E. none of the above.

21. The purpose of the detailed physical examination is to:
    A. identify any non-life-threatening injuries or physiological abnormalities.
    B. ensure that no life-threatening conditions were overlooked in the initial assessment and rapid physical examination.
    C. ensure the adequacy of initial interventions.
    D. review exam findings and diagnostic test results to ensure the accuracy of the diagnosis and treatment plan.
    E. all of the above.

22. Assessment of the head and neck conducted during the detailed physical exam that is not typically done during a rapid physical examination may include:
    A. palpating for facial fractures and skull fractures.
    B. symmetry of pupils and response to light.
    C. examination of the ears with an otoscope.
    D. palpation of the neck for cervical crepitus or deformities.
    E. assessing airway patency and/or endotracheal tube depth.

23. Assessment of the thorax conducted during the detailed physical exam that is not typically done during a rapid physical examination may include:
    A. inspection, auscultation, palpation and percussion of the chest.
    B. assessment of adequacy of ventilation.
    C. review of chest X-ray films for hemothoraces, pneumothoraces, mediastinal trauma, rib fractures, and endotracheal tube placement.
    D. auscultation for normal or abnormal heart tones.
    E. all of the above.

24. Assessment of the abdomen conducted during the detailed physical exam that is not typically done during a rapid physical examination may include:
    A. inspection for signs of retroperitoneal bleeding such as Grey Turner's sign.
    B. assessment of proper placement of the nasogastric or orogastric (NG or OG) tube.
    C. assessment of bowel sounds.
    D. review of abdominal X-rays.
    E. all of the above.

25. During the detailed physical examination of a patient with a Foley catheter in place, the critical care paramedic should:
    A. immediately empty full drainage bags to minimize the possibility of leakage during transport.
    B. inspect the contents of the drainage bag for color, clarity, and volume.
    C. remove the Foley catheter if gross hematuria is present.
    D. send any dark or cloudy urine to the laboratory for analysis before transport.
    E. all of the above.

26. When assessing the extremities and posterior surface during the detailed physical examination, the critical care paramedic should:
    A. ensure the patency of all peripheral and central IV lines, aspirating and flushing each if necessary.
    B. assess distal perfusion and motor and sensory function in all extremities.
    C. ensure the proper placement of any splinting devices already in place.
    D. gently palpate for crepitus, deformity or areas of warmth.
    E. all of the above.

27. According to EMTALA/COBRA guidelines, which of the following is NOT considered documentation required prior to initiating transport?
    A. physician certification stating that the risks of the transport do not outweigh the expected benefits
    B. written request for transport and/or patient consent to transport
    C. precertification from the patient's insurance company
    D. advanced acceptance by the receiving hospital, including name of the accepting physician
    E. copies of all medical records, diagnostic tests, or X-rays, unless the delay in providing them may jeopardize the patient

28. Patient packaging prior to transport may include:
    A. placement of a cervical collar on intubated patients, thus minimizing head movement and the chance of tube dislodgement.
    B. placement of a chest tube and chest drainage device.
    C. "bundling" of all cords, tubes, and leads that may snag on parts of the aircraft or ground transport unit.
    D. endotracheal intubation of the patient, "just in case."
    E. A and C.

29. In dealing with a patient's family members prior to transport, the critical care paramedic should:
    A. delay transport long enough to allow all family members to say goodbye to the patient.
    B. brief any family members accompanying the patient on safety procedures and the behavior expected of them during transport.
    C. assure the family that the patient will be fine.
    D. give the family a copy of the patient's chart, along with a detailed map to the destination.
    E. all of the above.

30. Family members following the critical care ground transport unit to the receiving hospital should be:
    A. instructed to follow the transport unit as closely as possible to avoid getting lost.
    B. given a detailed map to the receiving facility.
    C. given a portable radio so they can receive updates on patient condition during transport.
    D. encouraged to accompany the patient in the transport unit if possible, especially if there is a possibility that the patient will not survive the transport.
    E. towed behind the ambulance using a suitable chain or rope while listening to Bob Dylan's "Knocking on Heaven's Door."

CHAPTER 7
Airway Management and Ventilation

DIRECTIONS Each of the questions or incomplete statements below is followed by suggested answers or completions. Select the **one answer** that is best in each case.

1. What is the most important critical care paramedic skill?
   A. airway management
   B. patient assessment
   C. CPR
   D. IV line placement
   E. rapid transport

2. Which of the following is NOT a laryngeal cartilage?
   A. epiglottal cartilage
   B. cuneiform cartilage
   C. arytenoid cartilage
   D. corniculate cartilage
   E. none of the above

3. Which of the following cells produce surfactant?
   A. septal cells
   B. alveolar macrophages
   C. ciliated columnar epithelial cells
   D. goblet cells
   E. none of the above

4. Each lung contains approximately how many alveoli?
   A. 150,000
   B. 15,000
   C. 1,500,000
   D. 15,000,000
   E. 150,000,000

5. Which of the lungs contains three lobes?
   A. left
   B. right
   C. both
   D. neither
   E. none of the above

6. As compliance increases, which of the following occurs?
   A. The lungs become easier to ventilate.
   B. Energy demand increases.
   C. Lung elasticity is less.
   D. B and C
   E. A and C

7. Which of the following is the formula for alveolar minute volume?
   A. $V_T - V_D$
   B. $V_T \times$ respiratory rate
   C. $(V_T - V_D) \times$ respiratory rate
   D. $V_A \times$ respiratory rate
   E. C and D

8. Carbon dioxide is primarily transported by which of the following methods?
   A. bound to hemoglobin
   B. dissolved in plasma
   C. converted to carbonic acid
   D. bound to chromatin in neutrophils
   E. none of the above

9. Oxygen is primarily transported by which of the following methods?
   A. bound to hemoglobin
   B. dissolved in plasma
   C. converted to carbonic acid
   D. bound to chromatin in neutrophils
   E. none of the above

10. The respiratory rhythmicity center is located in which portion of the brain?
    A. pons
    B. cerebellum
    C. thalamus
    D. medulla oblongata
    E. hypothalamus

11. The reflex that prevents hyperexpansion of the lungs is known as:
    A. Cushing's reflex.
    B. carcinoid reflex.
    C. Hering-Breuer reflex.
    D. Frank-Starling reflex.
    E. none of the above.

12. Respiratory rate can be affected by activation of centers in the brain associated with which of the following?
    A. sexual arousal
    B. eating
    C. rage
    D. A and C
    E. A, B and C

13. A proprietary laryngoscope blade that features an optical system that refracts light 20 degrees from horizontal is:
    A. Grandview™.
    B. Viewmax™.
    C. Grandmax™.
    D. Welch-Allyn™.
    E. none of the above.

14. Arrange the following airway management techniques from least frequently used to most frequently used.
    1. rescue airways
    2. basic mechanical airways
    3. basic airway maneuvers
    4. surgical airways
    5. endotracheal intubation

    A. 3, 2, 5, 1, 4
    B. 3, 4, 2, 1, 5
    C. 4, 1, 5, 2, 3
    D. 4, 2, 5, 3, 1
    E. 4, 1, 5, 3, 2

15. How can you determine that a gum elastic bougie is properly placed in the trachea?
    A. direct visualization
    B. lack of phonation
    C. presence of condensation inside the tube
    D. "bumps" are felt as the tip passes over the tracheal rings
    E. tip of bougie exits the patient's nose

16. In regard to the Beck Airway Airflow Monitor (BAAM):
    A. whistling will be heard with inhalation.
    B. whistling will be heard with exhalation.
    C. the light will illuminate with any air movement.
    D. A and B.
    E. none of the above.

17. Which of the following can assist the critical care paramedic in intubating a patient with a difficult airway?
    A. gum elastic bougie
    B. valsalva maneuver
    C. BURP maneuver
    D. all of the above
    E. A and C

18. You have responded to a motor vehicle collision where a patient remains trapped in the wreckage. The patient's GCS is 8 and falling and you elect to attempt intubation before the fire department can remove the roof. Which of the following techniques would most likely be the most effective?
    A. sky-hook technique
    B. lighted stylet
    C. nasotracheal intubation
    D. intubating LMA
    E. none of the above

19. When attempting retrograde intubation, the needle should be placed into which of the following structures?
    A. arytenoid membrane
    B. cricothyroid membrane
    C. cricohyoid membrane

    D. thyroid isthmus
    E. cricoarytenoid membrane

20. Which of the following would NOT be an indication for RSI?
    A. impending respiratory failure
    B. paralysis of a combative patient who threatens personnel
    C. acute airway disorder that threatens airway patency
    D. altered mental status with significant risk of vomiting or aspiration
    E. GCS ≤8

21. Which of the following drugs does NOT affect mental status?
    A. thiopental sodium
    B. midazolam
    C. vecuronium
    D. etomidate
    E. methohexital

22. The induction dose for etomidate is:
    A. 0.2–0.3 mg/kg.
    B. 2.0–3.0 mg/kg.
    C. 0.01–0.02 mg/kg.
    D. 20–30 mg/kg.
    E. none of the above.

23. A typical induction dose for fentanyl is:
    A. 2–10 mcg/kg.
    B. 0.1–0.2 mcg/kg.
    C. 1–2 mg/kg.
    D. 1 mg.
    E. none of the above.

24. Which of the following is classified as a dissociative agent?
    A. methohexital
    B. midazolam
    C. lorazepam
    D. thiopental sodium
    E. ketamine

25. The pediatric dose of atropine sulfate as a premedication for succinylcholine administration is:
    A. 1 mg.
    B. 0.01 mg/kg.
    C. 1 mg/kg.
    D. 0.001 mg/kg.
    E. none of the above.

26. The defasiculating dose of vecuronium as a premedication for succinylcholine administration in adults is:
    A. 0.1 mg/kg.
    B. 100 mg.
    C. 1.0 mg/kg.
    D. 0.1 mcg/kg.
    E. none of the above.

27. During which phase of succinylcholine's effects are muscle fasiculations seen?
    A. Phase I
    B. Phase II
    C. Phase III
    D. all of the above
    E. A and B

28. Succinylcholine is metabolized in what tissue?
    A. muscle
    B. kidney
    C. liver
    D. spleen
    E. bone marrow

29. Acetylcholine is metabolized by which of the following enzymes?
    A. catechol-o-methyl transferase (COMT)
    B. 5-hydroxytryptophan
    C. vecuronium
    D. curare
    E. none of the above

30. Which of the following substances result(s) from the action of the enzyme discussed in question 29?
    A. acetic acid
    B. methecholine
    C. choline
    D. A and B
    E. A and C

31. Which of the following neuromuscular blocking agents is the shortest acting?
    A. pancuronium
    B. succinylcholine
    C. vecuronium
    D. rocuronium
    E. mivacurium

32. Which of the following drugs readily crosses the blood-brain barrier?
    A. mivacurium
    B. rocuronium
    C. vecuronium
    D. pancuronium
    E. none of the above

33. Which of the following agents CANNOT be reversed by the administration of neostigmine?
    A. pancuronium
    B. succinylcholine
    C. vecuronium
    D. rocuronium
    E. atracurium

34. The following steps are a part of the RSI process. Place them in the order in which they are typically performed:
    1. release Sellick's maneuver
    2. paralyze
    3. perform induction
    4. confirm placement
    5. apply Sellick's maneuver
    6. intubate
    A. 3, 2, 5, 6, 4, 1
    B. 3, 1, 5, 1, 2, 6
    C. 3, 5, 2, 6, 4, 1
    D. 2, 3, 5, 6, 1, 4
    E. 2, 5, 3, 6, 1, 4

35. Esophageal Tracheal Combitubes (ETCs) are supplied in which of the following sizes?
    A. 37 F
    B. 52 F
    C. 41 F
    D. A and C
    E. A and B

36. When the Combitube has been inserted into the trachea, which tube must be ventilated?
    A. either
    B. blue tube (#1)
    C. clear tube (#2)
    D. red tube (#3)
    E. none of the above

37. The Combitube should NOT be used in patients less than _____ tall.
    A. 48 inches
    B. 54 inches
    C. 122 centimeters
    D. A and C
    E. none of the above

38. Which of the following airways most effectively isolates the trachea?
    A. Pharyngotracheal Lumen Airway (PtL)
    B. Esophageal Tracheal Combitube (ETC)
    C. Laryngeal Mask Airway (LMA)
    D. Ambu Laryngeal Mask (ALM)
    E. none of the above

39. Endotracheal intubation can be performed with which of the following rescue airways in place?
    A. Cobra PLA
    B. Ambu Laryngeal Mask (ALM)
    C. LMA Fastrach
    D. A and B
    E. A and C

40. Which of the following is/are true of the King LT airway?
    A. It is a supraglottic airway.
    B. It stabilizes the airway at the base of the tongue.
    C. It allows up to 30 cm/H_2O ventilation pressure.
    D. all of the above
    E. none of the above

41. Which of the following is NOT a complication of needle cricothyrotomy?
    A. excessive bleeding
    B. barotrauma
    C. subcutaneous emphysema
    D. hypoventilation
    E. none of the above

42. Which of the following is true with regard to the cricoid cartilage?
    A. It is inferior to the thyroid cartilage.
    B. It is superior to the thyroid cartilage.
    C. It is responsible for the palpable "Adam's apple."
    D. A and C
    E. none of the above

43. When performing a needle cricothyrotomy, which of the following is true?
    A. The needle should be directed 45° caudally.
    B. The needle should be inserted 45° in a cephalad direction.
    C. The needle should be inserted at a 90° angle.
    D. all of the above
    E. none of the above

44. Which of the following is NOT a complication of open cricothyrotomy?
    A. laryngeal nerve damage
    B. thyroid gland damage
    C. vagus nerve damage
    D. excessive bleeding
    E. infection

45. All of the following physical findings would suggest the potential for a difficult airway EXCEPT:
    A. small mouth.
    B. long neck.
    C. anterior larynx.
    D. obesity.
    E. thick neck.

46. The illustration in Figure 7–1 suggests which Mallampati class?
    A. class I
    B. class II
    C. class III
    D. class IV
    E. none of the above

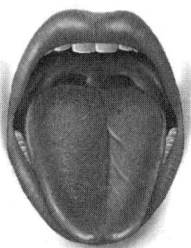

Figure 7–1

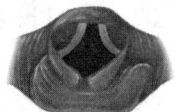

Figure 7–2

47. The illustration in Figure 7–2 suggests which Cormack and Lehane grade?
    A. grade I
    B. grade II
    C. grade III
    D. grade IV
    E. none of the above

48. The term POGO in airway management refers to:
    A. a procedure to improve intubation chances in patients with an anterior larynx.
    B. a mnemonic to help remember how to troubleshoot a malfunctioning mechanical ventilator.
    C. an airway that isolates the esophagus, thus allowing endotracheal intubation.
    D. an airway maneuver that facilitates mechanical ventilation.
    E. a scoring system that reflects the percentage of glottis that can be visualized.

49. Which of the following airways can be used in a patient with facial trauma?
    A. endotracheal tube
    B. Laryngeal Mask Airway (LMA)
    C. King LT airway
    D. Cobra PLA
    E. all of the above

50. In regard to pulse oximetry, which of the following statements is true?
    A. The oximeter measures the amount of oxygen dissolved in plasma.
    B. The oximeter measures the amount of carbon dioxide dissolved in plasma and, from that, calculates the oxygen saturation.
    C. The oximeter measures the number of red blood cells and calculates the oxygen saturation from a complex formula.
    D. The oximeter directly measures the amount of oxygen bound to hemoglobin through the use of near-red and infrared light.
    E. The oximeter obtains initial data from the patient and communicates it to a server in Fargo where it is interpreted and the results returned to the unit.

51. Your patient has an $ETCO_2$ level of 6%. What is the partial pressure of exhaled CO_2 at sea level?
    A. 38 mmHg
    B. 46 mmHg
    C. 50 mmHg
    D. 35 mmHg
    E. 28 mmHg

52. When using capnography, exhalation of dead space gases and alveolar gases with the shortest transport time is seen in which of the following phases?
    A. phase I
    B. phase II
    C. phase III
    D. phase IV
    E. phase V

53. The ventilators most commonly used in prehospital care are:
    A. negative pressure.
    B. positive pressure.
    C. intermittent positive-pressure/negative pressure.
    D. high frequency.
    E. none of the above.

54. Which of the following parameters are a good starting point when initially setting tidal volume for a patient?
    A. 0.5–0.15 mL/kg
    B. 1.0–1.5 mL/kg

C. 5.0–15 mL/kg
D. 20–25 mL/kg
E. none of the above

55. In regard to setting the sigh rate on a mechanical ventilator, which of the following statements is **NOT** true?
    A. The rate should be set to 10–15 times per minute.
    B. The sigh should be 1.5–2.0 times the tidal volume.
    C. The sigh helps to re-expand collapsed alveoli.
    D. The rate should be set to 10–15 times per hour.
    E. none of the above

CHAPTER 8

The Shock Patient: Assessment and Management

DIRECTIONS Each of the questions or incomplete statements below is followed by suggested answers or completions. Select the **one answer** that is best in each case.

1. When glucose metabolism is functioning normally, how many molecules of adenosine triphosphate (ATP) are generated from one molecule of glucose?
   A. 2
   B. 16
   C. 24
   D. 32
   E. 36

2. Where does glycolysis primarily occur?
   A. cell nucleus
   B. Golgi apparatus
   C. mitochondria
   D. cytoplasm
   E. ribosomes

3. The normal end product of glycolysis is:
   A. pyruvic acid.
   B. adenosine triphosphate (ATP).
   C. lactic acid.
   D. acetic acid.
   E. none of the above.

4. Where does the tricarboxylic acid (TCA) cycle primarily occur?
   A. cell nucleus
   B. Golgi apparatus
   C. mitochondria
   D. cytoplasm
   E. ribosomes

5. What is the net gain in ATP from glycolysis?
   A. 2
   B. 16
   C. 24
   D. 32
   E. 36

6. The phenomenon in which the energy yield from glucose falls because of an inadequate supply of oxygen is termed:
   A. dysoxia.
   B. hypoxia.
   C. hypoxemia.
   D. all of the above.
   E. none of the above.

Match the following:

Column A

7. ____C____ MRO_2
8. ____D____ SvO_2
9. ____E____ VO_2
10. ____A____ DO_2
11. ____B____ CO

Column B
A. amount of measurable oxygen delivered to tissues
B. cardiac output
C. the tissues metabolic requirement for oxygen
D. venous oxygen saturation
E. amount of oxygen withdrawn at the capillary level

12. Which of the following factors does NOT affect the VO_2?
    A. cardiac output
    B. arterial oxygen saturation
    C. venous oxygen saturation
    D. amount of hemoglobin present.
    E. amount of phagocytes present

13. The majority of energy produced by the cell is used for which of the following functions?
    A. protein production
    B. sodium/potassium pump
    C. cellular reproduction
    D. glycolysis
    E. DNA replication

14. Which of the following statements is true?
    A. Extracellular sodium levels are normally 140 mEq/L.
    B. Intracellular sodium levels are normally 10 mEq/L.
    C. Intracellular potassium levels are normally 140 mEq/L.
    D. Extracellular potassium levels are normally 4 mEq/L.
    E. all of the above

15. In shock, the failure of what system ultimately leads to cell lysis?
    A. glycolysis
    B. protein synthesis
    C. cell membrane lipid repair
    D. sodium/potassium pump
    E. RNA-mediated protein production

16. In regard to lactic acid production during anaerobic metabolism, which of the following is/are true?
    A. Hydrogen ions increase.
    B. pH increases.
    C. NADH is converted to NAD+.
    D. A and C.
    E. B and C.

17. Which of the following is NOT an action of angiotensin II?
    A. vasodilation
    B. vasoconstriction
    C. promotes ADH release
    D. increases blood pressure
    E. none of the above

18. Which neurohumoral agent causes renal sodium and water retention?
    A. cortisol
    B. epinephrine
    C. antidiuretic hormone
    D. angiotensin II
    E. aldosterone

19. Which neurohumoral agent increases blood sugar?
    A. cortisol
    B. norepinephrine
    C. antidiuretic hormone
    D. angiotensin II
    E. aldosterone

20. The sequential and significant derangement of function of two or more organ systems is called:
    A. DIC.
    B. SAS.
    C. MODS.
    D. ARDS.
    E. SIR.

21. The hallmark of decompensated shock is which of the following?
    A. fall in blood pressure
    B. tachycardia
    C. tachypnea
    D. altered mental status
    E. decreased urine output

22. Studies suggest that in trauma where the source of bleeding cannot be adequately controlled, fluids should be administered to maintain the systolic blood pressure in which of the following ranges?
    A. < 120 mmHg
    B. 100–120 mmHg
    C. 70–85 mmHg
    D. > 70 mmHg
    E. none of the above

23. The process by which hemoglobin-based oxygen carrying solutions (HBOCs) are manufactured is called:
    A. polymerization.
    B. genetic engineering.
    C. recombinant DNA technology.
    D. lipolysis.
    E. none of the above.

24. PolyHeme™ is manufactured from which source?
    A. bovine blood
    B. porcine blood
    C. simian blood
    D. human blood
    E. none of the above

25. When comparing HBOCs to human blood, which of the following is NOT true?
    A. HBOCs require blood typing.
    B. HBOCs are filtered to remove any infectious agents.
    C. HBOCs have a longer shelf life.
    D. Some HBOCs do not require refrigeration.
    E. none of the above

26. In which of the following shock types is central venous pressure (CVP) decreased?
    A. cardiogenic
    B. hypovolemic
    C. obstructive
    D. distributive
    E. all of the above

27. In which of the following shock types is systemic vascular resistance (SVR) decreased?
    A. cardiogenic
    B. hypovolemic
    C. obstructive
    D. distributive
    E. none of the above

28. In which of the following shock types is cardiac output (CO) increased?
    A. cardiogenic
    B. hypovolemic
    C. obstructive
    D. distributive
    E. all of the above

29. Which of the following is a normal urine output level for an adult?
    A. 5–10 mL/kg/hour
    B. 0.5–1.0 mL/kg/hour
    C. 0.1–0.4 mL/kg/hour
    D. 10–20 mL/hour
    E. none of the above

30. The sympathetic nervous system arises from which of the following neurological regions?
    A. cranial nerves and lumbar spinal cord
    B. cranial nerves and sacral spinal cord
    C. thoracic and lumbar spinal cord
    D. cervical and thoracic spinal cord
    E. none of the above

CHAPTER 9

Cardiac and Hemodynamic Monitoring

1. When using a 15-Lead ECG, which of the following leads are added to the standard 12-Lead configuration?
   A. V4R, V8, and V9
   B. V4R, V5R, and V6R
   C. V7, V8, and V9
   D. MCL1, V7 and V8
   E. none of the above

2. The proper placement for lead V9 is:
   A. right anterior axillary line.
   B. right mid-axillary line.
   C. left posterior axillary line.
   D. left paravertebral line.
   E. none of the above.

3. The sounds heard over an artery when pressure is released from a blood pressure cuff are referred to as:
   A. Boborygmy sounds.
   B. Khrushchev sounds.
   C. Korotkoff's sounds.
   D. Einthoven's sounds.
   E. Starling sounds.

4. A device that changes energy from one form to another is called a:
   A. transformer.
   B. rheostat.
   C. transducer.
   D. transistor.
   E. toddler.

5. A patient has a blood pressure of 160/70 mmHg. What is the mean arterial pressure?
   A. 70 mmHg
   B. 80 mmHg
   C. 100 mmHg
   D. 90 mmHg
   E. none of the above

6. The phlebostatic axis can be defined as:
   A. the QRS vector in Lead MCL1.
   B. the point at which the pressure transducer is at the level of the right and left atrium.
   C. the difference between the systolic and diastolic blood pressure.
   D. the notch on the arterial waveform that results from back flow of blood following closure of the aortic valve.
   E. none of the above.

7. Which of the following is useful in determining patency of circulation distal to the wrist?
   A. Marshall's test
   B. Weber test
   C. Rinne's test
   D. Chvostek's test
   E. Allen's test

8. The technique whereby a needle or guide wire is inserted into a vessel through a needle is called:
   A. Salinger technique.
   B. LaSalle's technique.
   C. Seldinger technique.
   D. Pierre's technique.
   E. none of the above.

9. Your patient has a CVP of 8 cm/H_2O. What is the pressure in millimeters of mercury?
   A. 5.9 mmHg
   B. 10.1 mmHg
   C. 7.8 mmHg
   D. 3.2 mmHg
   E. 5.0 mmHg

10. All of the following are complications of arterial catheter placement EXCEPT:
    A. pain.
    B. bleeding.
    C. vasospasm.
    D. distal ischemia.
    E. vagal stimulation.

11. Which of the following information CANNOT be determined from central venous pressure (CVP) monitoring?
    A. coronary perfusion pressure
    B. intravascular blood volume
    C. right ventricular end-diastolic pressure
    D. preload
    E. none of the above

12. Which of the following is an indication for central venous catheter (CVP) placement?
    A. patient requiring inotropic infusions
    B. measurement of left atrial pressure
    C. continuing hypovolemia secondary to fluid shifts
    D. A and C
    E. A and B

13. Which of the following tests is essential following subclavian central line placement?
    A. 12-Lead ECG
    B. complete blood count
    C. serum osmolality
    D. chest x-ray
    E. none of the above

14. Which of the following medications can be administered locally in case of vasopressor extravasation?
    A. lidocaine (Xylocaine)
    B. phentolamine (Regitine)
    C. neostigmine
    D. bupivicaine
    E. none of the above

15. A patient had a subclavian line placed approximately 1 hour ago by a surgical resident. The patient now has dyspnea, tachypnea, hypoxia, and chest discomfort. What is the most likely etiology?
    A. infection
    B. acute pulmonary embolism
    C. pericardial tamponade
    D. pneumothorax
    E. none of the above

Scenario

Questions 16–18 refer to the following scenario:
You are called to transport a patient from a community hospital to a major medical center. The patient has had several bowel surgeries. He has a blood pressure of 88/50 mmHg, a pulse of 122 per minute, and a CVP of 2 mmHg. His hematocrit is 56%.

16. Which of the following treatments is indicated?
    A. administer 2 units packed red blood cells
    B. initiate pressor support with dopamine
    C. initiate a vasopressin (Pitressin) infusion
    D. administer isotonic saline bolus
    E. none of the above

17. What is the patient's mean arterial pressure?
    A. 63 mmHg
    B. 56 mmHg
    C. 66 mmHg
    D. 38 mmHg
    E. none of the above

18. What is the most likely cause of the patient's problem?
    A. cardiogenic shock
    B. gastrointestinal fluid losses
    C. hemorrhage
    D. disseminated intravascular coagulopathy (DIC)
    E. none of the above

19. Which of the following hemodynamic parameters CANNOT be measured with a Swan-Ganz catheter?
    A. cardiac output
    B. right atrial pressure

C. coronary perfusion pressure
D. pulmonary artery pressure
E. pulmonary artery wedge pressure

20. Positive-end-expiratory pressure (PEEP) would have what effect on right atrial pressure?
    A. none
    B. increased
    C. decreased
    D. both increased and decreased
    E. none of the above

21. The tracing in Figure 9–1 represents:
    A. arterial blood pressure.
    B. right atrial pressure.
    C. pulmonary artery pressure.
    D. right ventricular pressure.
    E. none of the above.

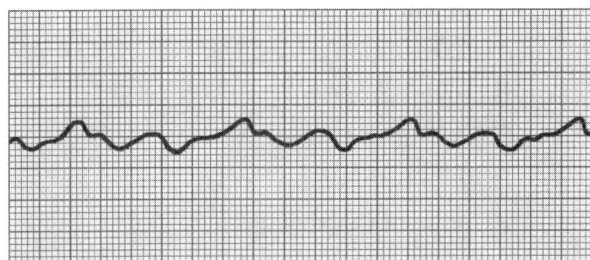

Figure 9–1

22. The tracing in Figure 9–2 above represents:
    A. arterial blood pressure.
    B. right atrial pressure.
    C. pulmonary artery pressure.
    D. right ventricular pressure.
    E. none of the above.

23. Which of the following would **NOT** result in low right ventricular pressures?
    A. hypovolemia
    B. right ventricular failure
    C. transducer above the phlebostatic axis
    D. pulmonary infarction
    E. none of the above

24. The tracing in Figure 9–3 represents:
    A. arterial blood pressure.
    B. right atrial pressure.
    C. pulmonary artery wedge pressure.
    D. right ventricular pressure.
    E. none of the above.

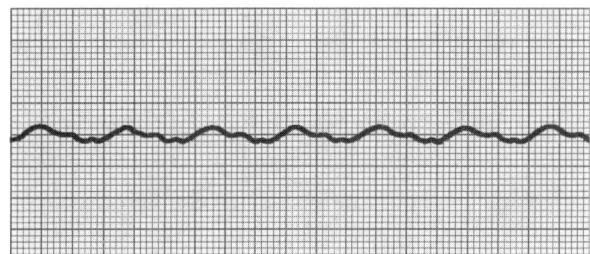

Figure 9–3

25. The tracing in Figure 9–4 represents:
    A. arterial blood pressure.
    B. right atrial pressure.
    C. pulmonary artery wedge pressure.
    D. right ventricular pressure.
    E. none of the above.

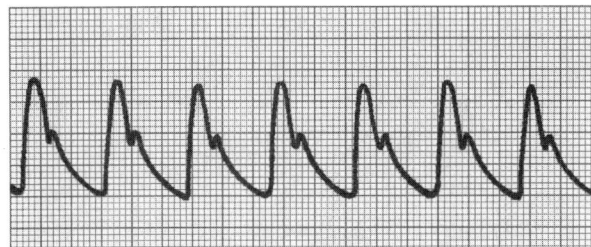

Figure 9–2

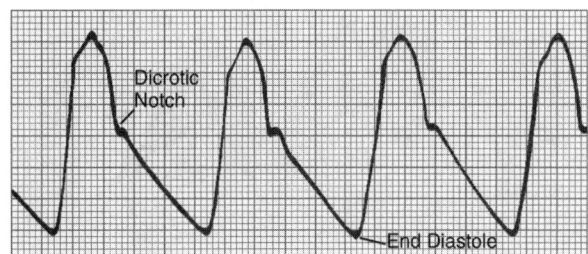

Figure 9–4

26. Your patient has pericardial tamponade as determined by bedside ultrasound. The cardiothoracic surgeon is preparing to perform a bedside pericardiocentesis under ultrasound guidance. You decide to quickly examine the patient and measure all of the Swan-Ganz pressures. Which of the following Swan-Ganz findings would you expect?
    A. low pulmonary artery wedge pressure
    B. high pulmonary artery wedge pressure
    C. muffled heart tones
    D. distended neck veins
    E. none of the above

27. The two tracings in Figure 9–5 were taken from the same patient 3 hours apart. Clinically, the patient appears unchanged. What is the likely explanation for the difference?
    A. The patient has suffered a right ventricular infarction.
    B. The patient has suffered a hemorrhage.
    C. The system is overdamped.
    D. The system is underdamped.
    E. none of the above

28. Which of the following is a complication of Swan-Ganz catheterization?
    A. pneumothorax
    B. ventricular dysrhythmias
    C. infection
    D. pulmonary artery rupture
    E. all of the above

29. Your patient is 5 feet 8 inches tall and weighs 200 pounds. What is her body surface area?
    A. 2.1 m^2
    B. 4.0 m^2
    C. 4.4 m^2
    D. 5.2 m^2
    E. 0.1 m^2

30. The patient in question 29 has a measured cardiac output of 4.6 Liters/minute. What is the patient's cardiac index?
    A. 1.05 L/min/m^2
    B. 0.95 L/min/m^2
    C. 2.19 L/min/m^2
    D. 7.90 L/min/m^2
    E. none of the above

31. Which of the following conditions does NOT typically decrease systemic vascular resistance?
    A. anaphylaxis
    B. spinal cord injury
    C. gram-negative sepsis
    D. aortic stenosis
    E. none of the above

32. In neurogenic shock, the cardiac output is typically:
    A. low
    B. normal
    C. high
    D. any of the above
    E. none of the above

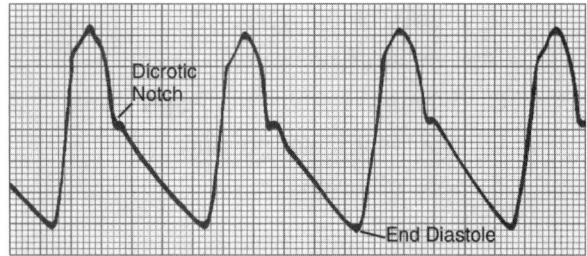
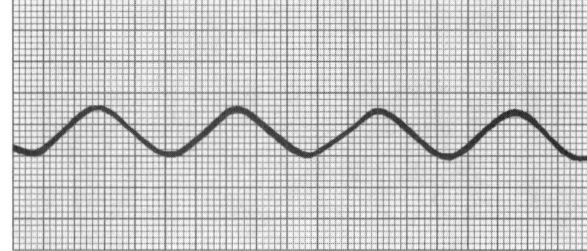

Figure 9–5

Scenario

Questions 33–36 refer to the following scenario:
You are transporting an ICU patient who is noted to have the following hemodynamic parameters:

    Blood pressure: 110/68 mmHg
    Pulse rate: 100 per minute
    Cardiac output: 3.8 L/min
    Central venous pressure (CVP): 2 mmHg
    Right atrial pressure (RAP): 6 mmHg (mean)
    Right ventricular pressure (RVR): 20/6 mmHg
    Pulmonary artery pressure (PAP): 24/8 mmHg
    Pulmonary artery wedge pressure (PAWP): 8 mmHg (mean)
    Weight: 140 pounds
    Height: 5 feet

33. What is the patient's systemic vascular resistance?
    A. 21.05 Wood's units
    B. 23.65 Wood's units
    C. 19.55 Wood's units
    D. 0.15 Wood's units
    E. none of the above

34. What is the patient's cardiac index?
    A. 1.0 L/min/m²
    B. 1.8 L/min/m²
    C. 4.1 L/min/m²
    D. 2.4 L/min/m²
    E. none of the above

35. What is the patient's stroke volume index?
    A. 0.4 L/beat × m²
    B. 0.02 L/beat × m²
    C. 4.1 L/beat × m²
    D. 0.0041 L/beat × m²
    E. none of the above

36. What is the patient's stroke volume?
    A. 55 mL
    B. 32 mL
    C. 22 mL
    D. 38 mL
    E. none of the above

37. If the transducer is above the level of the phlebostatic axis, which of the following will occur?
    A. Readings will be normal.
    B. Readings will be high.
    C. Readings will be low.
    D. Readings will be impossible.
    E. none of the above

38. As the Swan-Ganz catheter is advanced, it proceeds through which of the following heart valves?
    A. aortic valve
    B. tricuspid valve
    C. pulmonic valve
    D. A and C
    E. B and C

39. When it is functioning normally, which of the following statements describes the intra-aortic balloon pump (IABP)?
    A. It inflates at the beginning of ventricular systole.
    B. It deflates at the end of ventricular systole.
    C. It inflates at the end of ventricular systole.
    D. It deflates at the beginning of ventricular systole.
    E. none of the above

40. Which gas is routinely used to inflate an IABP?
    A. oxygen
    B. hydrogen
    C. nitrogen
    D. argon
    E. helium

CHAPTER 10

ECG Monitoring and Critical Care

DIRECTIONS
Each of the questions or incomplete statements below is followed by suggested answers or completions. Select the **one answer** that is best in each case.

1. The Modified Central Leads (MCL) are analogous to:
   A. bipolar limb leads.
   B. corresponding precordial leads.
   C. augmented voltage leads.
   D. posterior chest leads.
   E. right-sided chest leads.

2. To monitor Modified Central Lead 1 (MCL$_1$), the positive ("red" or "left leg") electrode should be placed on the:
   A. left midaxillary line in the 5th intercostal space.
   B. right upper arm.
   C. left upper arm.
   D. right sternal border in the 4th intercostal space.
   E. left sternal border in the 4th intercostal space.

3. If the critical care paramedic does not have a 12-Lead ECG available, one useful purpose of continuous monitoring of the MCL Leads is to:
   A. recognize early ST-segment elevation.
   B. distinguish ventricular tachycardia from supraventricular tachycardia with aberrant conduction.
   C. recognition of pre-excitation syndromes.
   D. recognition of left ventricular hypertrophy.
   E. none of the above.

4. For continuous monitoring of MCL Leads, the ECG monitor should either have the capability of displaying multiple leads simultaneously or should be:
   A. set to monitor Lead III.
   B. set to monitor Lead II.
   C. set to monitor Lead I.
   D. set to monitor Lead AVL.
   E. none of the above.

5. When monitoring Lead MCL$_1$, normal typical P-QRS-T morphology is:
   A. P waves usually positive, QRS usually biphasic, T waves negative or positive.
   B. P waves usually negative, QRS usually positive, T waves negative or positive.
   C. P waves usually negative, QRS usually negative, T waves negative or positive.
   D. P waves usually positive, QRS usually positive, T waves usually biphasic.
   E. P waves usually positive, QRS usually positive, T waves usually positive or biphasic.

6. The pre-transport ECG evaluation is performed to assess for ECG findings that indicate potential risks for deterioration of the patient's cardiovascular and hemodynamic status during transport. Which of the following indicates a risk for hemodynamic compromise?
   A. physiologic left axis deviation
   B. right ventricular infarction
   C. first-degree atrioventricular block
   D. left ventricular hypertrophy
   E. B and D

7. The three broad categories of conduction system blocks are:
   A. sinoatrial blocks, hemifascicular blocks, bundle branch blocks.
   B. interventricular blocks, sinoatrial blocks, hemifascicular blocks.
   C. sinoatrial blocks, atrioventricular blocks, interventricular blocks.
   D. first-degree heart block, second-degree heart block, third-degree heart block.
   E. none of the above.

8. Which of the following is **NOT** considered a risk factor for complete heart block?
   A. first- or second-degree atrioventricular blocks
   B. sinoatrial block
   C. hemifascicular block
   D. left bundle branch block
   E. combination of two or more types of conduction blocks

9. Hemifascicular blocks occur in which part of the conduction system?
   A. atrioventricular node
   B. bundle of His
   C. left bundle branch
   D. right bundle branch
   E. Purkinje system

10. One of the most accurate indicators of a left anterior hemiblock is:
    A. wide (greater than 0.12 seconds) QRS complex.
    B. pathologic left axis deviation.
    C. pathologic right axis deviation.
    D. larger than normal R wave in Lead III.
    E. none of the above.

11. The left anterior fascicle receives its blood supply from which coronary artery?
    A. circumflex branch of the left coronary artery
    B. left anterior descending branch of the left coronary artery
    C. proximal right coronary artery
    D. marginal branch of the right coronary artery
    E. none of the above

12. In the setting of acute myocardial infarction, the presence of a hemiblock indicates:
    A. mortality rate four times higher than uncomplicated MI.
    B. predisposition for ventricular tachycardia.
    C. greater potential for complete heart block.
    D. impending cardiogenic shock.
    E. A and C.

13. The Leads needed for rapid axis determination are:
    A. II, III, AVF.
    B. MCL_1, MCL_6, III.
    C. I, II, III.
    D. I, II, AVL.
    E. II, III, MCL_1.

14. Presence of a left bundle branch block:
    A. always indicates hemodynamic instability.
    B. is indicated by a QRS width of less than 0.12 seconds.
    C. is most commonly a side effect of high frequency radio ablation.
    D. makes diagnosing ST segment elevation very difficult.
    E. all of the above.

15. To accurately differentiate a left from a right bundle branch block, one may:
    A. determine which "rabbit ear" points higher in Lead II.
    B. utilize the "turn signal" criteria in Lead II.
    C. utilize the "turn signal" criteria in MCL_1 or V_1.
    D. look for an RSR^1 in MCL_1 or V_1.
    E. none of the above.

16. The 12-Lead ECG tracing shown in Figure 10–1 represents:
    A. right bundle branch block.
    B. left posterior hemiblock.
    C. accelerated idioventricular rhythm.
    D. left bundle branch block.
    E. anterior wall ST-segment elevation.

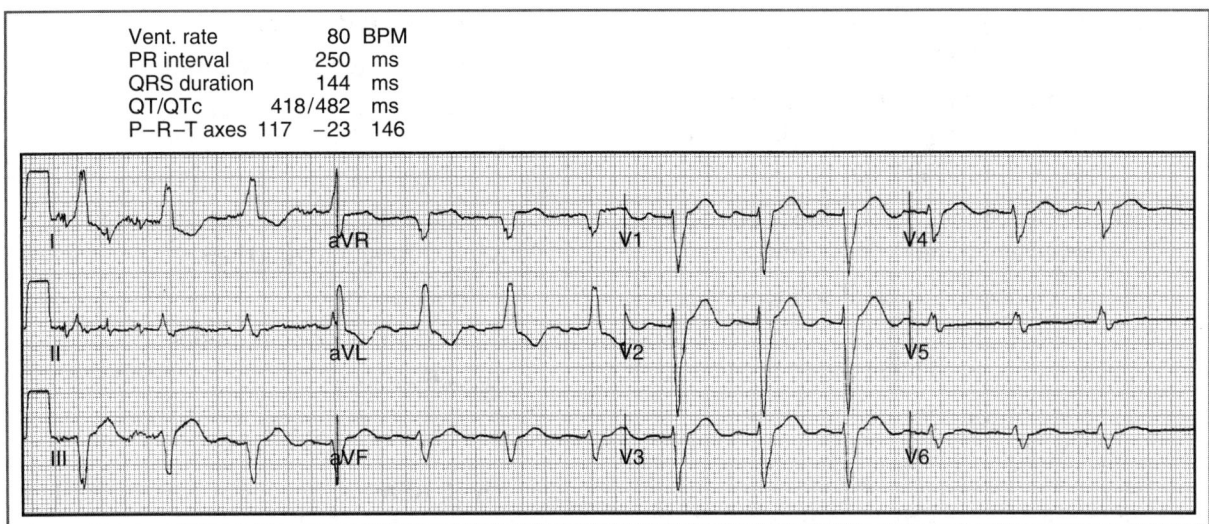

Figure 10–1

17. A wide-complex tachycardia that has mostly positive QRS complexes in V_1 and mostly negative QRS complexes in V_6 is most likely to be:
    A. sinus tachycardia with left bundle branch block.
    B. ventricular tachycardia.
    C. Wolff-Parkinson-White syndrome.
    D. Lown-Ganong-Levine syndrome.
    E. none of the above.

18. The best leads to appreciate the characteristic Delta waves of Wolff-Parkinson-White syndrome are:
    A. inferior leads such as II, III and AVF.
    B. anteroseptal leads such as V_1 and V_2.
    C. anterior and lateral leads such as V_4–V_6, Lead I and AVL.
    D. right-sided chest lead V_4R.
    E. none of the above.

19. You are transporting an 18-year-old male from a community hospital to the CCU at the regional tertiary care center. The patient was seen at the referring hospital's Emergency Department complaining of nausea, palpitations, and near-syncope, which had spontaneously resolved prior to your arrival to transfer the patient. The patient's 12-Lead ECG revealed a previously undiagnosed WPW syndrome. During transport to the tertiary care center, the patient suddenly complains of chest pain and dyspnea. He exhibits jugular venous distension and markedly labored respirations and hypotension at 96/60 mmHg. The ECG reveals a narrow-complex tachycardia at a rate of 230 with characteristic Delta waves in V_6. The most appropriate treatment for this patient at this time is:
    A. IV bolus of adenosine to terminate the re-entry tachycardia.
    B. IV infusion of procainamide.
    C. emergency overdrive pacing.
    D. emergency synchronized cardioversion.
    E. IV infusion of amiodarone.

20. In Wolff-Parkinson-White syndrome, electrical impulses travel down an accessory conduction pathway known as:
    A. Bundle of Kent
    B. James Fibers
    C. Mahaim Fibers.
    D. left anterior fascicle.
    E. left posterior fascicle.

21. Lown-Ganong-Levine syndrome is characterized clinically by:
    A. shortened PR interval (less than .04 seconds) and slurred QRS complexes with Delta waves.
    B. shortened PR interval (less than .04 seconds) and normal QRS complexes.
    C. shortened PR interval and RSR^1 in Lead II.
    D. delta waves in Lead II and RSR^1 in V$_1$.
    E. none of the above.

22. Hypokalemia can have adverse cardiac side effects and is defined as an abnormally low serum potassium level. Normal serum potassium level is:
    A. 2.5–4.5 mEq/L.
    B. 35–45 mmHg.
    C. 5.0–7.5 mEq/L.
    D. 3.5–5.0 mEq/L.
    E. 4.0–6.0 mEq/L.

23. ECG findings in hypokalemia include:
    A. ST-segment elevation.
    B. tall, peaked T waves.
    C. ST-segment depression and flattening of T waves.
    D. sine waves.
    E. prominent U waves.

24. ECG changes usually present in mild hyperkalemia (serum potassium 5.0-6.5 mEq/L) are:
    A. sine waves.
    B. high-degree AV blocks.
    C. flattened P waves.
    D. tall, peaked T waves.
    E. left axis deviation.

25. ECG changes usually present in severe hyperkalemia (serum potassium greater than 8.0 mEq/L) are:
    A. sine waves.
    B. high-degree AV blocks.
    C. flattened P waves.
    D. tall, peaked T waves.
    E. left axis deviation.

26. Hyperkalemia is a common complication in patients with:
    A. vomiting and diarrhea.
    B. renal failure.
    C. CHF and taking diuretics.
    D. dehydration.
    E. none of the above.

27. Which of the following is NOT typically an option available for the critical care paramedic for emergency management of life-threatening hyperkalemia?
    A. hemodialysis
    B. intracellular shift of serum K$^+$ using sodium bicarbonate, insulin and dextrose, or large doses of albuterol
    C. cation exchange using Kayexalate
    D. cellular membrane stabilization using calcium chloride or calcium gluconate
    E. none of the above

28. ECG findings indicating hypocalcemia include:
    A. prolonged PR interval.
    B. widened QRS complex.
    C. prolonged QT interval.
    D. delta waves.
    E. none of the above.

29. Prolongation of QT interval increases likelihood of:
    A. high-degree atrioventricular blocks.
    B. torsades de pointes.
    C. sinus tachycardia.
    D. Wolff-Parkinson-White syndrome.
    E. bundle branch blocks.

30. You are transporting a 60-year-old female to the CCU at the tertiary care center for treatment of chest pain and acute onset of

atrial fibrillation. The patient received a bolus of diltiazem at the community hospital ED, which subsequently relieved her chest pain and reduced her heart rate from 170 to 76. The patient is currently receiving a heparin infusion for anticoagulation and an infusion of procainamide for rate control. During transport, your patient experiences several short runs of polymorphic ventricular tachycardia that resembles torsades de pointes. You should:
   A. perform synchronized cardioversion the next time it happens.
   B. increase the procainamide infusion to suppress the ventricular tachycardia.
   C. carefully evaluate the ECG to determine if the corrected QT interval (QT_c) is prolonged, and consider discontinuing the procainamide infusion if it is.
   D. begin an amiodarone infusion.
   E. none of the above.

31. Right ventricular infarction (RVI) often presents with:
   A. lateral wall myocardial infarction.
   B. occlusion of the left anterior descending (LAD) artery.
   C. inferior wall myocardial infarction.
   D. anterior wall myocardial infarction.
   E. septal infarction.

32. Many patients with RVI are also especially susceptible to reduction in preload; thus the critical care paramedic should be cautious in administering:
   A. dopamine.
   B. nitrates.
   C. oxygen.
   D. aspirin.
   E. albuterol.

33. The triad of clinical findings that indicate preload dependency are:
   A. hypertension, bradycardia, altered respiratory pattern.
   B. hypotension, jugular venous distension, narrowed pulse pressure.
   C. hypotension, jugular venous distension, clear lung sounds.
   D. hypotension, jugular venous distension, syncope.
   E. none of the above.

34. The diagnostic lead for recognizing right ventricular infarction (RVI) is:
   A. MCL_1.
   B. Lead II.
   C. V_4.
   D. AVF.
   E. V_4R.

35. Which of the following is NOT an indication for obtaining a 15-lead ECG?
   A. normal 12-lead ECG findings in a patient exhibiting cardiovascular symptoms
   B. anteroseptal myocardial infarction
   C. inferior wall infarction
   D. ST Segment depression in Leads V_1–V_4, indicating reciprocal changes from posterior myocardial infarction
   E. lateral wall myocardial infarction

36. Correct electrode placement for Lead V_4R is:
   A. 5th intercostal space, left midclavicular line.
   B. 4th intercostal space, right sternal border.
   C. 5th intercostal space, right midclavicular line.
   D. halfway between V_3 and V_5.
   E. none of the above.

37. The right ventricle and inferior wall of the left ventricle receive blood supplied by which artery?
   A. right coronary artery
   B. left coronary artery
   C. left anterior descending branch of the left coronary artery
   D. circumflex branch of the left coronary artery
   E. none of the above

38. Cardiac output is determined by:
   A. stroke volume multiplied by heart rate.
   B. preload multiplied by myocardial activity.
   C. preload multiplied by afterload.
   D. stroke volume multiplied by systemic vascular resistance (SVR).
   E. none of the above.

39. The part of the ECG tracing that reflects ventricular repolarization is:
   A. P Wave.
   B. QRS Complex.
   C. T Wave.
   D. ST Segment.
   E. PR interval.

40. Lack of tension in papillary muscles or *chordae tendonae* may result in:
   A. mitral regurgitation and a resultant heart murmur.
   B. aortic stenosis.
   C. congestive heart failure.
   D. aortic regurgitation.
   E. A and C.

Interpret the following 12-lead ECGs.

41.

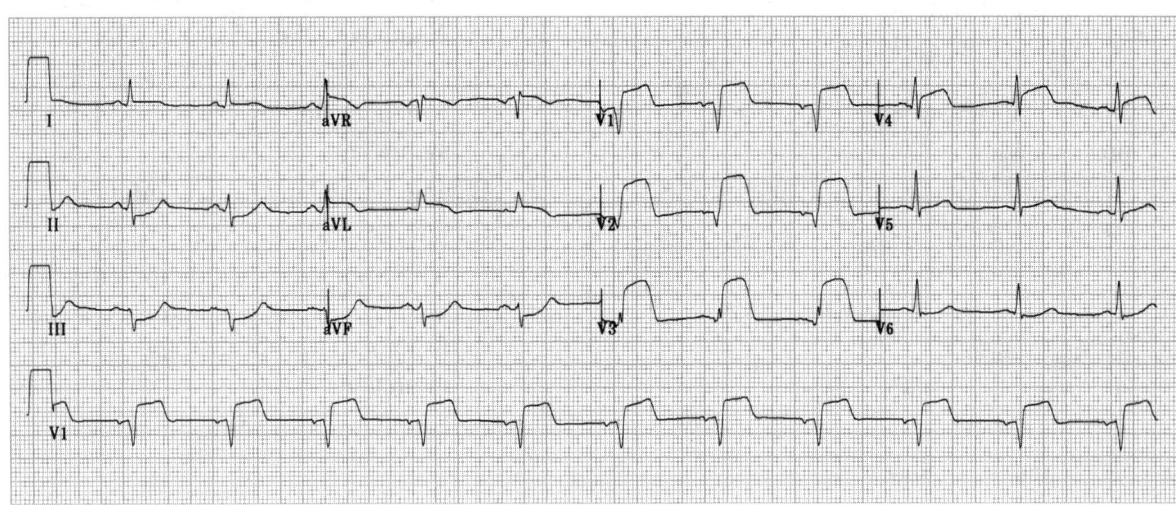

Figure 10–2

42.

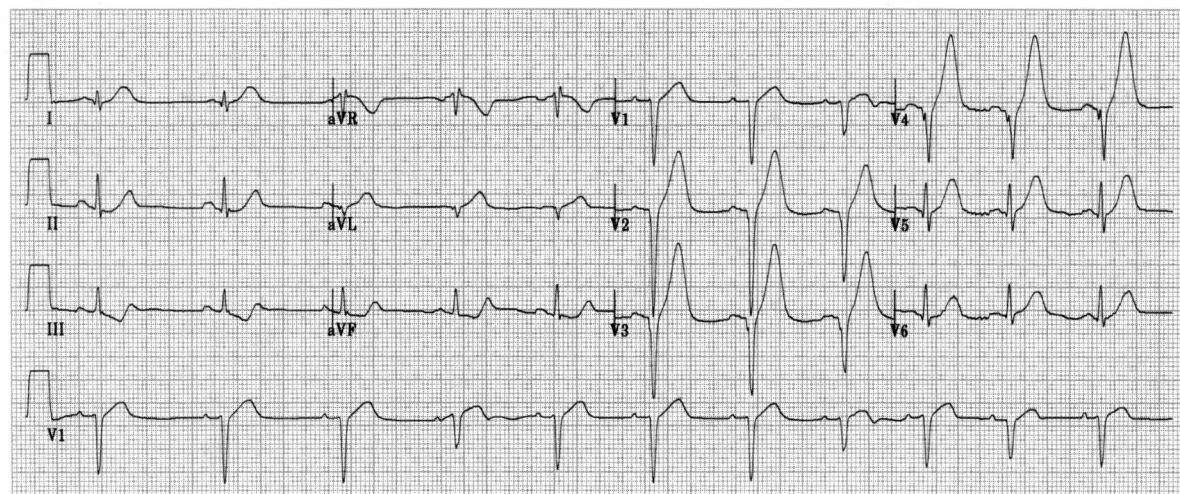

Figure 10–3

43.

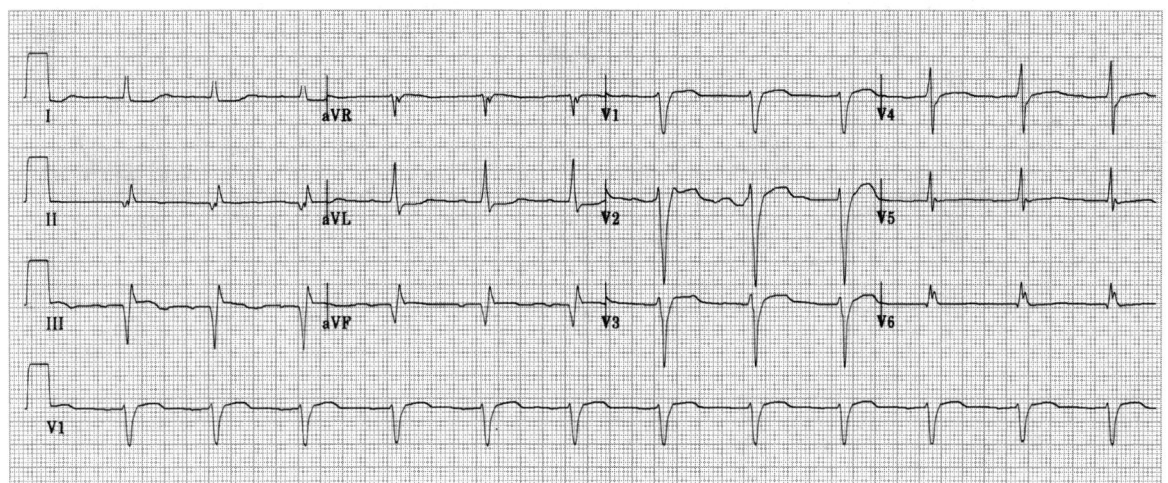

Figure 10–4

44.

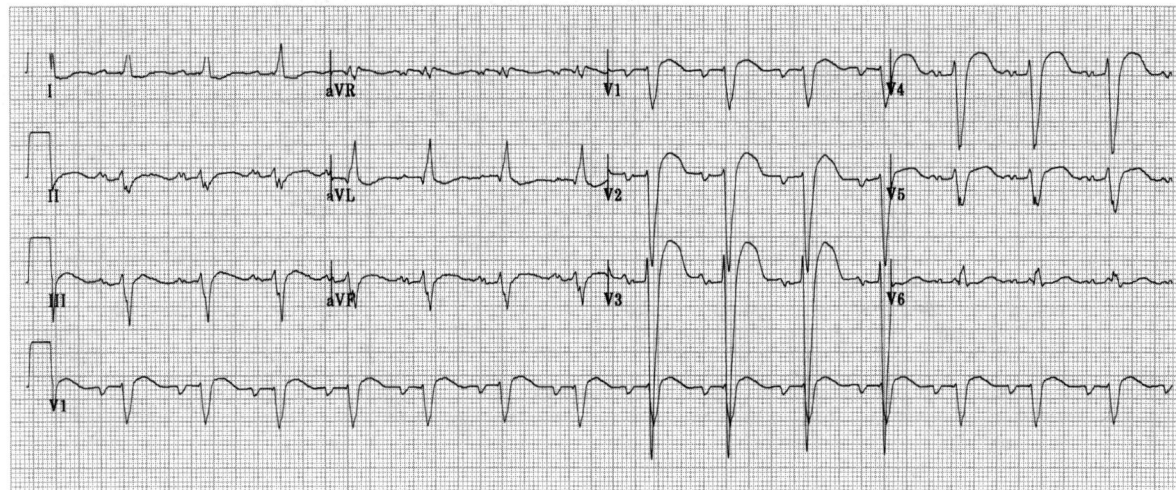

Figure 10–5

45.

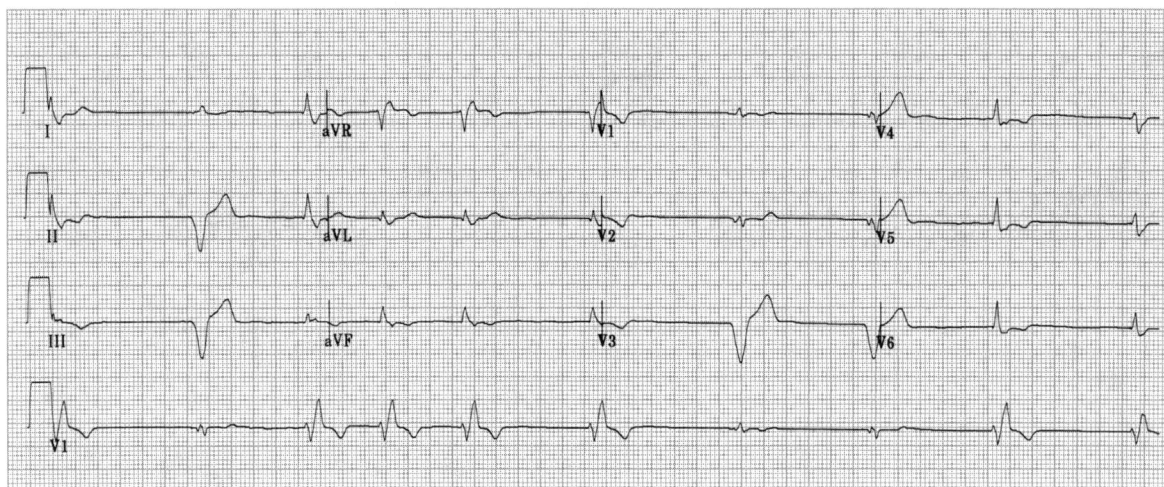

Figure 10–6

46.

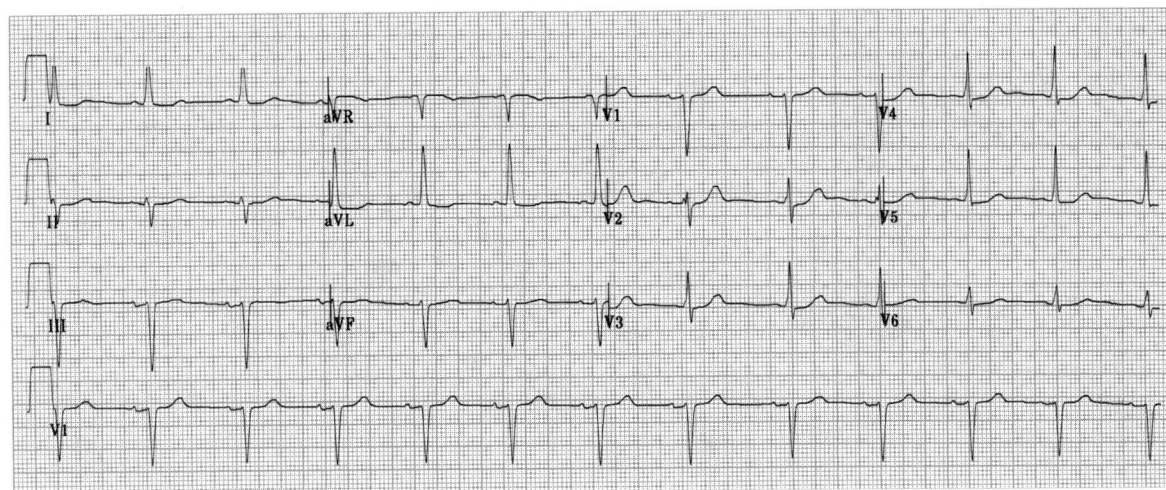

Figure 10–7

47.

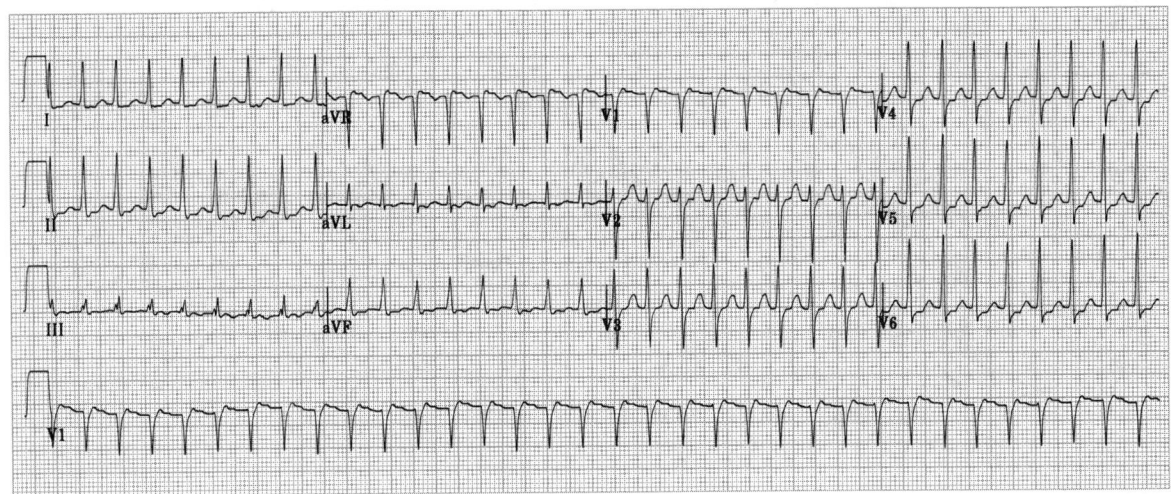

Figure 10–8

48.

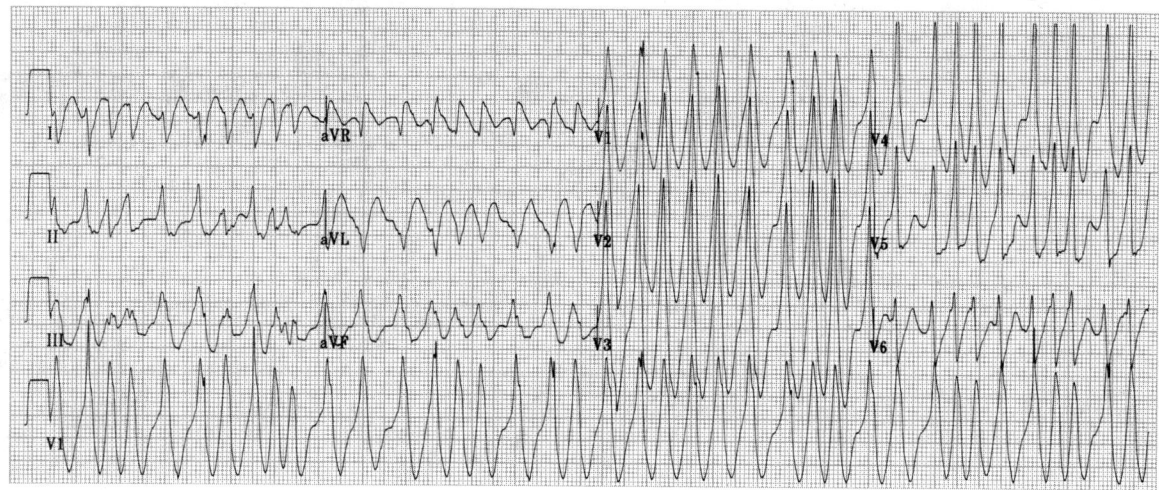

Figure 10–9

49.

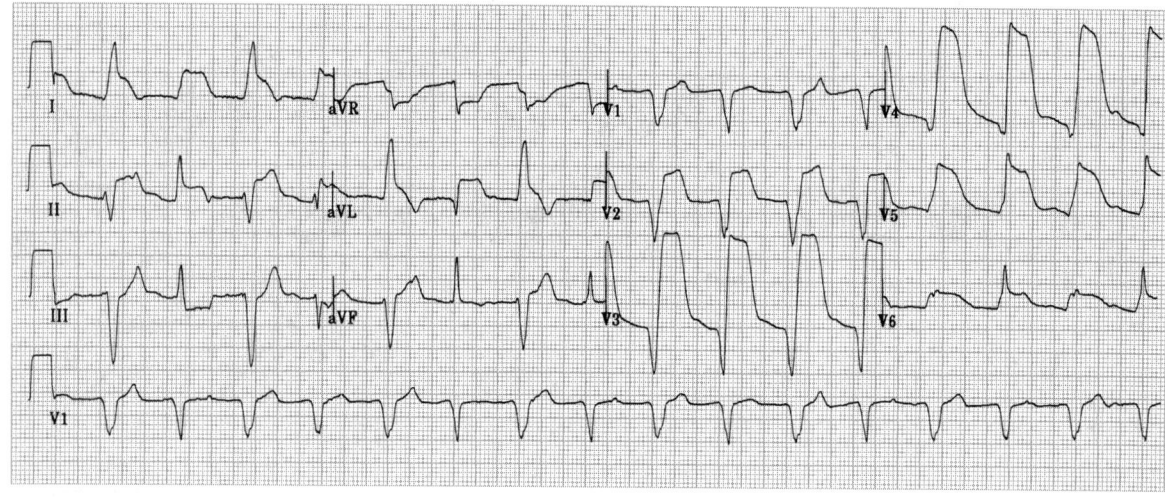

Figure 10–10

50.

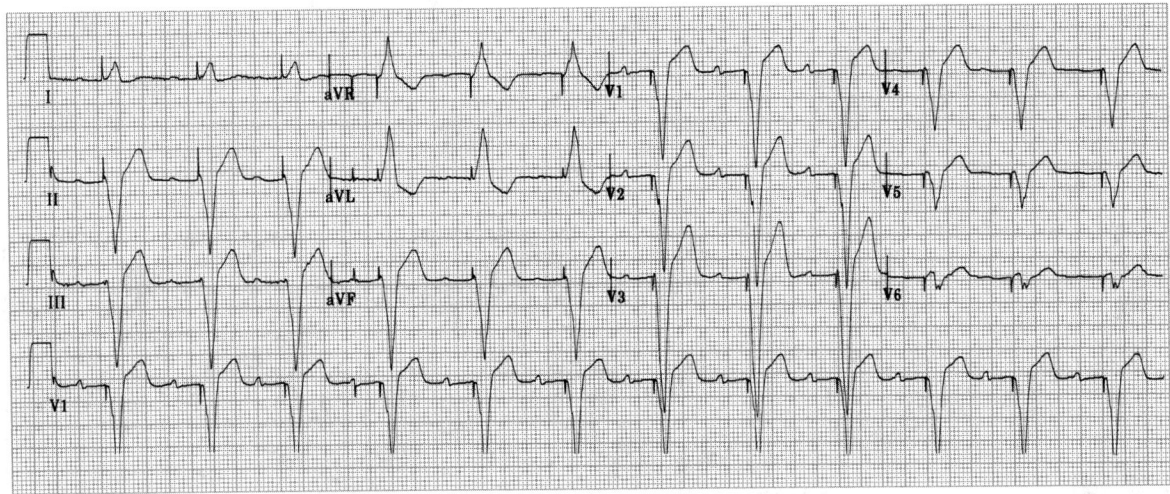

Figure 10–11

CHAPTER 11

Critical Care Pharmacology

DIRECTIONS Each of the questions or incomplete statements below is followed by suggested answers or completions. Select the **one answer** that is best in each case.

1. The role of pharmacology in critical care medicine is:
   A. to maintain a standard of education and promoting our cause.
   B. to identify disease processes and beginning definitive treatment.
   C. to implement ACLS guidelines for the American Heart Association.
   D. to prevent patients from overdosing themselves on medications.
   E. to treat emergent or ongoing disease processes and injuries.

2. A pharmacological agonist is generally defined as:
   A. a drug that stimulates receptor sites on cells in order to cause an effect.
   B. a drug that stimulates receptor sites on cells in order to inhibit an effect.
   C. a drug that blocks receptor sites on cells in order to cause an effect.
   D. a drug that blocks receptor sites on cells in order to inhibit an effect.
   E. none of the above.

3. A pharmacological antagonist is generally defined as:
   A. a drug that stimulates receptor sites on cells in order to cause an effect.
   B. a drug that stimulates receptor sites on cells in order to inhibit an effect.
   C. a drug that blocks receptor sites on cells in order to cause an effect.
   D. a drug that blocks receptor sites on cells in order to inhibit an effect.
   E. none of the above.

4. Drug administration by a critical care paramedic is generally done:
   A. because it is expected by their employer.
   B. in order to affect cellular activity.
   C. as a means of controlling the patient.
   D. in order to affect patient billing.
   E. as a means of altering mental status.

5. The science of pharmacology requires the critical care paramedic to:
   A. recognize the risks inherent in drug therapy.
   B. understand the pharmacokinetics involved in biotransformation.
   C. understand the pharmacodynamics involved at the cellular level.
   D. all of the above.
   E. A and C.

6. Pharmacology is generally defined as:
   A. the scientific study of medications.
   B. the scientific study of plant-based chemicals and their uses.
   C. the scientific study of drugs and how they alter body chemistry.
   D. the scientific study of how chemicals alter body and cellular activity.
   E. none of the above.

7. The study of how the body absorbs, distributes, transports, inactivates, and eliminates drugs is generally referred to as:
   A. pharmacology.
   B. pharmacokinetics.
   C. pharmacodynamics.
   D. bioavailability.
   E. biotransformation.

8. The study of what a drug does to the body as it alters cellular and tissue activity is generally referred to as:
   A. pharmacology.
   B. pharmacokinetics.
   C. pharmacodynamics.
   D. bioavailability.
   E. biotransformation.

9. Bioavailability is generally defined as:
   A. the study of drugs.
   B. the study of biotransformation in the body.
   C. the free, unbound state of a drug that allows it to exert an action on the body.
   D. the bound state of a drug that allows it to exert an action on the body.
   E. the method by which a drug changes into an inactive state.

10. Biotransformation is generally defined as:
    A. the study of drugs.
    B. the study of biotransformation in the body.
    C. the free, unbound state of a drug that allows it to exert an action on the body.
    D. the bound state of a drug that allows it to exert an action on the body.
    E. the method by which a drug changes into an inactive state.

11. The half-life of a drug is generally defined as:
    A. the time it takes one-half of a drug to be eliminated from the body.
    B. the time it takes one-half of a drug to be utilized by the body.
    C. the time it takes the body to make use of half a drug dose.
    D. the time it takes the body to eliminate half of a drug dose.
    E. none of the above.

12. Drug toxicity can be defined as harmful levels of a drug in the blood stream that can:
    A. cause only short-term damage.
    B. cause only moderate brain damage.
    C. cause only hallucinations.
    D. cause only unconsciousness.
    E. cause various outcomes.

13. In cardiac emergencies, pharmacologic agents can be used to:
    A. restore blood pressure.
    B. increase myocardial contractility.
    C. decrease myocardial oxygen demand.
    D. all of the above.
    E. A and B.

14. A positive chronotropic drug is one that:
    A. increases myocardial contractility.
    B. increases heart rate.
    C. decreases myocardial contractility.
    D. decreases heart rate.
    E. both increases heart rate and decreases myocardial contractility.

15. A negative inotropic drug is one that:
    A. increases myocardial contractility.
    B. increases heart rate.
    C. decreases myocardial contractility.
    D. decreases heart rate.
    E. both increases heart rate and decreases myocardial contractility.

16. The main reason for the use of an antihypertensive drug is:
    A. to increase afterload at the arterial level.
    B. to decrease preload at the arterial level.
    C. to increase afterload at the arterial and venous level.
    D. to decrease afterload at the arterial and venous level.
    E. none of the above.

17. Beta-blocking agents will introduce:
    A. negative inotropic effects.
    B. positive chronotropic effects.
    C. positive inotropic and negative chronotropic effects.
    D. negative inotropic and positive chronotropic effects.
    E. both negative inotropic and chronotropic effects.

18. Chronic hypertension can/will:
    A. decrease MVO$_2$.
    B. elevate metabolic demands of the myocardium.
    C. decrease end organ tissue perfusion.
    D. all of the above.
    E. B and C.

19. A drug's "action" can best be defined by:
    A. what bodily function(s) it affects.
    B. how it changes vital signs.
    C. how it changes pH.
    D. whether it has a positive or negative affect.
    E. all of the above.

20. A reason for the use of a drug is commonly referred to as a/an _____ for that drug.
    A. action
    B. control
    C. indication
    D. contraindication
    E. interaction

21. Side effects of a drug may be influenced by:
    A. medical conditions not associated with use of a particular drug.
    B. concomitant administration of other drugs.
    C. temperature at time of administration.
    D. all of the above.
    E. none of the above.

22. Vasodilatory drugs, such as sodium nitroprusside and hydralazine hydrochloride are designed to:
    A. increase cardiac output and preload.
    B. decrease systolic and diastolic pressures.
    C. increase left ventricular preload and afterload.
    D. decrease left ventricular preload and afterload.
    E. B and D.

23. Special considerations in the use of nitroprusside sodium include:
    A. monitoring patients with impaired hepatic or renal function.
    B. use of light-blocking containers.
    C. administration of less than 24 hours.
    D. all of the above.
    E. A and B.

24. Indications for the use of nesiritide may include:
    A. congestive heart failure.
    B. emphysema.
    C. hypotension.
    D. all of the above.
    E. none of the above.

25. _____ is the term for a drug that binds to receptor sites, causing relaxation of smooth vascular muscle.
    A. Peptide agent
    B. Beta-blocker
    C. Alpha-blocker
    D. Antihypertensive
    E. Antihistamine

26. The standard adult dosage for intravenous nitroglycerin is given as:
    A. 5–50 mcg/min as a continuous infusion.
    B. 5–25 mcg/min as a continuous infusion.
    C. 5–25 mg/min, bolused every 5 minutes for 24 hours.
    D. 5–50 mg/min as a continuous infusion.
    E. none of the above.

27. The contraindication(s) to the use of hydralazine hydrochloride may include:
    A. coronary artery disease.
    B. mitral stenosis.
    C. hypertension.
    D. persistent tachycardia.
    E. A, B and D.

28. Clonidine hydrochloride acts mainly on the:
    A. smooth vascular muscle.
    B. cardiac muscle.
    C. alpha-adrenergic receptors.
    D. all of the above.
    E. none of the above.

29. The term "ACE inhibitor" refers to a drug that acts on:
    A. altered-coronary events.
    B. angiotensin-converting enzymes.
    C. angiotensin-converging events.
    D. arterial-clogging enzymes.
    E. arterial-converting enzymes.

30. Angiotensin converting enzyme _____ the conversion of angiotensin I to angiotensin II in order to cause _____.
    A. metabolizes, vasodilation
    B. metabolizes, vasoconstriction
    C. catalyzes, vasodilation
    D. catalyzes, vasoconstriction
    E. catalyzes, metabolism

31. Beta blockers are generally designed to:
    A. decrease inotropic, dromotropic, and chronotropic effects on the heart.
    B. increase inotropic, dromotropic, and chronotropic effects on the heart.
    C. decrease inotropic and dromotropic, increase chronotropic effects on the heart
    D. increase dromotropic and chronotropic, decrease inotropic effects on the heart.
    E. decrease inotropic and chronotropic, increase dromotropic effects on the heart.

32. ACE Inhibitors should be used cautiously in patients with a known history of:
    A. renal impairment.
    B. arterial stenosis.
    C. dialysis or diuretic use.
    D. all of the above.
    E. none of the above.

33. Labetalol hydrochloride is contraindicated in patients with a history of:
    A. bronchial asthma.
    B. tachycardia.
    C. hypertension.
    D. Mobitz II heart block.
    E. A and D.

34. Vasopressor agents are used to:
    A. maintain end-organ perfusion.
    B. decrease afterload.
    C. increase blood pressure.
    D. all of the above.
    E. A and C.

35. The use of vasopressor drugs has a "risk/benefit" component that includes:
    A. increased MVO_2 demand and increased tissue necrosis.
    B. increased heart rate and decreased ischemia.
    C. increased cardiac complications and increased end-organ perfusion.
    D. decreased cardiac complications and decreased end-organ perfusion.
    E. none of the above.

36. Sympathomimetic drugs primarily affect the:
    A. autonomic nervous system.
    B. central nervous system.
    C. alpha- and beta-adrenergic receptors.
    D. central nervous system and alpha-adrenergic receptors.
    E. A and C.

37. You administer dopamine at 7 mcg/kg/min to a 42-year-old patient en route to a cardiac specialty center. What known side effects might you expect to see en route?
    A. tachycardia and hypertension
    B. hypotension and anxiety
    C. angina and decreased peripheral perfusion
    D. all of the above
    E. A and C

38. The generally accepted dosage range of pediatric dopamine is:
    A. 5–20 mcg/kg/min.
    B. 5–50 mcg/kg/min.
    C. 5–25 mg/kg/min.
    D. 5–50 mg/kg/min.
    E. none of the above.

39. Which of the following statements is true regarding the action of dopamine and dobutamine in the body?
    A. Dopamine acts on both the alpha- and beta-adrenergic receptors.
    B. Dobutamine acts on both the alpha- and beta-adrenergic receptors.
    C. Both act on the alpha- and beta-adrenergic receptors.
    D. Neither acts on the beta-adrenergic receptors.
    E. Neither acts on the alpha-adrenergic receptors.

40. You are transporting a 22-year-old trauma patient who is expected to undergo surgery upon arrival at a tertiary care center. Your patient persistently exhibits low blood pressure despite previous aggressive volume and vasoconstrictive drug therapy. During transport, you decide to introduce a sympathomimetic regimen in an attempt to maintain end-organ perfusion. Of the following choices, the best drug for this is:
    A. dopamine hydrochloride.
    B. phenylephrine hydrochloride.
    C. norepinephrine bitartrate.
    D. dobutamine hydrochloride.
    E. epinephrine hydrochloride.

41. The drug vasopressin has several effects that are beneficial in resuscitation. Among them are:
    A. elevated systemic vascular resistance.
    B. antidiuretic (ADH) properties.
    C. bronchoconstriction.
    D. all of the above.
    E. A and B.

42. In a perfusing patient, the contraindications to the use of vasopressin include:
    A. pheochromocytoma.
    B. epilepsy.
    C. hypertension.
    D. all of the above.
    E. A and C.

43. Procainimide is an antidysrhythmic that causes _____ blockade, whereas amiodarone is a drug that causes _____ blockade.
    A. calcium, sodium
    B. sodium, magnesium
    C. sodium, potassium
    D. potassium, calcium.
    E. none of the above.

44. Known actions of the drug lidocaine hydrochloride include:
    A. suppression of ischemic ectopic foci.
    B. increased intracranial pressure during rapid sequence intubation (RSI).
    C. decreased ventricular fibrillation threshold.
    D. all of the above.
    E. none of the above.

45. For lidocaine hydrochloride in perfusing patients, the standard adult and pediatric dosages are (respectively):
    A. 1.0–1.5 kg/mg IV and 0.5–1.0 kg/mg IV.
    B. 1.5–2.0 mg/kg IV and 0.5–1.0 mg/kg IV.
    C. 1.0–1.5 mg/kg IV and 0.5–1.0 mg/kg IV.
    D. 1.0–2.0 mg/kg IV and 0.5–1.0 mg/kg IV.
    E. 1.0–2.0 mcg/kg IV and 0.1–0.2 mg/kg IV.

46. The antidysrhythmic drug procainamide is considered to have _____ and _____ effects.
    A. negative inotropic, positive dromotropic
    B. positive dromotropic, negative inotropic
    C. negative conduction, positive dromotropic
    D. positive conduction, negative dromotropic
    E. negative dromotropic, negative inotropic

47. You are transporting a patient with a ventricular conduction defect that has been unresponsive to amiodarone and lidocaine. The patient is also being treated for digitalis toxicity and hypotension. Your continued therapeutic choices could include:
    A. procainamide infusion.
    B. supportive oxygen and fluid therapy.
    C. adenosine IV push.
    D. all of the above.
    E. none of the above.

48. Indications for the use of the Class III antidysrhythmic amiodarone include:
    A. initial treatment of atrial dysrhythmias.
    B. initial treatment of ventricular dysrhythmias.
    C. treatment of paroxysmal ventricular tachycardia refractory to other antidysrhythmics.
    D. all of the above.
    E. B and C.

49. Atropine sulfate is placed in what drug classification(s)?
    A. sympathomimetic, parasympathomimetic
    B. sympatholytic, parasympatholytic
    C. parasympatholytic, sympathomimetic
    D. parasympatholytic, antimuscarinic
    E. all of the above

50. You are treating a patient for chest discomfort concurrent with hypotension that has been unresponsive to oxygen and fluid replacement therapy. The patient is pale and cool to the touch, and ECG shows an apparent sinus bradycardia without ectopy. The patient tells you he has no known/previous cardiac disease. You decide to begin drug therapy and initiate administration of 1.0 mg IVP of atropine sulfate. Shortly after, your patient begins to exhibit signs and symptoms different from the initial complaint. Of the following, which would be considered a "normal" side effect of this drug?
    A. cardiac palpitations
    B. dilated pupils
    C. anxiety
    D. all of the above
    E. A and B

51. Adenosine works by blocking _____ channels in the heart and has the effect of _____ conduction through the _____ pathways.
    A. calcium, slowing, SA
    B. sodium, increasing, AV
    C. potassium, slowing, AV
    D. magnesium, increasing, SA
    E. none of the above

52. Drugs that may potentiate the effects of adenosine can include:
    A. theophylline.
    B. dipyridamole.
    C. benzodiazepine.
    D. albuterol.
    E. verapamil.

53. The use of magnesium sulfate in preterm labor relates to its _____ effects.
    A. anticonvulsant
    B. laxative
    C. tocolytic
    D. all of the above
    E. none of the above

54. The known mitigating agents for long-term use of magnesium sulfate include:
    A. glucagon.
    B. calcium gluconate.
    C. glycogen.
    D. calcium carbonate.
    E. calcium sulfate.

55. Magnesium sulfate for management of renal disease or failure is administered:
    A. administered 1–3 g diluted in 200 mL D5W, via IN infusion.
    B. administered 1–2 g diluted in 10 mL 0.9% NaCl, via IVP.
    C. administered 1–5 g diluted in 100 mL D5W, via IV infusion.
    D. administered 1–2 g diluted in 100 – 250 mL D5W, via IV infusion.
    E. contraindicated.

56. You are treating a 64-year-old female complaining of chest discomfort and palpitations. Interview and assessment reveal no apparent mechanism of trauma, and the patient denies previous cardiac medical history. Vital signs are: B/P=116/52 mmHg, RR=26 per minute and irregular, HR=130 per minute and irregular, and SpO_2=92%. Breath sounds are clear and 12-Lead ECG shows an apparent uncontrolled atrial fibrillation. After initial treatment with oxygen by NRB, you gain IV access and initiate therapy using adenosine. When you assess patient response 2 minutes later, she reports no relief.

    After a second dose of adenosine without response, it appears the patient is refractory to this drug. Your choice for continued drug therapy may include which of the following?
    1. magnesium sulfate
    2. propranolol hydrochloride
    3. diltiazem
    4. procainamide
    5. amiodarone

    A. 1, 3, and 5
    B. 1, 4, and 5
    C. 3 and 5
    D. 5
    E. 1, 2, 3, 4, and 5

57. Propranolol hydrochloride is a Class II antihypertensive and antidysrhythmic that acts as a sympatholytic affecting the _____ nervous system, as well as acting as a beta-adrenergic _____.
    A. central, agonist
    B. autonomic, agonist
    C. central, antagonist
    D. autonomic, antagonist
    E. none of the above

58. Contraindications to the use of propranolol hydrochloride would include:
    A. acute congestive heart failure.
    B. asthma.
    C. bradycardia.
    D. hypotension.
    E. all of the above.

59. The adult dose of propranolol hydrochloride is generally accepted as:
    A. 1–2 mg IVP every 2 min.
    B. 1–3 mg IVP every 5 min.
    C. 1–5 mg slow IVP every 2 min.
    D. 1–3 mg slow IVP every 5 min.
    E. 1–3 mg slow IVP every 2 min.

60. Administration of cardioprotective medications can:
    1. decrease mortality.
    2. eliminate risk of AMI.
    3. decrease infarction size.
    4. decrease atherosclerosis.
    5. eliminate risk of reinfarction.

    A. 1, 2, and 3
    B. 1 and 3
    C. 1, 3, and 5
    D. 2 and 4
    E. 3, 4, and 5

61. Aspirin acts to inhibit platelet aggregation by:
    A. decreasing synthesis of coagulation factors.
    B. decreasing calcium in blood.
    C. decreasing synthesis of sodium.
    D. increasing synthesis of potassium.
    E. all of the above.

62. Contraindications to the use of salicylates include:
    1. recent surgery.
    2. gastrointestinal bleeding.
    3. known allergic sensitivity.
    4. pregnancy.
    5. severe anemia.

    A. 1 and 2
    B. 1, 3 and 5
    C. 1, 2, 3 and 4
    D. 1, 2, 3, 4 and 5
    E. None of the above

63. The primary use of the sympathomimetic/sympatholytic drug metoprolol tartrate is:
    A. management of hypertension.
    B. preservation of myocardial tissue during AMI.
    C. mitigation of sudden cardiac death.
    D. decrease risk of reinfarction.
    E. all of the above.

64. Known side effects from use of metoprolol tartrate may include:
    A. hypertension.
    B. bronchodilation.
    C. hypoglycemia.
    D. A and B.
    E. B and C.

65. Inotropic agents are known to _____ peripheral perfusion, as well as _____ preload and afterload by _____ stroke volume and heart rate.
    A. decrease, increase, decreasing
    B. increase, decrease, increasing
    C. increase, increase, decreasing
    D. decrease, decrease, increasing
    E. none of the above

66. Inotropic agents include, but are not limited to:
    1. digoxin.
    2. milrinone lactate.
    3. inamrinone lactate.
    4. amiodarone.
    5. tirofiban hydrochloride.

    A. 1 and 2
    B. 1, 2, and 3
    C. 1, 2, 3, and 4
    D. 1, 2, 3, and 5
    E. 1, 2, 3, 4, and 5

67. You are treating a patient with digitalis toxicity, signs of congestive heart failure, and a history of aortic valve obstruction. Inotropic drug therapies of choice may include:
    A. milrinone lactate.
    B. inamironone lactate.
    C. digoxin.
    D. all of the above.
    E. none of the above.

68. Examples of anticoagulant/antiplatelet agents are:
    A. heparin sodium.
    B. warfarin sodium.
    C. clopidogrel bisulfate.
    D. enoxaparin.
    E. all of the above.

69. Your patient is exhibiting signs of altered mental status and hypertension. His past pertinent medical history includes atrial valve replacement and pulmonary embolus, as well as atrial fibrillation. His medications include digitalis and warfarin. After basic life support measures and IV access, you decide to institute additional

drug therapy. Your therapy should fall into which of the following drug classes?
   A. anticoagulant
   B. antihypertensive
   C. antiplatelet
   D. antianginal
   E. antidepressant

70. The generally recommended adult loading dose for heparin sodium is:
    A. 500–700 mg slow IVP.
    B. 500–700 mg IV infusion.
    C. 5,000–10,000 units slow IVP.
    D. 5,000–7,500 units IVP.
    E. 5,000–7,000 mg IVP.

71. Warfarin sodium is indicated for prophylaxis and treatment of acute:
    1. deep vein thrombosis.
    2. peripheral artery disease.
    3. pulmonary embolus.
    4. cerebral vascular disease.
    5. cerebral transient ischemic attacks.

    A. 1, 2, and 4
    B. 2, 3, and 5
    C. 1, 2, 3, and 4
    D. 1, 3, and 5
    E. 1, 2, 3, 4, and 5

72. Side effects of anticoagulant therapy include, but are not limited to:
    A. allergic reaction.
    B. hemorrhage.
    C. vitamin C or K deficiency.
    D. A and B.
    E. none of the above.

73. The agent eptifibatide immediately reverses and inhibits platelet aggregation by preventing the binding of _____ and _____.
    A. fibrinallation, glycoburide
    B. fibrinocide, glycogen
    C. fibrinogen, glycoprotein IIb/IIIa
    D. fibrin, glyburide IIa/IIIb
    E. fibrinogen, glycoprotein IIa/IIIb

74. Your patient is receiving abciximab therapy and begins to exhibit signs and symptoms of cardiac compromise and altered mental status. Her blood pressure has fallen from 110/62 mmHg to 96/48 mmHg, she is tachypneic, and she begins to bleed from the nose. Your response to this situation should be based upon your knowledge of:
    A. the patient's advance directives regarding this eventuality.
    B. the patient's "DNR," that directs no further therapy.
    C. the law and the certainty that your actions could not have harmed the patient.
    D. the known side effects of this drug and your ability to deal with them.
    E. the human body, pharmacology, and the patient's medical history.

75. Tirofiban hydrochloride and clopidogrel bisulfate share the following attributes. They:
    A. inhibit platelet aggregation of adenosine diphosphate (ADP).
    B. inhibit platelet aggregation at glycoprotein IAB/III receptor sites.
    C. inhibit coagulation of blood and aggregation of platelets.
    D. all of the above.
    E. none of the above.

76. Fibrinolytics are commonly used to treat patients during acute cardiac events such as myocardial infarction (AMI). Other uses for this class of agents may include:
    A. avoiding onset of congestive heart failure during AMI.
    B. treating pulmonary embolus.
    C. treating ischemic stroke.
    D. activating plasminogen in the body.
    E. all of the above.

77. Tenectaplase is a single-bolus medication administered:
    A. in a 40 mg dose over 15 seconds via IVP.
    B. in a 40 g dose over 15 seconds via IVP.
    C. in a weight related (30–50 mg) dose over 5 seconds via IVP.
    D. in a weight related dose (30 to 50 g) over 15 seconds via IVP.
    E. none of the above.

78. You are on duty in the Emergency Department at 3 A.M. The incoming BLS crew presents an unconscious 40-year-old patient with report of an apparent stroke. The crew states the patient was complaining of a severe headache upon their arrival, and the patient stated that after self-administration of 650 mg of aspirin he had called 911. The patient lost consciousness before the crew could obtain information about the time and type of onset; however, the patient did state he was a diabetic. Vital signs, reported as stable throughout contact and upon arrival, are: BP=210/104 mmHg bilaterally, HR/Pulse=54 beats per minute and irregular, RR=10 and assisted via BVM at 15 Lpm with 100% O_2, and SpO_2=95%. Prior to initiation of alteplase recombinant therapy, the ED resuscitation team should:
    1. attempt to gain more history from the patient's past records.
    2. wait for the results of a non-contrast CT scan.
    3. gain IV access and run an ABG, CBC, BMP and TOX Screen.
    4. secure the airway via ETT and obtain a 12-Lead ECG.
    5. perform a dextrostix and administer IV D5W PRN.

    A. 1, 3, and 5
    B. 1, 2, 3, and 5
    C. 1, 2, 4, and 5
    D. all of the above
    E. none of the above

79. The introduction of antiepileptic agents in status epilepticus may prevent onset of:
    A. cellular ischemia.
    B. rhabdomyolysis.
    C. orthopedic injury.
    D. all of the above.
    E. A and C.

80. The emergent use of phenytoin, fosphenytoin, and phenobarbital sodium may cause additional sequelae that includes:
    1. CNS depression.
    2. ataxia.
    3. nystagmus.
    4. hypertension.
    5. hyperglycemia.

    A. 1 and 5
    B. 1, 2, and 4
    C. 1, 2, and 3
    D. 2, 3, and 4
    E. 1, 2, 3, 4, and 5

81. The drug mannitol is primarily indicated for the management of:
    A. increasing intracranial pressure.
    B. increasing mean arterial pressure.
    C. increasing cerebral perfusion pressure.
    D. decreasing intracranial pressure.
    E. decreasing systemic vascular resistance.

82. Methylprednisolone is a/an _____ used in the management of acute bronchospasm and chronic inflammatory diseases.
    A. osmotic diuretic
    B. glucocorticoid steroid
    C. diuretic steroid
    D. anabolic steroid
    E. none of the above

83. Indication(s) for the use of dexamethasone may include:
    A. adrenal insufficiency.
    B. chronic inflammatory disease states.

C. long-term therapy in rheumatic disorders.
D. A and B.
E. B and C.

84. You are treating a stroke patient with known renal disease who also suffers from diabetes. What drug regimen(s) may you consider for treatment of neurologic deficits?
   A. dexamethasone
   B. nimodipine
   C. mannitol
   D. methylprednisolone
   E. all of the above

85. In patients with reactive airway disease, the use of _____ agents is indicated for treatment of acute hypoxia.
   A. sympatholytic
   B. alpha-adrenergic
   C. sympathomimetic
   D. beta-antagonist
   E. all of the above

86. You are transporting a pediatric patient with new-onset asthma, exacerbated by acute bronchospasm. After two nebulized albuterol treatments, he is not responding. What secondary agent(s) could be considered?
   A. ipatropium bromide
   B. levalbuterol hydrochloride
   C. hydrocortisone gluconate
   D. A, B, and C
   E. A and C

87. Known side effects of sympathomimetics can include:
   1. tachycardia.
   2. hypotension.
   3. palpitations.
   4. hypertension.
   5. thrombocytopenia.

   A. 2, 3, and 4
   B. 1, 3, and 4
   C. 1, 3, 4, and 5
   D. 1, 2, 4, and 5
   E. all of the above

88. Neuromuscular blocking agents are used, in conjunction with sedation, primarily to help:
   1. decrease oxygen demands.
   2. decrease intracranial pressure.
   3. suppress the gag reflex.
   4. decrease ventricular response.
   5. increase mentation.

   A. 1 and 2
   B. 1, 2, and 3
   C. 1, 2, 3, and 4
   D. 1, 2, 3, 4, and 5
   E. none of the above

89. Actions of succinylcholine are described as:
   A. Depolarization produced by neuromuscular blockade of anticholinergic motor end plate receptors.
   B. Depolarization produced by neuromuscular blockade of adrenergic motor end plate receptors.
   C. Repolarization produced by neuromuscular blockade of anticholinergic motor end plate receptors.
   D. Depolarization produced by neuromuscular blockade of the cholinergic motor end plate receptors.
   E. Depolarization produced by neuromuscular blockade of the parasympathomimetic system.

90. You have used succinylcholine to facilitate intubation of a comatose patient. Several minutes later your partner tells you that the patient is very cold to the touch. Assessment by rectal probe reveals that the patient's core temperature is now reading 90 degrees F. This event is:
   A. of no concern, since you have warm IV fluids.
   B. a known side effect of the drug.
   C. an untoward reaction you did not expect.
   D. all of the above.
   E. none of the above.

91. Vecuronium, pancuronium and cisatracurium are best classified as:
    A. depolarizing paralytic agents.
    B. nondepolarizing parasympathetic agents.
    C. nondepolarizing sympatholytic agents.
    D. nondepolarizing sympathomimetic agents.
    E. nondepolarizing paralytic agents.

92. Narcotic analgesics are primarily used to:
    1. mitigate anxiety disorders.
    2. mitigate debilitating pain.
    3. increase systemic oxygen demand.
    4. decrease metabolic demand.
    5. increase cellular oxygen supply.

    A. 1 and 3
    B. 1, 2, and 4
    C. 2, 4, and 5
    D. 1, 2, and 5
    E. 2, 3, and 4

93. Hydromorphone hydrochloride, morphine sulfate, and meperidine hydrochloride are examples of:
    A. CNS narcotic agonists.
    B. ANS narcotic antagonists.
    C. CNS narcotic antagonists.
    D. ANS narcotic agonists.
    E. none of the above.

94. Contraindications for the use of narcotic agonists include:
    1. hypertension.
    2. respiratory depression.
    3. altered mental status.
    4. constipation.
    5. seizures.

    A. 1 and 3
    B. 2, 3, and 4
    C. 1, 2, 3, and 4
    D. 2, 4, and 5
    E. 2, 3, 4, and 5

95. Narcotic agonist agents are primarily indicated for patients suffering from:
    A. short-term management of acute pain.
    B. long-term management of chronic pain.
    C. myasthenia gravis.
    D. active labor pain.
    E. all of the above.

96. Narcotic agonist-antagonist combination agents are contraindicated for patients suffering from:
    A. angioedema.
    B. renal impairment.
    C. pulmonary edema.
    D. A and B.
    E. none of the above.

97. Administration of ketorolac tromethamine in the emergent setting is most appropriately accomplished via the _____ route:
    A. oral
    B. buccal
    C. rectal
    D. intravenous
    E. endotracheal

98. What is the primary difference between narcotics and sedatives?
    A. Narcotics abolish pain; sedatives lessen pain.
    B. Narcotics alleviate pain; sedatives alleviate stress and anxiety.
    C. Narcotics alleviate pain and stress; sedatives abolish stress and anxiety.
    D. Narcotics alleviate stress and anxiety; sedatives alleviate pain.
    E. none of the above

99. The benzodiazepines most commonly used in emergency medicine are:
    1. midazolam.
    2. lorazepam.

3. estazolam.
4. diazepam.
5. chloral hydrate.

A. 1 and 2
B. 2 and 3
C. 1, 2, and 4
D. 1, 2, 4, and 5
E. 1, 2, 3, 4, and 5

100. You are treating a 32-year-old female patient suffering from extreme pain secondary to muscle spasm following a trip-and-fall accident. You decide to administer 5 mg of diazepam, IVP. Shortly thereafter the patient becomes hypotensive and apneac. Your next action(s) to consider would be:

A. ventilations via BVM with 100% O_2, consider orotracheal intubation.
B. administration of 2.0 mg IVP flumazenil every 5 min, titrated to effect.
C. administration of 0.2 mg IVP flumazenil every 1 min, max dose 1.0 mg.
D. A and B.
E. A and C.

101. Caution should be used in the administration of propofol in patients with:

A. allergy to eggs.
B. administration of inhaled anesthetics.
C. simultaneous use of benzodiazepines.
D. all of the above.
E. A and B.

102. Barbiturate hypnotics include all of the following agents EXCEPT:

A. propofol.
B. etomidate.
C. pentobarbital.
D. thiopental sodium.
E. A and B.

103. The narcotic/benzodiazepine antagonists most often used in the emergent setting are:

A. naloxone and flumazenil.
B. aminocaproic acid and disulfiram.
C. edetate disodium and ipecac syrup.
D. naltrexone hydrochloride and pralidoxime chloride.
E. none of the above.

104. Cefazolin sodium and ceftriaxone sodium are classified as:

A. antivirals.
B. antibiotics.
C. antiemetics.
D. antifungals.
E. none of the above.

105. Cephalosporin-based medications specifically treat _____ bacteria:

A. gram-positive
B. gram-negative
C. aerobic
D. anaerobic
E. all of the above

106. The terms VRSA and MRSA specifically refer to a bacterial organism that is resistant to treatment with vancomycin and methicillin. That organism is:

A. *staphylococcus auriana*.
B. *staphylococcum aurius*.
C. *staphylococcus aureus*.
D. all of the above.
E. none of the above.

107. A drug most often used in the pediatric setting to combat systemic bacteremia and also found in the critical care setting is:

A. imipenem-cilastatin sodium.
B. ampicillin sodium.
C. fluconazole.
D. gentamicin sulfate.
E. clindamycin hydrochloride.

108. The drug fluconazole is most often administered in the critical care setting for the treatment of:
    A. candidemia or candidiasis.
    B. fungal pneumonia.
    C. cryptococcal meningitis.
    D. all of the above.
    E. none of the above.

109. You are transporting a 68-year-old patient in acute congestive heart failure. He has no history of CHF but is status-post 4-vessel CABG 3 months ago. The patient is tachycardic, hypertensive, and tachypneic with +4 edema to the lower extremities as well as obvious crackles in all lung fields. After oxygen administration and IV access, you begin consideration of drug therapy. Your patient is known to have a sensitivity to nitrates. Your immediate choice is administration of a loop diuretic, such as furosemide or bumetanide. The recommended dosage for bumetanide is:
    A. 1.5–2.5 mg IVP over 2 minutes, every 4 to 5 hours.
    B. 0.5–2.0 mg slow IVP over 1–2 minutes, every 4 to 5 hours.
    C. 0.5–2.5 mg slow IVP over 2–4 minutes, max dose 10 mg.
    D. 0.5–1.0 mg IVP over 1–2 minutes, every 4 hours.
    E. none of the above.

110. Ranitidine, cimetidine, and famotidine are classified as:
    A. H1 receptor site agonists.
    B. H1 receptor site antagonists.
    C. H2 receptor site agonists.
    D. H2 receptor site antagonists.
    E. H1 and H2 receptor site antagonists.

111. You are treating a 20-year-old female patient who has been vomiting almost continuously for 4 hours and is awaiting CT scan to rule out CNS etiology. In order to treat her dehydration, you begin intravenous therapy. Additionally, per physician order, you administer 2.5 mg prochlorperazine slow IVP for nausea. Several minutes later your patient begins to drool and complain of severe neck pain. You recognize this as an extrapyramidal reaction and request orders to administer:
    A. 1 mg diphenhydramine, PO.
    B. 1.5 mg diphenhydramine IM.
    C. 12.5–25 mg diphenhydramine slow IVP.
    D. 50–100 mg diphenhydramine slow IVP.
    E. none of the above.

112. Your 52-year-old male patient is being transported by air to another facility for CT scan. He complains of severe headache and is hypertensive as well as mildly disoriented. Prior to transport, oxygen therapy was initiated by nasal cannula, an IV was started with 0.9% NaCl, and 0.1 mg of clonidine was administered PO. En route, his blood pressure increases to 210/112 mmHg and his headache becomes more severe. You make the decision to initiate therapy to decrease the B/P. Your choice of drug intervention would most likely be:
    A. clonidine, 0.1 mg PO.
    B. nitroprusside, 0.5 mcg/kg/min, titrated.
    C. labetalol, 2 mg, IM.
    D. fentanyl, 1000 mcg, slow IVP.
    E. nalbuphine, 5 mg PO.

Scenario

Questions 113–115 refer to the following scenario:

You are transporting a 60-year-old male from a community hospital ICU to an ICU at a university hospital. The patient has renal failure and MODS following an out-of-hospital cardiac arrest from which he was resuscitated. He is receiving IV dopamine (800 mg/250 mL D_5W) at 8 mcg per minute and IV nitroglycerin (50 mg/250 mL D_5W) at 20 mcg per minute. He weighs 132 pounds.

113. At what rate is the dopamine infusing?
   A. 0.9 mL/hour
   B. 18.0 mL/hour
   C. 9.0 mL/hour
   D. 60 mL/hour
   E. none of the above

114. At what rate is the nitroglycerin infusing?
   A. 6.0 mL/hour
   B. 9.0 mL/hour
   C. 60 mL/hour
   D. 100 mL/hour
   E. none of the above

115. The patient develops chest pain, so you increase the dosage of nitroglycerin to 15 mL/hour. How many mcg per minute is he now receiving?
   A. 5 mcg/minute
   B. 0.5 mcg/minute
   C. 25 mcg/min
   D. 50 mcg/min
   E. none of the above

CHAPTER 12
Interpretation of Lab and Basic Diagnostic Tests

DIRECTIONS Each of the questions or incomplete statements below is followed by suggested answers or completions. Select the **one answer** that is best in each case.

1. The measure of how well a test detects a disease without giving a false-positive result is called:
   A. sensitivity.
   B. standard deviation.
   C. mean.
   D. specificity.
   E. none of the above.

2. In order to have in excess of a 99% confidence interval, the curve must extend out how far?
   A. −1 standard deviation from the mean
   B. 1 standard deviation from the mean
   C. 2 standard deviations from the mean.
   D. 3 standard deviations from the mean
   E. none of the above

3. A person does not have the disease in question and tests negative for the disease. This is referred to as:
   A. true negative.
   B. false negative.
   C. true positive.
   D. false positive.
   E. none of the above.

4. The term "nanogram" means:
   A. one millionth of a gram.
   B. one billionth of a gram.
   C. one thousandth of a gram.
   D. one million grams.
   E. one billion grams.

5. The CBC for your patient reveals a hematocrit of 28%, a hemoglobin of 8.5 g/dL, an MCV 125 µm^3, an MCH of 45 pg, and an MCHC of 45%. Which of the following is least likely a cause for these abnormal lab values?
   A. alcoholism
   B. iron deficiency
   C. folate deficiency
   D. vitamin B$_{12}$ deficiency
   E. none of the above

6. Which of the following white cell types would you expect to see elevated in a bacterial infection?
   A. lymphocyte
   B. eosinophil
   C. basophil
   D. monocyte
   E. neutrophil

7. You are transporting a recent arrival from Africa who became ill shortly after arrival. On the CBC differential you note that the percentages of monocytes and eosinophils are elevated. What is the most likely cause?
   A. allergies
   B. malaria
   C. parasites
   D. A and C
   E. B and C

8. A measure of less mature forms of red blood cells is:
   A. band count.
   B. sed rate.
   C. C-reactive protein.
   D. reticulocyte count.
   E. none of the above.

9. The cell type in the marrow that gives rise to all blood cell types is:
   A. hemocytoblast.
   B. myeloid stem cell.
   C. prosynthroblast.
   D. myeloblast.
   E. none of the above.

10. In leukemia, white blood cell values are:
    A. normal.
    B. elevated.
    C. reduced.
    D. absent.
    E. none of the above.

11. A "left shift" in the CBC differential is associated with:
    A. appendicitis.
    B. bacterial infection.
    C. pyelonephritis.
    D. all of the above.
    E. none of the above.

12. Which of the following lab values is used to monitor heparin therapy?
    A. partial thromboplastin time (PTT)
    B. D-dimer
    C. prothrombin time (PT)
    D. internationalized normalized ratio (INR)
    E. none of the above

13. Which of the following is a normal anion gap?
    A. 12–14 mEq/L
    B. 1–2 mEq/L
    C. 20–24 mEq/L
    D. 0 mEq/L
    E. none of the above

14. Which of the following is a bivalent cation?
    A. Na^+
    B. K^+
    C. Cl^-
    D. Mg^{++}
    E. none of the above

15. A BUN/creatinine ratio of 23:1 points to:
    A. prerenal causes
    B. renal causes
    C. postrenal causes
    D. A and C
    E. none of the above

16. Which of the following is characteristic of gout?
    A. decreased uric acid
    B. increased uric acid
    C. decreased serum osmolality
    D. increased serum osmolality
    E. B and D

Scenario

Questions 17–20 refer to the following scenario:

Your patient has the following basic metabolic profile (BMP):

Na^+ = 151 mEq/L
K^+ = 4.9 mEq/L
Cl^- = 110 mEq/L
HCO_3^- = 24 mEq/L
BUN = 31 mg/dL
creatinine = 1.1 mg/dL
glucose = 128 mg/dL

17. What is the BUN/creatinine ratio?
    A. 28:1
    B. 1:28
    C. 30
    D. 15
    E. none of the above

18. What is the calculated anion gap?
    A. 15 mEq/L
    B. 22 mEq/L
    C. 31 mEq/L
    D. 19 mEq/L
    E. none of the above

19. Which of the following ECG changes would you expect to see in this patient?
    A. peaked T-waves
    B. delta waves

C. Osborne waves
D. inverted P waves
E. none of the above

20. These lab values are most consistent with:
    A. moderate overhydration.
    B. normal hydration.
    C. dehydration.
    D. acute pulmonary edema.
    E. none of the above.

21. Which of the following is NOT associated with hypochloremia?
    A. vomiting
    B. gastric suctioning
    C. diarrhea
    D. diuretic use
    E. renal failure.

22. A patient tells you his Hemoglobin A_1C was 12%. What does this indicate?
    A. The patient is a heavy smoker.
    B. The patients has diabetes under excellent control.
    C. The patient has markedly elevated cholesterol levels.
    D. The patient has diabetes under poor control.
    E. none of the above

23. Which of the following is NOT associated with increased risk for heart disease?
    A. elevated HDL
    B. elevated cholesterol
    C. elevated triglycerides
    D. elevated LDL
    E. none of the above

Match each following LDH isoenzyme with its source:

24. _____ LDH_1
25. _____ LDH_2
26. _____ LDH_3
27. _____ LDH_4
28. _____ LDH_5

A. placenta, kidney, pancreas
B. reticuloendothelial system
C. heart, erythrocytes, renal cortex
D. lung tissue
E. skeletal muscle, liver

Match each following CK isoenzyme with its source:

29. _____ CK-I (BB)
30. _____ CK-II (MB)
31. _____ CK-III (MM)

A. heart
B. skeletal muscle
C. brain and smooth muscle

32. Which marker is the first to elevate following myocardial infarction?
    A. CK
    B. LDH
    C. myoglobin
    D. troponin
    E. none of the above

33. Which of the following tests of liver function is the first to elevate during alcohol abuse?
    A. ALP
    B. GGT
    C. ALT
    D. AST
    E. aldolase

34. Your patient has a total bilirubin of 3.1 mg/dL of which 2.9 mg/dL is direct bilirubin. Which of the following is the most likely cause?
    A. sickle cell disease
    B. autoimmune disease
    C. drug toxicity
    D. gallstones
    E. none of the above

35. Which of the following is a serological marker for *Neisseria gonorrhea* infection?
    A. VDRL
    B. RPR
    C. FTA-ABS
    D. MHA-TP
    E. none of the above

36. Which of the following blood types is safest to administer in an emergency when the patient's blood type is not known?
    A. AB⁺
    B. AB⁻
    C. O⁺
    D. O⁻
    E. none of the above

37. You are transporting a patient between hospitals. A quick look at his chart reveals the following:

    Anti-HAV = Negative
    Anti-HBV = Positive
    HBsAg = Positive

    Which of the following statements is true?
    A. The patient has been immunized against hepatitis A.
    B. The patient has hepatitis A.
    C. The patient has hepatitis B.
    D. The patient has hepatitis C.
    E. none of the above

38. Which of the following findings on a urinalysis would point to a urinary tract infection?
    A. positive leukocyte esterase
    B. positive nitrite
    C. 10–12 WBC/HPF
    D. all of the above
    E. A and B

39. In a concentrated urine sample, one would expect the specific gravity to be:
    A. elevated.
    B. low.
    C. normal.
    D. not impacted by concentration.
    E. none of the above.

40. Which of the following tests uses ionizing radiation?
    A. computed tomography
    B. magnetic resonance imaging
    C. positron emission tomography
    D. ultrasound
    E. none of the above

41. Which of the following findings is inconsistent with a diagnosis of respiratory acidosis?
    A. pH = 7.25
    B. increased PaCO₂
    C. decreased PaCO₂
    D. decreased HCO₃⁻
    E. none of the above

42. A patient is suffering diabetic ketoacidosis and being treated in an ICU with oxygen and a heparin drip. Which of the following laboratory findings would NOT be expected?
    A. PO₂ = 158 mmHg
    B. PCO₂ = 23 mmHg
    C. HCO₃⁻ = 12 mEg/L
    D. pH = 7.48
    E. none of the above

Scenario

Questions 43–44 refer to the following scenario:
You are transporting a patient with fulminant pancreatitis. He is receiving IV H₂ blockers and has an NG tube in place. He is also on a morphine drip. His ABGs are:

pH = 7.5, PO₂ = 101 mmHg, PCO₂ = 38 mmHg, HCO₃⁻ = 36 mEq/L, HgB = 13.0 g/dL, and SaO₂ = 99%

43. Which acid-base derangement is present?
    A. respiratory acidosis
    B. respiratory alkalosis

C. metabolic acidosis
  D. metabolic alkalosis
  E. none of the above

44. What is the most likely cause of the patient's condition?
  A. severe vomiting
  B. NG suctioning
  C. diarrhea
  D. A and B
  E. A and C

45. Which of the following statements about blood gases is true?
  A. An abnormally decreased amount of bicarbonate is called "base deficit."
  B. An abnormally high pH is called "base deficit."
  C. An abnormally low pH is called "base deficit."
  D. An abnormally increased amount of carbon dioxide is called "base excess."
  E. An abnormally decreased amount of carbon dioxide is called "base excess."

CHAPTER 13

Introduction to Trauma

DIRECTIONS: Each of the questions or incomplete statements below is followed by suggested answers or completions. Select the **one answer** that is best in each case.

1. Trauma is the _____ leading cause of death for all patients.
   A. first
   B. second
   C. third
   D. fourth
   E. fifth

2. The number one cause of trauma deaths in the United States is:
   A. falls.
   B. aviation accidents.
   C. medical malpractice.
   D. homicide.
   E. none of the above.

3. Trauma is a particularly costly disease because of:
   A. total years of productive life lost (YPLL).
   B. medical costs.
   C. future transportation costs.
   D. age-adjusted inflation index.
   E. total years of life lost (YLL).

4. The landmark "white paper" *Accidental Death and Disability: The Neglected Disease of Modern Society* was published in what year?
   A. 1963
   B. 1966
   C. 1973
   D. 1978
   E. 2006

5. The first civilian special care unit devoted specifically to trauma was in:
   A. Baltimore (Johns Hopkins Hospital).
   B. New York (Montefiore Medical Center).
   C. San Antonio (Bexar County Medical Center).
   D. Los Angeles (Rampart Receiving Hospital).
   E. Baltimore (University of Maryland).

6. A hospital can appropriately manage most seriously injured patients but does not have an active residency program or research center. According to the American College of Surgeons, this hospital would be categorized as:
   A. Level I.
   B. Level II.
   C. Level III.
   D. Level IV.
   E. Level V.

7. Which of the following statements about trauma is FALSE?
   A. Approximately 50% of trauma deaths die immediately or within several minutes.
   B. Approximately 30% of trauma deaths die within several hours of their injuries.
   C. Approximately 80% of trauma deaths die either immediately or within several hours of their injuries.
   D. Approximately 50% of trauma deaths die either immediately or within several hours of their injuries.
   E. Approximately 20% of trauma deaths die within days to weeks of their injuries.

8. Death following trauma has a _____ distribution
   A. unimodal
   B. bimodal
   C. trimodal
   D. pentamodal
   E. bipedal

9. The greatest number of trauma deaths can be saved by:
   A. helicopter transport.
   B. the "Golden Hour."
   C. prevention.
   D. intraosseous lines.
   E. suspended animation.

10. Which of the following is often used in injury prevention to detail the relationship between variables that can be altered before, during, and after an event?
    A. Haddon matrix
    B. sample matrix
    C. NHTSA matrix
    D. relativity matrix
    E. Bon Secours matrix

11. Which of the following would be a type of PASSIVE injury prevention?
    A. buckling of a seat belt
    B. installing a stop sign
    C. putting on a helmet
    D. placing a child in a safety seat.
    E. none of the above

Scenario

Questions 12–13 refer to the following scenario:
You are called to treat an adult multiple trauma patient with the following parameters:

Blood pressure: 80/50 mmHg
Pulse: 120 per minute
Respiratory rate: 30 per minute
Eye opening: to pain
Best motor response: withdraws to pain
Best verbal response: inappropriate words

12. What is the patient's Glasgow Coma Score (GCS)?
    A. 7
    B. 8
    C. 9
    D. 10
    E. 11

13. What is his Revised Trauma Score?
    A. 4
    B. 8
    C. 9
    D. 10
    E. 11

14. The TRISS scoring system combines patient age with:
    A. the Injury Severity Score.
    B. the Pediatric Trauma Score.
    C. the Revised Trauma Score.
    D. A and B.
    E. A and C.

Scenario

Questions 15–16 refer to the following scenario:
A 7-year-old child, who was a restrained passenger in a high-speed freeway collision, has the following parameters:

Blood pressure: 92/70 mmHg
Weight: 22 kg
Airway: patent, crying
Mental status: alert, appropriate, interacts
Exam: fractured right forearm, no other injuries, normal movement.
Open wounds: none

15. What is the patient's Glasgow Coma Score (GCS)?
    A. 8
    B. 9
    C. 11
    D. 14
    E. 15

16. What is his Pediatric Trauma Score?
    A. 4
    B. 8

C. 9
D. 10
E. 11

17. The physical results of a mechanism of injury are called:
    A. biomechanics of trauma.
    B. injuries from trauma.
    C. Newtonian effects.
    D. tertiary aggregate.
    E. none of the above.

18. You are called in the middle of the night to a bar where you find a 22-year-old male victim of a gunshot wound. Your chief concern should be:
    A. identifying the shooter.
    B. managing the patient's airway.
    C. safety of the bystanders.
    D. preserving evidence.
    E. your safety and that of your crew.

19. Which of the following types of energy can cause injury?
    A. radiation
    B. thermal
    C. electrical
    D. all of the above
    E. A and C

20. Which of the following findings IS NOT indicative of Class III hemorrhagic shock?
    A. 26–39% blood volume loss
    B. coma
    C. moderate tachypnea
    D. significant tachycardia
    E. none of the above

21. Which of the following findings IS indicative of Class I hemorrhagic shock?
    A. blood volume loss 15–25%
    B. normal heart rate
    C. metabolic acidosis
    D. oliguria
    E. none of the above

Scenario

Questions 22–23 refer to the following scenario:
You are called to treat a patient who was stabbed in the abdomen. She has tachycardia, decreased peripheral pulses, normal BP, confusion, and cool extremities.

22. According to hemorrhagic shock classifications, what approximate blood volume loss would you expect?
    A. < 15%
    B. > 40%
    C. 15–25%
    D. 26–39%
    E. cannot tell from the data provided

23. The patient would be categorized as Class _____ hemorrhagic shock.
    A. I
    B. II
    C. III
    D. IV
    E. V

24. Place the following trauma patient management priorities in the proper order (highest priority first):
    1. maintenance of body temperature
    2. pain control
    3. patient safety
    4. management of the airway
    5. rescuer safety
    6. protection from spinal cord injury

    A. 3, 4, 5, 6, 1, 2
    B. 5, 4, 3, 2, 6, 1
    C. 5, 3, 4, 6, 1, 2
    D. 3, 5, 2, 1, 4, 6
    E. none of the above

25. CCP agencies have a responsibility to practice evidence-based trauma care. Which of the following would be effective in achieving this goal?
    A. Track patient outcomes by type of patient and care received during transport.
    B. Review research published in scholarly trauma journals.
    C. Participate in receiving hospitals' research regarding efficacy of patient management techniques.
    D. all of the above
    E. A and B

CHAPTER 14
Neurologic Trauma

DIRECTIONS: Each of the questions or incomplete statements below is followed by suggested answers or completions. Select the **one answer** that is best in each case.

1. Neurologic injuries are often difficult to manage because:
   A. significant secondary injury can take hours to days to manifest.
   B. autoregulatory functions can be compromised.
   C. histopathologic changes can occur.
   D. edema can affect all tissues in the body.
   E. all of the above.

2. The most valuable tool a critical care paramedic has when dealing with neurologic injuries is:
   A. a penlight.
   B. a hammer.
   C. clinical assessment skills.
   D. a magnetic resonance imager.
   E. a CT scanner.

3. The Glasgow Coma Scale (GCS) is an assessment tool that, in part, places numeric value on a patient's ability to:
   A. respond to pain or move their extremities voluntarily.
   B. respond to voice commands or speak comprehensible words.
   C. withdraw from pain or describe and physically locate pain.
   D. all of the above.
   E. A and C.

4. During your assessment of an unrestrained passenger in a motor vehicle collision, you find that your patient opens his eyes in response to verbal stimuli but is unable to articulate speech or move his lower extremities. As you assess his back, he cries out in pain when you palpate in the area of T-10, T-11, and T-12, but he exhibits no ability to withdraw his lower extremities from painful stimuli. What is this patient's apparent GCS?
   A. 5
   B. 7
   C. 11
   D. 13
   E. 15

5. A detailed neurological examination of a conscious patient may involve assessment of:
   A. extraocular movements.
   B. facial symmetry.
   C. ataxia.
   D. arm drift.
   E. all of the above.

6. Hand grasps are a/an _____ indicator of gross motor strength.
   A. objective
   B. deductive
   C. subjective
   D. intuitive
   E. palpable

7. The purpose of a lumbar puncture is to:
   A. obtain cerebral spinal fluid for laboratory examination.
   B. release pressure in the spinal cord.
   C. evaluate intracranial pressure.
   D. assess spinal nerve response.
   E. A or C.

8. The use of CT scan may be indicated for evaluation of _____ injuries, whereas MRI is more sensitive in evaluating _____ injuries.
   A. brain, liver
   B. bone, soft tissue
   C. brain, bone
   D. cardiovascular, muscular
   E. none of the above

9. The electroencephalogram is a device that is intended to record and document:
   1. brain wave activity.
   2. cardiac muscle electrical activity.

3. brain electrical emissions.
4. sacral area spinal cord impulses.
5. seizure activity.

A. 1 and 2
B. 1, 2, and 3
C. 1, 3, and 5
D. 1, 3, 4, and 5
E. 1, 2, 3, 4, and 5

10. The term _____ refers to a state in which a patient has no meaningful response to external stimuli for an extended period of time.
    A. lucid interval
    B. somnolence
    C. concussion
    D. coma
    E. altered mental state

11. The part of the brain responsible for maintaining waking consciousness is called the:
    A. reticular activating system.
    B. ocular activating system.
    C. vascular cortex system.
    D. responsive activating system.
    E. none of the above.

12. Factors in a determination of brain death may include lack of:
    A. motor response to stimulation.
    B. corneal reflexes.
    C. spontaneous respirations.
    D. occulovestibular reflexes.
    E. all of the above.

13. Your patient is suffering from a brain tumor and is unable to articulate speech, move her body, or breathe on her own. She does, however, track your movements and appears to hear sounds. This type of brain lesion leaves the patient in a neurological state known as:
    A. "locked out."
    B. "locked up."
    C. "locked in."
    D. "comatose."
    E. none of the above.

14. The range of measurement for a normal intracranial pressure (ICP) is:
    A. 10–20 mm.
    B. 0–10 mm.
    C. 10–20 mL.
    D. 0–10 mmHg.
    E. 10–20 mmHg.

15. The potential damage caused by elevated ICP is based on which of the following factors?
    1. duration of the elevated pressure
    2. rate of elevation
    3. age of patient
    4. reason for elevation
    5. level of pressure achieved

    A. 1, 2, and 3
    B. 1, 2, and 4
    C. 1, 2, and 5
    D. 1, 2, 3, and 4
    E. 1, 2, 3, 4, and 5

16. Mass effect, an early compensatory mechanism associated with ICP and cerebral edema, is a result of _____ in the cranial vault.
    A. compression of the arterial system
    B. compression of the venous system
    C. compression of both venous and arterial systems
    D. expansion of the arterial system
    E. expansion of the venous system

17. Signs and symptoms of tentorial (or uncal) herniation may include:
    A. contralateral dilated pupil.
    B. constricted pupils.
    C. ipsilateral dilated pupil.
    D. A and C.
    E. B and C.

18. _____ may result from diffuse or midline lesions. The most common presentation is decreased level of consciousness coupled with bilaterally constricted, fixed-at-midpoint pupils.
    A. Uncal herniation
    B. Central tentorial herniation
    C. Subfalcine herniation
    D. Tonsillar herniation
    E. None of the above

19. Midline shift is another name for:
    A. uncal herniation.
    B. central tentorial herniation.
    C. subfalcine herniation.
    D. tonsillar herniation.
    E. none of the above.

20. The herniation of the brain involves a recognized cascade of events. Components of this cascade are known to include:
    1. uncal herniation over the edge of the tentorium.
    2. tentorial cingulated herniation into the falx.
    3. cingulated herniation under the falx.
    4. cerebellar tonsillar herniation into the foramen magnum.
    5. downward transtentorial herniation.

    A. 1, 2, and 3
    B. 2, 3, and 4
    C. 1, 3, and 5
    D. 1, 2, 3, and 4
    E. 1, 3, 4, and 5

21. _____ describes the abnormal accumulation of cerebrospinal fluid in the brain.
    A. Hydrotentorius
    B. Hydrocerebellus
    C. Hydrocephalus
    D. Hydroencephalus
    E. Hydroencerebullus

22. An endocrine disorder that may result from compression to the hypothalamus or posterior pituitary gland during central herniation is:
    A. diabetes mellitus.
    B. renal failure.
    C. diabetes insipidus.
    D. hepatic failure.
    E. diabetic ketoacidosis.

23. During insertion of a pressure transducer, the external auditory meatus (EAM) is used as a landmark for the _____ of the brain.
    A. precentral gyrus
    B. occipital lobe
    C. pons
    D. temporal lobe
    E. lateral ventricle

24. The most common placement of intracranial pressure monitor devices is:
    1. epidural.
    2. subarachnoid.
    3. ventricular.
    4. subdural.
    5. intraparenchymal.

    A. 1 and 2
    B. 2 and 3
    C. 1, 2, and 3
    D. 1, 2, 3, 4, and 5
    E. 2, 3, 4, and 5

25. You are caring for an ICU patient who has an extraventricular drain (EVD) in place. The patient was repositioned to facilitate loading into your aircraft for transfer to another facility. Shortly after loading and take-off, the ICP monitor alarm sounds. After ensuring that the patient is still breathing and has a pulse, you should immediately:
    A. change patient position and reopen the drainage port.
    B. recharge the EVD transducer and restart the monitor.

C. ensure that the EVD drain is at the level of the pons and recharge the system.

D. ensure that the EVD transducer is at the level of the EAM and rebalance.

E. none of the above.

26. Place in order the following steps for "zeroing" an extraventricular drain (EVD):
    1. don BSI and turn off stopcock to drainage system.
    2. press the "zero" button and wait for monitor to read zero.
    3. turn stopcock between the collection burette and bag upward.
    4. unscrew the line cap next to transducer, empty burette, and replace cap.
    5. turn all stopcocks to original position and check waveform.

    A. 1, 2, 3, 4, 5
    B. 1, 3, 4, 2, 5
    C. 1, 3, 2, 4, 5
    D. 1, 2, 4, 3, 5
    E. none of the above

27. When flushing an EVD, failure to close the stopcock appropriately prior to introducing the saline can cause:
    A. cerebrospinal fluid (CSF) to drain into the pons.
    B. saline to be flushed directly into the ventricles.
    C. saline to contaminate the CSF.
    D. CSF to drain inappropriately into the saline bag.
    E. none of the above.

28. Advantage(s) and disadvantage(s) of using a fiber-optic bolt (FOB) vs. an EVD for interfacility transport include which of the following?
    A. The FOB is easily placed and not dependent upon ventricular size.
    B. The FOB is not dependent upon positioning.
    C. The FOB is easily broken if not handled correctly.
    D. all of the above
    E. A and C

29. In addition to monitoring intracranial pressure with an EVD or FOB, it is also advisable to monitor _____ in the seriously head-injured patient.
    A. central venous pressure
    B. peripheral arterial pressure
    C. central arterial pressure
    D. peripheral venous pressure
    E. all of the above

30. Subdural and epidural hematomas are most often surgically managed by means of:
    A. vacuum evacuation.
    B. hemicraniotomy.
    C. lobectomy.
    D. intracranial suctioning.
    E. No intervention is necessary.

31. Hemicraniectomy may include removal of _____ and is most commonly done over the _____ lobe:
    A. brain tissue, frontal
    B. skin, occipital
    C. bone, temporal
    D. vessels, parietal
    E. none of the above

32. During transport of patient with a head injury, the critical care paramedic can do several things to manage intracranial pressure that do not involve drugs or monitors. Among these are:
    A. placing the patient in semi-Fowler's position, arms and legs extended.
    B. keeping head and neck in neutral alignment with a cervical collar.
    C. placing the patient in supine position, arms and legs flexed.
    D. B and C.
    E. A and B.

33. A _____ body core temperature can result from hypothalamic compression, as well as from stress and injury.
    A. hypothermic
    B. hyperthermic
    C. normothermic
    D. all of the above
    E. none of the above

34. One current controversy in management of head injuries regards:
    A. decreasing mean arterial pressure to decrease intracranial pressure.
    B. increasing mean arterial pressure to control intracranial perfusion.
    C. permissive hypotension without regard to adequate intracranial pressure.
    D. all of the above.
    E. none of the above.

35. You are asked to manage the airway of a semiconscious patient with a head injury who has just arrived at the Emergency Department by private vehicle after a fall from construction scaffolding. His friend tells you the patient was conscious at the scene and refused ambulance transport but later started to act "tired," so he brought him in.
    Post intubation, you are directed by the anesthesiologist to ventilate the patient to chest rise at a rate no faster than 12 breaths per minute, an order contrary to your own protocols.
    When you question the order, the anesthesiologist tells you current research has shown that hyperventilating patients with intracranial hypertension may, in fact, harm them because:
    A. hypercapnia results in cerebral vasoconstriction, increasing CBF and ICP.
    B. hypercapnia results in cerebral vasodilation, increasing CBF and ICP.
    C. hypocapnia decreases ICP but increases vasoconstriction and ischemia.
    D. A and C.
    E. B and C.

36. A controversial therapy, therapeutic hypothermia, is thought to benefit the patient by:
    A. decreasing cerebral perfusion.
    B. decreasing cerebral edema.
    C. maintaining intracranial pressure.
    D. all of the above.
    E. none of the above.

37. The intracranial compartment is a rigid structure that contains certain elements in proportion. They are:
    A. brain tissue–80%, blood–10%, CSF–10%.
    B. brain tissue–75%, blood–15%, CSF–10%.
    C. brain tissue–75%, blood–20%, CSF–5%.
    D. brain tissue–90%, blood–5%, CSF–5%.
    E. none of the above.

38. Monroe-Kellie presents a two-part hypothesis. Part one states pressure is normally well controlled through alterations in blood and CSF volume. The second part states:
    A. to maintain normal ICP, the volume of all compartments must be maintained in normal proportions.
    B. to maintain normal ICP, the volume of one compartment must be offset by a reciprocal change in the volume of another compartment.
    C. to maintain normal ICP, the volume of the fluid must be decreased in relation to the brain tissue.
    D. to maintain normal ICP, the volume of all compartments must be equal.
    E. none of the above.

39. You are assisting a team in the treatment of a patient with a severe head injury. The ICP is dangerously high and the brain appears to be herniating through the foramen magnum. The patient is being ventilated with 100% oxygen via BVM. Among pharmacological choices, the only appropriate drug

you carry in your aircraft is mannitol. You open the drug box and note that all the vials of mannitol appear crystallized. Your immediate action should be to:
- A. continue hyperventilation and do not use the drug; it is ruined.
- B. warm the vial(s) gently with hot packs to liquefy the crystals.
- C. inject 1 mL normal saline into the vial and shake it to liquefy the crystals.
- D. inject the mannitol as is via IVP; it will dissolve in the bloodstream.
- E. none of the above.

40. Osmotic draw of fluid from the brain can be accomplished by use of:
- A. hypertonic saline.
- B. hypotonic saline.
- C. $D_{50}W$.
- D. D_5W.
- E. none of the above.

41. The use of pentobarbital and thiopental to manage ICP is an alternative therapy when the patient is refractory to other drug-based therapies. Its efficacy is in question, however, because it has side effects that include:
- A. severe hypotension.
- B. vasodilation.
- C. decreased MAP.
- D. all of the above.
- E. none of the above.

42. The four classes of drugs used most often in management of head injuries are:
  1. osmotics
  2. analgesics
  3. barbiturates
  4. sedatives
  5. paralytics

- A. 1, 2, 3, and 4
- B. 1, 2, 4, and 5
- C. 2, 3, 4, and 5
- D. 1, 3, 4, and 5
- E. 1, 2, 3, and 5

43. The spinal cord is subject to the same histopathologic injuries as the brain. Of the following, which are among the most common?
- A. concussion
- B. infarction
- C. compression
- D. all of the above
- E. A and C

44. Your patient has experienced loss of pain and thermal sensation below T-10. You know that this type of presentation is most likely a result of:
- A. central cord syndrome.
- B. anterior cord syndrome.
- C. Brown-Sequard syndrome.
- D. Kellie-Monroe syndrome.
- E. none of the above.

45. Which of the following statements are true of central cord injury?
  1. Damage to the central cord is usually the result of hematoma formation, infarction, or hypoxia.
  2. Central cord injury is most often noted with hyperextension injuries.
  3. Motor deficits associated with central cord injury are more severe in the upper extremities than in the lower extremities.
  4. Sensory deficits associated with central cord injury are more severe in the lower extremities than in the upper extremities.
  5. For central cord injury to occur, there must first be an injury to the overlying vertebrae.

- A. 1, 2, and 3
- B. 1, 2, and 5
- C. 1, 2, 4, and 5
- D. 1, 3, 4, and 5
- E. 2, 3, 4, and 5

46. The syndrome that describes the lateral partial injury to one-half the horizontal plane of the spinal cord is:
    A. anterior cord syndrome.
    B. Brown–Sequard syndrome.
    C. posterior cord syndrome.
    D. autonomic dysreflexia.
    E. central cord syndrome.

47. The hallmark signs and symptoms of neurogenic shock include:
    A. hypotension and bradycardia.
    B. warm, dry skin above the lesion and cool, diaphoretic skin below the lesion.
    C. warm, dry skin below the lesion and cool, diaphoretic skin above the lesion.
    D. A and B.
    E. A and C.

48. The most common cause(s) of autonomic dysreflexia is/are:
    A. fecal impaction or urinary retention.
    B. aberrant stimulation of the stretch receptors in the visceral bowel.
    C. aberrant response of the injured sympathetic autonomic nervous system.
    D. all of the above.
    E. A and C.

49. Diagnosis of spinal cord injury can be accomplished without technology by use of hands-on assessment techniques. Among them are:
    A. pain response.
    B. loss of sensation below a palpated "step-off."
    C. loss or impairment of the Babinski reflex.
    D. all of the above.
    E. A and B.

50. X-ray and CT-scan technology illuminate:
    A. all potential injuries to the spine.
    B. only osseous injuries.
    C. only soft-tissue injuries.
    D. all of the above.
    E. none of the above.

51. Options for management of spinal cord injury could include:
    A. drug therapy.
    B. positional fixation.
    C. surgical decompression.
    D. physical therapy.
    E. all of the above.

52. The algorithm decision tree for prehospital assessment of traumatic brain injury (TBI) includes specific recommendations for assessing pain and pupillary response using the:
    A. Trauma Severity Score.
    B. Trauma Brain Injury Score.
    C. Glasgow Coma Score.
    D. all of the above.
    E. none of the above.

53. You are transferring a postneurosurgery patient with an ICP monitor. His ICP is 12 mmHg. His blood pressure is 110/60 mmHg. What is his most likely cerebral perfusion pressure (CPP)?
    A. 10–12 mmHg
    B. 50–52 mmHg
    C. 64–66 mmHg
    D. 72–74 mmHg
    E. 89–90 mmHg

54. In regard to question number 53, the resulting CPP:
    A. would suggest hypoperfusion in an adult.
    B. would suggest hypoperfusion in a child.

C. is relatively normal.
D. is markedly elevated.
E. none of the above.

55. The sympathetic nervous system arises from which regions of the central nervous system?
    A. cervical spinal cord
    B. thoracic spinal cord
    C. lumbar spinal cord
    D. A and C
    E. B and C

CHAPTER 15

Thoracic Trauma: Assessment and Management

DIRECTIONS: Each of the questions or incomplete statements below is followed by suggested answers or completions. Select the **one answer** that is best in each case.

1. Thoracic trauma is directly responsible for approximately _____ of all trauma deaths.
   A. 50%
   B. 25%
   C. 30%
   D. 75%
   E. 90%

2. The first step in assessment of the thoracic trauma patient is to:
   A. assess adequacy of breathing.
   B. evaluate the ABG report for evidence of hypoxia, hypercarbia, acidosis, or ventilation/perfusion mismatch.
   C. ensure airway patency.
   D. examine chest radiographic films.
   E. none of the above.

3. Which of the following is NOT a clinical sign of tension pneumothorax?
   A. mediastinal shift to the ipsilateral side
   B. widened pulse pressure
   C. collapse of the ipsilateral lung
   D. distended neck veins
   E. hypotension

4. Early signs of tension pneumothorax include:
   A. jugular venous distension.
   B. hypotension.
   C. tracheal deviation.
   D. increasing respiratory distress despite supplemental oxygen.
   E. lethargy or coma.

5. In the patient suffering from tension pneumothorax, breath sounds will be:
   A. decreased or absent on the ipsilateral side.
   B. wheezing on the affected side.
   C. increased on the contralateral side.
   D. unequal only if the patient is receiving positive pressure ventilation.
   E. none of the above.

6. Initial emergency management of tension pneumothorax requires:
   A. positive pressure ventilation.
   B. placement of a chest tube.
   C. needle pleural decompression.
   D. careful review of the chest radiographs before intervention.
   E. thoracic drainage and suction.

7. When performing needle pleural decompression, placement of the needle should be at a:
   A. 90-degree angle in the 5th intercostal space, over the superior rib border in the midclavicular line.
   B. 45-degree angle in the 3rd intercostal space, under the inferior rib border in the midclavicular line.
   C. 90-degree angle in the 3rd intercostal space, over the superior rib border in the midclavicular line.
   D. 45-degree angle in the 3rd intercostal space, over the superior rib border in the midclavicular line.
   E. none of the above.

8. Clinical signs of hemothorax include:
   A. hyporesonance to percussion on the affected side.
   B. hyperresonance to percussion on the affected side.
   C. hyporesonance to percussion on the contralateral side.
   D. hyperresonance to percussion on the contralateral side.
   E. none of the above.

9. Which of the following is NOT a typical clinical finding in the patient with massive hemothorax?
   A. absent or decreased breath sounds on the affected side
   B. tracheal deviation toward the contralateral side
   C. hypotension and tachycardia
   D. distended neck veins
   E. dyspnea

10. Massive hemothorax usually presents with _____, followed by _____.
    A. dyspnea, shock
    B. shock, dyspnea
    C. dyspnea, narrowed pulse pressure
    D. narrowed pulse pressure, shock
    E. none of the above

11. Management of the patient with massive hemothorax should include:
    A. low-concentration oxygen.
    B. needle thoracentesis.
    C. tube thoracotomy.
    D. whole blood infusion.
    E. all of the above.

12. You are transporting a 20-year-old male gunshot victim from a community hospital to the tertiary care center 30 minutes away, where a surgical team awaits your arrival. The patient was shot in the left lower chest with a large-caliber handgun, and brought to the community hospital by bystanders. The referring hospital's ED staff has intubated the patient and placed him on a mechanical ventilator, inserted a thoracostomy tube in the left lateral chest, and placed bilateral large-bore IV accesses. The patient has received nearly 1000 mL of IV crystalloids on your arrival, and his blood pressure is 86/50 mmHg. Halfway through your transport, you note that the chest drainage system has collected 1300 mL of blood from the thoracostomy, and it is still steadily draining. You should:
    A. increase the IV infusion rate to compensate for the blood loss.
    B. continue to monitor the chest drainage and take no further intervention.
    C. administer vasopressors.
    D. clamp the thoracostomy tube and carefully monitor the patient for compromise in ventilatory status for the rest of the transport.
    E. none of the above.

13. Which of the following is NOT considered an indication for insertion of a chest tube?
    A. pneumomediastinum
    B. hemothorax with >200 mL/hr blood loss
    C. pneumothorax of >20%
    D. cardiac tamponade
    E. hemomediastinum

14. Which of the following is NOT typically a step performed prior to insertion of the chest tube?
    A. Administer a local anesthetic to the skin, muscle tissue, and periosteum surrounding the insertion site.
    B. Clamp the tube with padded hemostats or a plastic tube clamp.
    C. Prep the site with an antiseptic solution and sterile drapes.
    D. Attach the chest tube to a suction/chest drainage system.
    E. Make a 3–4 cm incision over the inferior rib border below the insertion site, and "tunnel" an insertion tract over the superior rib border, using curved hemostats and a gloved finger.

15. Following insertion of the chest tube, the critical care paramedic should:
    A. sedate and paralyze the patient, intubate and place the patient on a mechanical ventilator.
    B. secure the tube with sutures and/or tape, apply an occlusive dressing, and attach the tube to a drainage system.
    C. place the patient in a 30°–60° reverse Trendelenburg position.
    D. perform follow-up chest radiography to confirm tube placement and lung re-expansion, if time permits.
    E. B and D.

16. The amount of suction applied by the chest drainage system is determined by the:
    A. vacuum pressure of the suction unit.
    B. length and diameter of the drainage tube, according to Poiseuille's Law.
    C. water level in the suction chamber.
    D. size of the pneumothorax.
    E. none of the above.

17. Continuous bubbling in the water chamber during inspiration indicates:
    A. an air leak or loss of seal in the chest drainage system.
    B. proper operation of the chest drainage system.
    C. reexpansion of the lung.
    D. a kink or blood clot in the chest tube.
    E. none of the above.

18. Fluctuations in the long tube of the water-seal chamber usually indicate:
    A. a clotted or kinked chest tube.
    B. a patent, closed chest drainage system.
    C. re-expansion of the lung.
    D. an air leak or loss of seal in the chest drainage system.
    E. none of the above.

19. Unless contraindicated, patients with chest tubes should be transported:
    A. supine.
    B. in semi-Fowler's position.
    C. in reverse Trendelenburg position.
    D. with the unaffected side down on the bed.
    E. either B or D.

20. To free the chest drainage system tube of clots in the tubing, the critical care paramedic should:
    A. inject 10,000 units of heparin directly into the tubing proximal to the clot.
    B. "strip" the tubing.
    C. replace the chest tube.
    D. squeeze the tubing in a hand-over-hand fashion, working from the proximal end to the distal end of the tube.
    E. use the suction unit's vacuum pressure to pull the clot through the tubing.

21. An open pneumothorax or "sucking chest wound" requires:
    A. that air moves more freely through the wound than through the trachea.
    B. a large-caliber gunshot wound.
    C. a "through-and-through" gunshot wound.
    D. positive pressure ventilation to produce the sucking sound.
    E. none of the above.

22. An open pneumothorax should initially be managed with:
    A. a chest tube.
    B. needle thoracentesis.
    C. an improvised or commercially available occlusive dressing.
    D. 100% oxygen via positive pressure ventilation.
    E. none of the above.

23. A flail chest is defined as:
    A. three or more rib fractures.
    B. three or more ribs broken in two or more places.
    C. two or more ribs broken in three or more places.
    D. four or more rib fractures.
    E. four or more ribs broken in two or more places.

24. A flail chest produces a "floating segment" that often moves in a direction opposite to the rest of the chest. This is called:
    A. the bellows system.
    B. parallel motion.
    C. paradoxical motion.
    D. "see-saw" breathing.
    E. none of the above.

25. Signs of flail chest include:
    A. pain and muscle spasm in the affected area.
    B. respiratory distress or failure.
    C. paradoxical motion.
    D. use of accessory muscles.
    E. all of the above.

26. Management of uncomplicated flail chest (with no pneumothorax) may include all of the following EXCEPT:
    A. supplemental oxygen.
    B. analgesia, unless otherwise contraindicated.
    C. needle thoracentesis or tube thoracostomy.
    D. gentle splinting of the flail segment using pillows or bulky dressings.
    E. continuous positive airway pressure (CPAP).

27. Pericardial tamponade is defined as:
    A. blood in the pericardial sac.
    B. serous fluid in the pericardial sac.
    C. accumulation of blood or serous fluid in the pericardial sac that results in decreased cardiac output.
    D. inflammation and scarring of the endocardium.
    E. weakening of the interventricular septum resulting from myocardial infarction.

28. The degree of instability associated with pericardial tamponade is directly related to the:
    A. amount of accumulated blood in the pericardial sac.
    B. size of the patient's heart.
    C. systemic vascular resistance.
    D. rapidity of the accumulation.
    E. A and D.

29. The hallmark sign of pericardial tamponade is called:
    A. Cushing's triad.
    B. Beck's triad.
    C. Asherman's trinity.
    D. Frank-Starling mechanism.
    E. Kussmaul's sign.

30. Which of the following is NOT a sign of pericardial tamponade?
    A. narrowed pulse pressure
    B. *pulsus paradoxus* or *electrical alternans*
    C. absent or decreased breath sounds on one side
    D. shock
    E. distended neck veins

31. *Pulsus paradoxus* is defined as:
    A. narrowed pulse pressure.
    B. a fall in systolic blood pressure >15 mmHg during inspiration.
    C. a fall in systolic blood pressure >15 mmHg during expiration.

D. QRS complexes of alternating amplitude on the ECG.
E. none of the above.

32. Definitive treatment for pericardial tamponade is:
    A. needle thoracentesis.
    B. tube thoracostomy.
    C. needle pericardiocentesis with subsequent placement of a pericardial window.
    D. coronary artery bypass graft (CABG).
    E. none of the above.

33. To perform an ECG-guided pericardiocentesis, the clinician should:
    A. using a parasternal approach, advance the needle until blood can be aspirated.
    B. using a subxiphoid approach, advance the needle at a 30-degree angle until blood can be aspirated.
    C. using a subxiphoid approach, advance the needle at a 30-degree angle while aspirating continuously, stopping advancement of the needle if a depolarization wave is observed on the ECG monitor.
    D. with the patient in Trendelenberg position, advance a lumber puncture needle through the 4th intercostal space on the left sternal border until blood can be aspirated.
    E. none of the above.

34. Pericardiocentesis should usually be:
    A. performed as soon as pericardial tamponade is suspected in the field.
    B. deferred until arrival at the receiving facility or done in the ER of the referring facility.
    C. performed only after the patient has been intubated.
    D. performed if there is evidence of an enlarged cardiac shadow and widened mediastinum on the chest radiograph.
    E. performed en route to the receiving facility.

35. Which of the following is NOT typically a finding indicative of traumatic aortic rupture?
    A. hypertension or unequal pulses in upper extremities
    B. shock
    C. severe chest or midscapular pain
    D. an MOI of rapid deceleration
    E. distended neck veins

36. The clinical presentation of a patient suffering from myocardial rupture is usually:
    A. respiratory failure and shock.
    B. hemoptysis and shock.
    C. cardiopulmonary arrest.
    D. engorged neck veins, florid face, and severe respiratory distress.
    E. none of the above.

37. Management of the hypotensive patient with traumatic aortic rupture includes:
    A. application of PASG.
    B. tube thoracostomy.
    C. endotracheal intubation.
    D. rapid transport to surgical intervention.
    E. none of the above.

38. Which of the following is NOT a diagnostic finding indicative of traumatic aortic rupture on the chest radiograph?
    A. widening of the superior mediastinum
    B. fractures of the first two sets of ribs
    C. enlarged cardiac shadow
    D. depression of the left mainstem bronchus
    E. tracheal deviation to the right

39. Clinical signs of myocardial contusion may mimic:
    A. acute coronary syndromes.
    B. aortic rupture.
    C. pericardial tamponade.
    D. myocardial rupture.
    E. none of the above.

40. Which of the following is NOT a common finding in the patient with a pulmonary contusion?
    A. crackles or rhonchi in the affected area
    B. tachypnea and respiratory distress
    C. tachycardia
    D. loss of breath sounds on the affected side
    E. anxiety

41. Management of the patient with pulmonary contusion and a PO_2 of less than 80 mmHg on supplemental oxygen includes:
    A. needle thoracentesis.
    B. beta-agonist bronchodilators.
    C. endotracheal intubation and positive pressure ventilation.
    D. tube thoracostomy.
    E. all of the above.

42. Which of the following is NOT a typical clinical finding indicative of diaphragmatic rupture?
    A. scaphoid abdomen
    B. presence of bowel sounds in the chest
    C. chest and abdominal pain radiating into the shoulder
    D. distended abdomen
    E. decreased breath sounds on the side of the injury due to compression of the ipsilateral lung

43. Clinical findings of tracheobronchial disruption include:
    A. pneumothorax that does not re-expand following insertion of a chest tube.
    B. tension pneumothorax.
    C. subcutaneous emphysema.
    D. severe dyspnea.
    E. all of the above.

44. Management of tracheobronchial disruption includes:
    A. careful endotracheal intubation, using chest radiography to assist in placing the tube below the injury site if possible.
    B. pericardiocentesis.
    C. continuous positive airway pressure (CPAP).
    D. placement of a chest tube.
    E. A and D.

45. You are called to transport a 50-year-old female to the ICU at the tertiary care center. Your patient was admitted to the community hospital 4 days prior for epigastric pain and difficulty swallowing food. Forty-eight hours ago she was taken to the endoscopy lab for esophageal dilatation and has since presented with frequent hematemesis, fever, elevated WBC count, and hypotension. You suspect:
    A. esophageal perforation.
    B. bleeding esophageal varices.
    C. Mallory-Weiss tear.
    D. perforated gastric ulcer.
    E. none of the above.

46. Blunt trauma to the chest can cause sudden cardiac death, even without detectable injury to the myocardium. This phenomenon is known as:
    A. myocardial contusion.
    B. *commotio cordis*.

C. occult traumatic arrest.
D. acute coronary syndrome.
E. Chagas disease.

47. Needle thoracentesis should be performed over the superior rib border because:
    A. intercostal blood vessels and nerve bundles lie under the inferior rib border.
    B. the musculature is thinner near the top of the rib, making entry into the pleural space easier.
    C. during deep inspiration, the intercostals spread the ribs apart.
    D. the superior rib borders are usually less calcified, allowing the needle to pass easily.
    E. the superior rib borders are more calcified, making it easier to palpate the correct landmark.

48. A traumatic dissecting aneurysm of the aorta results from:
    A. shearing of the base of the aorta from the heart.
    B. traumatic separation of the tunica intima from the tunica media, resulting in a false lumen.
    C. shearing of the aorta from the *ligamentum teres*.
    D. compression of the heart, resulting in a "blowout" of a congenital malformation in the aorta.
    E. advanced atherosclerosis.

49. Which of the following is NOT commonly affected in a myocardial contusion?
    A. right anterior ventricle
    B. inferior wall of left ventricle
    C. anterior interventricular septum
    D. left anterior ventricle
    E. none of the above

50. When performing a needle thoracentesis, it is helpful to remember that the 2nd intercostal space is approximately level with what easily palpable landmark?
    A. the xiphoid process
    B. the costal margin
    C. the angle of Louis
    D. the suprasternal notch
    E. none of the above

CHAPTER 16

Abdominal and Genitourinary Trauma

DIRECTIONS: Each of the questions or incomplete statements below is followed by suggested answers or completions. Select the **one answer** that is best in each case.

1. Organs or structures located within the retroperitoneal space include:
   A. gall bladder.
   B. pancreas.
   C. urethra.
   D. liver.
   E. spleen.

2. Organs or structures located within the pelvic cavity include:
   A. ureters.
   B. kidneys.
   C. sigmoid colon.
   D. rectum.
   E. spleen.

3. Organs or structures located within the peritoneal space include:
   A. kidneys.
   B. urethra.
   C. gall bladder.
   D. ureters.
   E. distal duodenum.

4. The serous membrane that lines the peritoneal space is called the:
   A. visceral peritoneum.
   B. mesentery.
   C. serosa.
   D. parietal peritoneum.
   E. greater omentum.

5. The _____ can be found in parts of all four abdominal quadrants.
   A. large intestine
   B. stomach
   C. urinary bladder
   D. small intestine
   E. none of the above

6. The liver is suspended in the abdominal cavity by the:
   A. *ligamentum arteriosum.*
   B. ligament of Trietz.
   C. falciform ligament and *ligamentum teres.*
   D. greater omentum.
   E. lesser omentum.

7. The hepatic artery supplies the liver with a blood supply comprising nearly _____ of cardiac output.
   A. 10%
   B. 25%
   C. 40%
   D. 50%
   E. 5%

8. Abdominal organs most susceptible to the diffuse pressure extremes of blunt trauma are:
   A. hollow organs.
   B. fluid-filled organs.
   C. solid organs.
   D. retroperitoneal organs.
   E. pelvic organs.

9. Loss of blood supply to a particular organ or body part due to trauma is known as:
   A. ischemia.
   B. infarct.
   C. devascularization.
   D. exsanguination.
   E. none of the above.

10. According to the Liver Injury Scale of the American Academy of Surgery for Trauma (AAST), the most common category of liver trauma, comprising 70–80% of all liver injuries, is:
    A. grades I–II.
    B. grade III.
    C. grades IV–V.
    D. grade VI.
    E. none of the above.

11. On the AAST Liver Injury Scale, the category of liver injury characterized by lacerations greater than 3 cm deep and hematomas involving greater than 50% of the liver's surface area is:
    A. grade I.
    B. grade II.
    C. grade III.
    D. grade IV.
    E. grade V.

12. On the AAST Spleen Injury Scale, Grade V injuries are described as:
    A. shattering and/or complete devascularization of the spleen.
    B. subcapsular hematomas involving less than 50% of spleen surface area.
    C. small subcapsular hematomas and shallow capsular lacerations.
    D. subcapsular hematomas involving greater than 50% of spleen surface area.
    E. none of the above.

13. Of the following, which is the most likely mechanism of injury to result in stomach rupture?
    A. acute deceleration, resulting in the stomach tearing loose from the greater omentum
    B. blunt trauma to the abdomen
    C. contrecoup injury
    D. penetrating trauma to the abdomen
    E. eating the 72-ounce sirloin in Amarillo

14. Referred pain to the left shoulder resulting from intraperitoneal bleeding that irritates the diaphragm is referred to as:
    A. Cullen's sign.
    B. Grey Turner's sign.
    C. Kehr's sign.
    D. Kussmaul's sign.
    E. McBurney's point.

15. Flank bruising resulting from retroperitoneal hemorrhage is referred to as:
    A. Cullen's sign.
    B. Grey Turner's sign.
    C. Kehr's sign.
    D. Kussmaul's sign.
    E. McBurney's point.

16. Periumbilical bruising resulting from intraperitoneal hemorrhage tracking down the *ligamentum teres* to the umbilicus is known as:
    A. Cullen's sign.
    B. Grey Turner's sign.
    C. Kehr's sign.
    D. Kussmaul's sign.
    E. McBurney's point.

17. Laparotomy is considered the "gold standard" therapy for intra-abdominal trauma because it allows for thorough visual assessment and immediate repair of injuries. However, it is usually reserved for:
    A. patients with significant abdominal distension.
    B. patients with injuries to the liver or spleen.
    C. stable trauma patients with diffuse abdominal pain where the location of injury is not easily appreciated during the physical examination.
    D. hemodynamically unstable patients.
    E. patients with retroperitoneal hemorrhage.

18. Which of the following is NOT a positive finding for intra-abdominal trauma in diagnostic peritoneal lavage (DPL)?
    A. 10 mL or more of aspirated blood
    B. RBC count in aspirated fluid of greater than 100,000
    C. presence of bile
    D. cloudy fluid
    E. fecal matter or food particles present

19. Diagnostic peritoneal lavage is an effective diagnostic technique for:
    A. determining presence of retroperitoneal bleeding.
    B. determining presence of continuing bleeding.
    C. determining presence of blood in the peritoneal space.
    D. differentiation between solid (liver, spleen) and hollow (stomach, intestines) organ injury.
    E. none of the above.

20. Critical care paramedics will sometimes be:
    A. asked to perform a diagnostic peritoneal lavage at the referring facility before transferring the patient.
    B. asked to complete a lavage that was started prior to their arrival, while en route with the patient to the tertiary care center.
    C. required to close the incision after an open diagnostic peritoneal lavage has been performed.
    D. required to utilize the results of a diagnostic peritoneal lavage in their decision making process.
    E. B and D.

21. Recordings of sound waves as they strike organs of varying density to produce an image of those organs is known as:
    A. sonar.
    B. radar.
    C. echolocation.
    D. sonography.
    E. roentgenogram.

22. The specific ultrasound technique used to detect blood in the pericardium or abdomen is known as:
    A. a venous Doppler study.
    B. an arteriogram.
    C. focused assessment with sonography for trauma (FAST).
    D. positron emission tomography (PET).
    E. none of the above.

23. The hepatorenal space, evaluated for presence of blood in the FAST exam, is also known as:
    A. McBurney's point.
    B. Grey Turner's cavity.
    C. Morrison's pouch.
    D. Pyriform sinus.
    E. none of the above.

24. Advantages of the FAST exam include:
    A. lack of complications.
    B. ease of use for providers of varying levels of education and training.
    C. portability.
    D. very high (98%) diagnostic accuracy.
    E. A, C, and D.

25. Advantages of computed tomography (CT) over other diagnostic techniques such as diagnostic peritoneal lavage and sonography include:
    A. CT is faster than other techniques.
    B. CT allows diagnosis of specific injuries.
    C. CT is less expensive.
    D. CT does not require radiologist interpretation for identification of subtle injury patterns.
    E. none of the above.

26. Metabolic acidosis and high lactate levels in the trauma victim usually indicate:
    A. anaerobic metabolism and inadequate tissue perfusion.
    B. liver injury.
    C. stomach rupture and release of stomach acid into the bloodstream.
    D. renal insufficiency.
    E. none of the above.

27. Patients with renal trauma and significantly impaired kidney function often present with:
    A. elevated lipase and serum amylase.
    B. elevated BUN and creatinine levels.
    C. elevated serum bilirubin.
    D. low BUN and creatinine levels.
    E. none of the above.

28. The use of sublingual capnometry to monitor the PCO_2 level is of particular benefit to the critical care paramedic because:
    A. the sublingual mucosa is continuous with the intestinal mucosa, allowing indirect monitoring of abdominal organ perfusion.
    B. it provides early evidence of parenchymal lung trauma.
    C. elevated sublingual PCO_2 provides a very early indicator of shock, particularly in abdominal trauma.
    D. elevated sublingual PCO_2 provides specific diagnosis of respiratory insufficiency.
    E. A and C.

29. The first step for the critical care paramedic in assessment and treatment of the patient with acute abdominal trauma is to:
    A. review DPL findings (if any) and diagnostic imaging.
    B. evaluate and stabilize hemodynamic status.
    C. evaluate and stabilize airway and breathing.
    D. review lab results, especially hemoglobin, hematocrit, serum lactate, lipase, and serum amylase levels.
    E. inspect the wallet for an American Express platinum card or wad of large bills.

30. Purposeful maintenance of a lower systolic blood pressure sufficient to maintain sufficient perfusion of the heart, lungs, brain, and kidneys without "popping the clot" is known as:
    A. therapeutic dehydration.
    B. strict fluid limitation.
    C. permissive hypotension.
    D. titration to hemodynamic effect.
    E. none of the above.

31. The target for titration of crystalloid volume resuscitation in the patient with uncontrolled hemorrhage is:
    A. diastolic blood pressure of at least 70 mmHg.
    B. normotension.
    C. hypertension.
    D. systolic blood pressure of ¾ normal or 75–80 mmHg.
    E. none of the above.

32. Typed and cross-matched blood should be administered to the patient with abdominal trauma at what point?
    A. after isotonic crystalloid boluses of 2–3 liters have failed to maintain hemodynamic stability
    B. only after O-negative blood has been administered
    C. as soon as there is evidence that the patient has lost large quantities of blood volume

D. never in the patient with uncontrolled intra-abdominal hemorrhage
E. after colloids and vasopressors have failed to maintain hemodynamic stability

33. The renal artery supplies the kidneys with a blood supply comprising nearly _____ of cardiac output.
   A. 10%
   B. 25%
   C. 40%
   D. 50%
   E. 5%

34. Evaluation of the renal and genitourinary systems in the patient with abdominal trauma should include:
   A. exploratory laparotomy.
   B. urinalysis.
   C. diagnostic peritoneal lavage.
   D. CT with contrast dye.
   E. B and D.

35. Kidney injuries can be graded on the AAST Spleen Injury Scale. In this scoring system, renal lacerations greater than 1 cm in depth without rupture of the collection system or urinary extravasation would receive a rating of:
   A. grade I.
   B. grade II.
   C. grade III.
   D. grade IV.
   E. grade V.

36. The risk of severe renal hemorrhage and associated injuries rises significantly with:
   A. presence of renal lacerations greater than 1 cm in depth.
   B. presence of subcapsular hematomas.
   C. presence of perirenal hematomas.
   D. lacerations to the corticomedullary junction or the collection system.
   E. none of the above.

37. Intraperitoneal bladder rupture is most often the result of:
   A. penetrating trauma.
   B. blunt trauma in the patient with a full bladder.
   C. pelvic fracture.
   D. hyperflexion of the spine.
   E. none of the above.

38. Extraperitoneal bladder rupture usually occurs at the bladder neck and as such often results from:
   A. penetrating trauma.
   B. blunt trauma in the patient with a full bladder.
   C. pelvic fracture.
   D. hyperflexion of the spine.
   E. none of the above.

39. Severe injury to the renal and genitourinary systems can usually be identified by:
   A. physical exam only.
   B. hematuria.
   C. radiographic studies that show extravasation of contrast dye into surrounding tissues.
   D. inability to void.
   E. none of the above.

40. Reproductive system injuries in trauma patients most often involve the:
   A. ovaries.
   B. uterus.
   C. fallopian tubes.
   D. external genitalia.
   E. none of the above.

41. Which of the following is NOT a part of the classic triad indicating bladder rupture?
    A. gross hematuria
    B. polyuria
    C. abdominal pain
    D. inability to void
    E. none of the above

42. You are called to transport a 20-year-old male patient from the community hospital to the tertiary care center 40 minutes away. The patient fell 20 feet from construction scaffolding to the sidewalk below, landing on his back on a concrete planter. Local EMS transported the patient to the community hospital. Your patient has severe back and left flank pain, frank hematuria, and X-rays that reveal fractures of the 10th–12th posterior ribs as well as a vertebral body fracture of T-10, without neurological deficits. You should suspect:
    A. laceration or rupture of the left kidney.
    B. bladder rupture.
    C. urethral transection.
    D. injury to the spleen.
    E. A and D.

43. The diagnostic study that involves infusion of contrast media into the urethra and serial radiographs is called a:
    A. CT with contrast.
    B. retrograde cystogram.
    C. intravenous pyelogram.
    D. in-and-out catheterization.
    E. none of the above.

44. A Grade V injury to the kidneys resulting in renal devascularization and damage to the renal artery can result in:
    A. life-threatening internal hemorrhage.
    B. impairment of the body's ability to regulate blood volume and pressure.
    C. impairment of the body's ability to manage the blood pH.
    D. Grey Turner's Sign.
    E. all of the above.

45. Kidney position is maintained by contact with adjacent organs, the peritoneum, and supporting connective tissues. Blunt trauma resulting in displacement of the kidney, or "floating kidney," can result in:
    A. exsanguination.
    B. kinking of ureters or renal blood vessels.
    C. herniation of the kidney through the peritoneum, a condition known as abdominorenal herniation.
    D. kidney throat.
    E. none of the above.

46. The classic rebound tenderness associated with acute appendicitis is best appreciated at what topographic landmark?
    A. umbilicus
    B. symphysis pubis
    C. epigastrium just below the xiphoid process
    D. McBurney's Point
    E. lover's lookout

47. You are called to transport a 50-year-old male to the tertiary care center for treatment of a broken femur sustained in a motor vehicle collision. Upon your arrival at the community hospital, the Emergency Department nurse greets you with relief, stating, "Thank goodness you're here. He just started vomiting blood, and we think he may have a ruptured stomach." Examination of the patient reveals a rather thin male with jaundice, a firm liver palpable well below the right costal margin, and a distended abdomen that produces a positive fluid wave with percussion. Further examination of the abdomen is otherwise unremarkable. You suspect:
    A. ruptured stomach or duodenum.
    B. bleeding esophageal varices unrelated to his motor vehicle accident.

   C. gastric ulcers.

   D. diaphragmatic herniation.

   E. intra-abdominal hemorrhage.

48. In the renal collecting system, collecting ducts often merge to form a/the:

   A. papillary duct.

   B. minor calyx.

   C. major calyx.

   D. urinary bladder.

   E. none of the above.

49. The functional unit of the kidney is:

   A. the ureter.

   B. Bowman's capsule.

   C. the nephron.

   D. the loop of Henle.

   E. none of the above.

50. Which of the following is **NOT** a sympathetic effect on renal function?

   A. lowered glomerular filtration rate

   B. changing the regional pattern of blood circulation

   C. constricting afferent arterioles

   D. reducing blood flow to the glomerular capillaries

   E. none of the above

CHAPTER 17

Face/Ear/Ocular/Neck Trauma

DIRECTIONS Each of the questions or incomplete statements below is followed by suggested answers or completions. Select the **one answer** that is best in each case.

1. The major arteries that supply blood to the face are:
   A. maxillofacial.
   B. facial.
   C. temporal.
   D. A and C.
   E. B and C.

2. The cranial nerves (CN) that innervate the face are:
   A. CN V and VII.
   B. CN V and VI.
   C. CN VI and VII.
   D. CN IV and VII.
   E. none of the above.

3. The trigeminal nerve, also known as _____, provides sensory function to the face and controls _____.
   A. CN VI, lacrimation
   B. CN V, mastication
   C. CN VIII, salivation
   D. all of the above
   E. none of the above

4. The facial nerve, also known as _____, controls _____.
   A. CN V, lacrimation and salivation
   B. CN VII, lacrimation and salivation
   C. CN VII, facial muscles
   D. A and C
   E. B and C

5. Three types of salivary glands are located in the maxillofacial region. They are the:
   A. parotid, lacrimal, and temporal.
   B. parotid, sublingual, and submandibular.
   C. sublingual, parotid, and temporal.
   D. temporal, submandibular, and lacrimal.
   E. none of the above.

6. Salivary secretions _____ when the sympathetic system is stimulated and _____ when the parasympathetic system is stimulated
   A. decrease, increase
   B. increase, decrease
   C. activate, cease production
   D. cease production, activate
   E. none of the above

7. The gland that is located superior to the angle of the mandible, anterior to the auditory canal, and inferior to the zygomatic arch is the _____ gland.
   A. lacrimal
   B. sublingual
   C. parotid
   D. submandibular
   E. zygomatic

8. Lacrimal glands secrete fluid that moistens and lubricates the eye. The lacrimal glands are located in the _____ area.
   A. suprazygomatic orbital
   B. supramandibular orbital
   C. superolateral orbital
   D. supraorbital
   E. all of the above

9. The temporomandibular joint is the hinge joint for the mandible. It also acts as the articulation point for what landmark(s)?
   A. zygomatic arch
   B. condylar process
   C. mandibular fossae
   D. A and C
   E. B and C

10. The zygomatic bone articulates with the _____ bone to complete the lateral wall of the orbit.
    A. frontal
    B. maxillary
    C. sphenoid
    D. all of the above
    E. none of the above

11. The three branches of the trigeminal nerve are the _____ divisions:
    A. ophthalmic, temporal, and maxillary
    B. cranial, ophthalmic, and maxillary
    C. ophthalmic, cranial, and temporal
    D. temporal, maxillar, and mandibular
    E. ophthalmic, maxillary, and mandibular

12. The ophthalmic nerve (CN V_1) is responsible for transmission of sensory impulses from the:
    1. skin of the anterior scalp
    2. upper eyelid
    3. nose and nasal cavity mucosa
    4. cornea
    5. lacrimal gland

    A. 1, 2, and 3
    B. 1, 3, and 4
    C. 1, 2, 4, and 5
    D. 1, 2, 3, and 5
    E. 1, 2, 3, 4, and 5

13. The maxillary nerve (CN V_2) transmits sensory impulses from the:
    1. nasal cavity mucosa.
    2. palate and upper teeth.
    3. skin of the cheek.
    4. upper lip.
    5. lower eyelid.

    A. 1, 2, 3, 4, and 5
    B. 1, 3, and 4
    C. 1, 2, 3, and 5
    D. 1, 2, 4, and 5
    E. 1, 2, and 3

14. The mandibular nerve (CN V_3) provides motor fibers to and sensory fibers from the:
    A. anterior tongue.
    B. muscles of mastication.
    C. temporal region of the scalp.
    D. lower teeth.
    E. all of the above.

15. Nerves and blood vessels access the surface of the orbit by means of:
    A. foramens.
    B. fissures.
    C. canals.
    D. all of the above.
    E. B and C.

16. In addition to the ophthalmic vein, which of the following also pass through the superior orbital fissure at the posterior orbital wall?
    1. optic nerve (CN II)
    2. oculomotor nerve (CN III)
    3. trochlear nerve (CN IV)
    4. ophthalmic branch of the trigeminal nerve (CN V)
    5. abducens nerve (CN VI)

    A. 1, 3, and 5
    B. 2, 4, and 5
    C. 1, 2, 3, and 4
    D. 2, 3, 4, and 5
    E. 1, 2, 3, 4, and 5

17. The paranasal sinuses are located within the _____ bones:
    1. frontal
    2. orbital
    3. ethmoid
    4. sphenoid
    5. maxillary

    A. 1, 2, 3, and 4
    B. 2, 3, and 5

C. 1, 3, 4, and 5
D. 1, 2, 3, 4, and 5
E. none of the above

18. The pinna is the:
    A. inside of the ear.
    B. tip of the nose.
    C. "widow's peak."
    D. visible part of the ear.
    E. none of the above.

19. The _____, _____, and _____ comprise the auditory ossicles of the ear.
    A. malleus, incus, stapes
    B. vestibular, semicircular, cochlea
    C. malleolus, incus, staples
    D. malleua, cochlea, stapes
    E. vestiblular, incus, staples

20. The _____ transmit(s) vibrations of the tympanic membrane to the inner ear.
    A. vestibular complex
    B. auditory tube
    C. vestibulocochlear nerve
    D. auditory ossicles
    E. auricular complex

21. The vestibulocochlear complex is comprised of the:
    A. auditory tube, vestibule, and cochlea.
    B. vestibule, cochlea, and auditory tube.
    C. vestibule, cochlea, and semilunar canals.
    D. auditory tube, cochlea, and semilunar canals.
    E. none of the above.

22. The anatomy of the eye includes many structures. The orbit, or bony structure protecting the globe, consists of the:
    A. frontal, zygomatic, and temporal bones.
    B. ethmoid, lacrimal, and temporal bones.
    C. ocular, zygomatic, and frontal bones.
    D. all of the above.
    E. none of the above.

23. You are transporting a 17-year-old patient who fell while running on a cross-country trail through the woods and has a small stick impaled in his left eye. The globe appears intact, but there is profuse bleeding from the upper outside corner of the eye. Based on its location, you feel the stick has passed by the globe and impaled itself through the _____, near the _____ canthus.
    A. caruncle, medial
    B. ciliary, lateral
    C. neural tunic, medial
    D. palpebra, lateral
    E. caruncle, lateral

24. A 30-year-old female walks into your Emergency Department complaining of blurry vision and pain in her right eye. She tells you she was hit in the eye by a softball about 30 minutes earlier, and she also complains of a "headache that won't go away." During your examination, you notice a persistent drain of clear, gelatinous fluid from the medial canthus, and the globe itself appears somewhat flat. Your next action should be to:
    A. cover both eyes in order to lessen the chance of continued movement.
    B. send the patient home with an eye patch and orders to see her personal optometrist the next day.
    C. admit the patient, contact a specialist and request orders for a CT scan.
    D. A and B.
    E. A and C.

25. Of the cranial nerves, which of the following is directly involved with the eyes?
    A. CN X
    B. CN IV
    C. CN VII
    D. CN IX
    E. CN VIII

26. The laryngopharynx extends from the _____ to the entrance of the _____.
    A. lips, nasal plexus
    B. soft palate, hyoid bone superiorly
    C. hyoid bone inferiorly, esophagus
    D. parotid ducts, trachea
    E. none of the above

27. You are treating a 46-year-old male who has tripped on some stairs and struck his maxilla. His airway is patent and bleeding is under control, but he cannot articulate speech. Upon inspection, you find he is missing several incisors and seems to be suffering from severe malocclusion. From this examination and its position, you surmise the patient may have a fracture of the:
    A. hyoid bone.
    B. 17th and 32nd molars.
    C. temporomandibular joint.
    D. hypopharynx.
    E. all of the above.

28. Several critical structures are located within the anatomy of the neck. They include which of these cardiovascular structures?
    A. carotid arteries
    B. jugular veins
    C. carotid sinus
    D. all of the above
    E. A and B

29. The internal jugular vein descends lateral to the common carotid artery. Both of these structures, as well as the _____, are housed in a fascial layer known as the _____.
    A. vagus nerve, carotid sheath
    B. carotid nerve, parotid sheath
    C. tracheal nerve, vagal sheath
    D. all of the above
    E. none of the above

30. The external jugular veins drain blood from the face, scalp, and cranium into the:
    A. carotid canals.
    B. carotid bifurcation.
    C. jugular sinuses.
    D. subclavian veins.
    E. subclavian arteries.

31. The larynx is located at the level of:
    A. C-4, C-5, and C-6.
    B. C-2, C-3, and C-4.
    C. C-3 and C-4.
    D. C-5 and C-6.
    E. none of the above.

32. The _____ connects the posterior trachea to the anterior wall of the esophagus and serves to anchor the two structures together.
    A. triangular tendon
    B. intrinsic fascia
    C. annular ligament
    D. annular tendon
    E. triangular ligament

33. Structures in the neck that are of importance to the critical care paramedic include which of the following?
    1. thyroid glands
    2. CN IX
    3. brachial plexus
    4. parathyroid glands
    5. CN X

    A. 1, 3, and 5
    B. 2, 3, and 4
    C. 2, 3, 4, and 5
    D. 1, 4, and 5
    E. 1, 2, 3, 4, and 5

34. Your patient is exhibiting stridor and inability to swallow following blunt trauma to the neck during a martial arts class. You decide to initiate RSI and intubate the patient. You are successful in securing the airway, but

during the procedure you note severe swelling at the level of the vallecula. There is obvious ecchymosis to the area immediately inferior to the hyoid and superior to the trachea, and you know there is a potential for damage to the:
   A. carotid sinus.
   B. thyroid gland.
   C. hyoid bone.
   D. trachealis muscle.
   E. A and C.

35. The cervical plexus originates bilaterally from spinal nerves _____, and accounts for the entire innervation of the diaphragm via the _____ nerve.
   A. C-2 and C-5, frenic
   B. C-1 and C-3, phrenic
   C. C-1 through C-5, phrenic
   D. C-3 through C-5, frenic
   E. C-2 through C-4, phrenic

36. The _____ is of concern to the critical care paramedic because injury to it is cause for potential damage to deeper structures in the neck.
   A. CN III
   B. brachial plexus
   C. cervical plexus
   D. platysma
   E. CN IV

37. For purposes of assessment, the neck is divided into Zones I, II, and III. Which of the following describe the three zones?
   1. thoracic inlet to the cricoid cartilage
   2. sternocleidomastoid to the ethmothyroid
   3. cricoid cartilage to the angle of the mandible
   4. angle of the mandible to base of the skull
   5. larynx to the sternum

   A. 1, 2, and 3
   B. 2, 3, and 4
   C. 1, 3, and 4
   D. 1, 4, and 5
   E. 2, 3, and 5

38. Blunt force trauma to the face has a _____ incidence of life-threatening airway compromise than penetrating trauma.
   A. lower
   B. higher
   C. similar
   D. comparative
   E. disproportionate

39. A transverse fracture to the superior portion of the maxilla is classified as a:
   A. Le Fort III.
   B. Le Fort I.
   C. Le Fort II.
   D. Le Fort IV.
   E. none of the above.

40. _____ and _____ can be a result(s) of compression to the ophthalmic and oculomotor branches of the trigeminal nerve.
   A. Enophthalmos, apex syndrome
   B. Ptosis, enophthalmos
   C. Ptosis, glossoptosis
   D. Enophthalmos, glossoptosis
   E. Ptosis, apex syndrome

41. Of the following, which are common causes of tympanic membrane rupture?
   1. barotrauma
   2. otorrhea
   3. impact to the mandible
   4. temporal bone fracture
   5. basilar skull fracture

   A. 1 and 2
   B. 1, 2, and 3
   C. 1, 2, 3, and 4
   D. 1, 3, 4, and 5
   E. 1, 2, 4, and 5

42. Loss of hearing secondary to shearing forces or violent shaking is usually indicative of injury to:
    A. CN VIII.
    B. CN V.
    C. CN IV.
    D. CN IX.
    E. CN X.

43. Injuries to the lacrimal apparatus, tarsal plate, and levator muscle are normally associated with injuries to the:
    A. forehead.
    B. cheek.
    C. eyebrow.
    D. eyelid.
    E. nose.

44. Your patient is exhibiting signs of subconjunctival hemorrhage but denies blunt trauma to the face or eye. She also denies a headache or feeling lethargic. Her medical history does not include diabetes or hypertension, and her current vital signs are normal for age and condition. What other question(s) might you ask as part of your interview that could help explain this condition?
    A. Have you engaged in recreational behaviors that could restrict your breathing?
    B. Have you been sneezing, coughing, or vomiting recently?
    C. Have you been skin diving or sky diving recently?
    D. all of the above
    E. none of the above

45. Corneal abrasions can be manifested by the following symptom(s):
    1. significant pain.
    2. increased sensitivity to light.
    3. lack of associated pain.
    4. decreased sensitivity to light.
    5. excessive lacrimation and secretions.

    A. 1 and 4
    B. 1 and 5
    C. 1, 2, and 3
    D. 1, 2, and 5
    E. 1, 2, 3, 4, and 5

46. The most appropriate patient position for assessment of hyphema would be:
    A. left lateral recumbent.
    B. prone.
    C. supine.
    D. semi-Fowler's.
    E. full Fowler's.

47. _____ is the traumatic removal of the eye.
    A. Hyphema
    B. Rupture
    C. Enucleation
    D. Detachment
    E. None of the above

48. You have been called to a women's shelter to examine a 54-year-old patient who is complaining of "black spots" in her visual field and "shadows" that aren't there. Your patient appears to have tenderness, swelling, and ecchymosis around the right orbit consistent with blunt trauma, various other abrasions to the face, and a lacerated lower lip. During transport, you call ahead to the Emergency Department and request them to page in an ophthalmologist to examine the patient's eye injury, because you suspect that a _____ is the cause of her visual symptoms.
    A. corneal tear
    B. detached retina

C. corneal abrasion

D. hyphema

E. ruptured globe

49. The tongue-blade test is used to assess for the presence of what type of fracture?
    A. hyoid bone
    B. zygomatic
    C. mandibular
    D. nasal
    E. all of the above

50. A major contraindication to the removal of a contact lens in the field is:
    A. corneal tear.
    B. detached retina.
    C. corneal abrasion.
    D. hyphema.
    E. ruptured globe.

51. Clinical findings of Horner's syndrome would include:
    1. hemiparesis.
    2. ptosis.
    3. pupillary miosis.
    4. facial anhidrosis.
    5. nystagmus.

    A. 1 and 5
    B. 2, 3, and 4
    C. 1, 2, and 3
    D. 3, 4, and 5
    E. 1, 2, 3, 4, and 5

52. Trauma to the vertebral arteries may present with hemiparesis as well as:
    1. diplopia.
    2. nystagmus.
    3. carotid bruits.
    4. vertigo.
    5. dysarthria.

    A. 1 and 3
    B. 1, 2, and 4
    C. 1, 2, 3, and 4
    D. 1, 2, 4, and 5
    E. 1, 2, 3, 4, and 5

53. Dental avulsions should be treated by:
    A. locating the avulsed tooth.
    B. washing off the dirt.
    C. placing the tooth in saline.
    D. inserting the tooth back into its socket.
    E. A, B, and C.

54. Application of a _____ bandage after reduction of a mandibular dislocation is sometimes helpful.
    A. Galliazzi
    B. Barton
    C. Pitts
    D. skull cap
    E. none of the above

55. The best way to control hemorrhaging injuries of the neck is:
    A. direct pressure.
    B. tourniquet around the neck.
    C. application of pressure at the femoral artery.
    D. patient inversion.
    E. none of the above.

CHAPTER 18

Burns and Electrical Injuries

DIRECTIONS Each of the questions or incomplete statements below is followed by suggested answers or completions. Select the **one answer** that is best in each case.

1. Morbidity and mortality in burn patients are typically dependent on the:
   A. age of the patient.
   B. associated injuries.
   C. physical condition of the patient.
   D. all of the above.
   E. A and C.

2. Mortality among burn patients is highest among patients with:
   A. associated inhalation injury.
   B. associated traumatic injury.
   C. thermal burns.
   D. chemical burns.
   E. none of the above.

3. Which of the following is NOT a typical complication in the burn patient?
   A. severe fluid loss
   B. organ failure
   C. hyperthermia
   D. infection
   E. B and D

4. Common burn mechanisms include:
   A. electrical.
   B. sonic.
   C. thermal.
   D. all of the above.
   E. A and C.

5. Which of the following is NOT a skin function of crucial importance to the burn patient?
   A. barrier against infection
   B. regulation of fluid levels
   C. regulation of body temperature
   D. storage of nutrients
   E. sensory contact with the environment

6. Burn severity is influenced by which factor(s)?
   A. intensity of the energy source
   B. duration of exposure
   C. conductance of the exposed tissue
   D. all of the above
   E. A and B

7. Heat is best defined as the:
   A. energy of molecules in motion.
   B. energy produced in oxidation reactions.
   C. energy required to produce one calorie.
   D. byproduct of cellular metabolism.
   E. none of the above.

8. Breakdown of cellular proteins as a result of prolonged exposure to heat is called:
   A. catabolism.
   B. denaturing.
   C. lysis.
   D. melanism.
   E. coagulation.

9. The zone theory that reflects the effects of high heat on human tissue is known as:
   A. degree of burn theory.
   B. rule of nines.
   C. Jackson's theory of thermal wounds.
   D. total body surface area (TBSA).
   E. none of the above.

10. The area of a burn characterized by rupture of cell membranes and denaturation of structural proteins is known as the:
    A. zone of coagulation.
    B. zone of stasis.
    C. zone of hyperemia.
    D. zone of denaturation.
    E. none of the above.

11. The area of a burn characterized by cellular injury and decreased blood flow is known as the:
    A. zone of coagulation.
    B. zone of stasis.
    C. zone of hyperemia.
    D. zone of ischemia.
    E. none of the above.

12. The area of a burn characterized by erythema and inflammation is known as the:
    A. zone of coagulation.
    B. zone of stasis.
    C. zone of hyperemia.
    D. zone of redness.
    E. none of the above.

13. If the zone of coagulation penetrates the dermis, it is classified as a:
    A. partial thickness burn.
    B. full thickness burn.
    C. chemical burn.
    D. radiation burn.
    E. none of the above.

14. The body's response to burn trauma characterized by massive catecholamine release is known as the _____ phase.
    A. emergent
    B. fluid shift
    C. hypermetabolic
    D. resolution
    E. none of the above

15. Which of the following is NOT a characteristic of the emergent phase of the body's physiologic response to burns?
    A. tachycardia
    B. tachypnea
    C. pain
    D. inflammatory response
    E. anxiety

16. The peak of inflammatory response to a burn occurs:
    A. 24 hours postburn.
    B. one week postburn.
    C. immediately following the burn.
    D. 6–8 hours postburn.
    E. none of the above.

17. The body's response to burn trauma characterized by increased blood flow to the injured area, increased capillary membrane permeability, and release of mast cells is called the _____ phase.
    A. emergent
    B. resolution
    C. hypermetabolic
    D. fluid shift
    E. none of the above

18. Degranulation of mast cells results in:
    A. histamine release.
    B. release of IgE antibodies.
    C. prostaglandin synthesis.
    D. all of the above.
    E. A and C.

19. Hypoproteinemia secondary to increased capillary membrane permeability results in:
    A. fluid shift from the intravascular to the extravascular space.
    B. hypovolemia.
    C. fluid shift from the extracellular to the intravascular space.
    D. all of the above.
    E. A and B.

20. Renal failure in burn patients most often occurs as a result of:
    A. decreased cardiac output, which in turn leads to decreased renal perfusion.
    B. increased hematocrit and hemoglobinuria.
    C. excessive fluid resuscitation.

D. all of the above.
E. A and B.

21. Which of the following is **NOT** considered appropriate care for a patient with extensive burns?
    A. reverse isolation precautions
    B. wet dressings
    C. lining the stretcher and covering the patient with dry sterile sheets
    D. airway maintenance
    E. analgesia

Scenario

Questions 22–26 refer to the following scenario:
You are called to transport an 18-year-old volunteer firefighter to the burn unit at the tertiary care center. Your patient was burned in a structure fire and brought by ambulance to the local Emergency Department. He has sustained second- and third-degree burns to his anterior chest and posterior right shoulder, including burns to the right side of the neck and a nearly circumferential burn to the right upper arm. His nostrils are coated with soot and his respirations are markedly stridorous. The local BLS ambulance personnel had removed the patient's clothing and dressed his burns prior to transport and administered high-concentration oxygen via mask. The Emergency Department staff have performed X-rays of the cervical spine, chest, and right arm and have initiated bilateral large bore IV access. Ringer's lactate is being infused at 412 mL/hr. The patient is awake and extremely anxious, writhing on the stretcher in obvious pain. His vital signs are BP 140/84 mmHg, HR 124 per minute, RR 26 per minute, and SpO_2 99% on 100% oxygen. Despite this, he exhibits mild circumoral cyanosis.

22. Based upon the information presented, which of the following is your primary concern?
    A. potential for volume overload
    B. need for analgesia
    C. impending airway compromise
    D. potential cervical spine injury
    E. potential circulatory compromise of the distal right arm

23. The patient's mental status and level of anxiety can be attributed to:
    A. pain.
    B. shock.
    C. potential hypoxemia.
    D. all of the above.
    E. A and C.

24. Based upon your assessment findings, what is the first intervention you would take with this patient?
    A. placement of a Foley catheter
    B. administration of 0.5–1.0 mcg/kg of Fentanyl for analgesia
    C. sedation and neuromuscular blockade, followed by intubation and positive pressure ventilation with 100% oxygen
    D. escharotomy of the right upper arm
    E. none of the above

25. Based on the description of the patient's burns, which of the following best approximates the total body surface area (TBSA) burned, according to the rule of nines?
    A. 22.5%
    B. 35%
    C. 31.5%
    D. 18%
    E. none of the above

26. Clinical findings indicating impaired circulation in this patient's right arm may include:
    A. increased pain sensation.
    B. delayed capillary refill.
    C. weak or absent radial pulse.
    D. metabolic acidosis.
    E. B and C.

27. A previously healthy 20-year-old burn patient presents with a decreased level of consciousness but no other significant associated injuries. Emergency Department personnel inform you that the patient was trapped in his apartment until being rescued by local firefighters. The most likely cause for this patient's altered mental status is:
    A. closed head injury.
    B. substance abuse.
    C. carbon monoxide poisoning.
    D. acute myocardial infarction.
    E. none of the above.

28. You are interviewing a patient with THERMAL burns. Of the following which question is of LEAST importance when determining the mechanism of injury (MOI) and history of events?
    A. Did the burn occur indoors or outdoors?
    B. How were the flames extinguished?
    C. Was the patient unconscious at the scene?
    D. Is there any associated trauma?
    E. How many people were involved in the incident?

29. You are interviewing a patient with CHEMICAL burns. Of the following which question is of LEAST importance when determining the mechanism of injury (MOI) and history of events?
    A. What was the agent?
    B. How did the exposure occur?
    C. Is there a material safety data sheet (MSDS)?
    D. Were the patient's clothes disposed of properly?
    E. What decontamination procedures were initiated?

30. You are interviewing a patient with ELECTRICAL burns. Of the following which question is of LEAST importance when determining the mechanism of injury (MOI) and history of events?
    A. What was the estimated voltage?
    B. Was the patient wearing any metal jewelry?
    C. What was the duration of contact?
    D. What type of current (AC or DC)?
    E. Was CPR or defibrillation administered at the scene?

31. All of the following would be considered critical information for the critical care paramedic or receiving facility EXCEPT:
    A. tetanus immunization history.
    B. allergies.
    C. age of the patient.
    D. current medications, including alcohol, illicit drugs and over-the-counter (OTC) medications.
    E. full accounting of all past surgeries, if any.

32. A toddler pulled a pot of soup off of the stove, sustaining scald burns to her face, arms, and torso. She has blisters and peeling skin over her face and neck, the anterior surface of her right arm, the right side of her chest and abdomen, and her anterior right thigh. The percentage of total body surface area (TBSA) burned is approximately:
    A. 25%.
    B. 50%.
    C. 43%.
    D. 35%.
    E. 15%.

33. A firefighter was caught in a grass fire and sustained second- and third-degree burns. He was wearing fire-retardant turnout pants and boots, but only a tee shirt and suspenders covered his upper body. His burns consist of

circumferential burns to both arms and burns to the anterior chest, face, neck, and abdomen. The percentage of total body surface area (TBSA) involved is approximately:

A. 45%.
B. 41%.
C. 27%.
D. 36%.
E. 18%.

34. Burns resulting in blisters, weeping wounds, and significant pain are classified as:

A. superficial burns.
B. partial thickness burns.
C. third-degree burns.
D. second-degree burns.
E. B and D.

35. Third-degree burns typically:

A. appear leathery or charred.
B. involve significant pain in the burned areas.
C. involve injury to the epidermis, dermis and subcutaneous tissue.
D. all of the above.
E. A and C.

36. General treatment guidelines appropriate for all burn patients include all of the following EXCEPT which?

A. Assess for associated injuries.
B. Intubate all critical burn patients, regardless of the presence or absence of inhalation injury.
C. Remove all clothing and jewelry.
D. Protect from infection and hypothermia.
E. Perform a 12-Lead ECG and cardiac monitoring for electrical burn patients.

37. Which of the following is NOT an indication of the possible need for endotracheal intubation in the critical burn patient?

A. loss of protective airway reflexes
B. carbonaceous sputum and singed nasal hairs
C. agitation indicative of hypoxia
D. hypothermia
E. extended transport time

38. Intubation of the burn patient with elevated carboxyhemoglobin levels should always include:

A. postintubation monitoring of oxygen saturation using non-invasive pulse oximetry.
B. paralytics and sedation.
C. postintubation monitoring of end-tidal CO_2 levels, preferably via waveform capnography.
D. preintubation administration of intravenous lidocaine to blunt increase in intracranial pressure.
E. all of the above.

39. Adequate fluid resuscitation is best measured by:

A. the amount of fluids dictated by the Parkland burn formula.
B. the "volume infused" reading on the IV infusion pump.
C. skin turgor and capillary refill time.
D. adequate urinary output for the age and size of the patient.
E. none of the above.

Scenario

Questions 40–44 refer to the following scenario:
A 70-year-old man has sustained second- and third-degree burns to the anterior chest, abdomen, and anterior thighs. His spouse states that the patient frequently sleeps on the couch with an electric heater placed nearby for warmth, and his blankets caught fire. His medical history is remarkable only for hypertension, chronic renal insufficiency, and gout. His medication history includes furosemide, allopurinol, colchicine and metoprolol. He has no known drug allergies and weighs approximately 180 pounds.

40. The total body surface area (TBSA) burned for this patient is approximately:
    A. 27%.
    B. 36%.
    C. 54%.
    D. 18%.
    E. none of the above.

41. Using the Parkland burn formula, calculate the amount of fluids the patient should receive in the first 24 hours.
    A. 19.4 liters (19,440 milliliters)
    B. 8.8 liters (8,856 milliliters)
    C. 25.9 liters (25,920 milliliters)
    D. 11.8 liters (11,808 milliliters)
    E. none of the above

42. Half the 24-hour fluid total should be given during the first 8 hours. Calculate the hourly infusion rate for the first 8 hours of fluid resuscitation.
    A. 1,200 mL/hour
    B. 550 mL/hr
    C. 1,600 mL/hr
    D. 738 mL/hr
    E. none of the above

43. IV fluids for this patient should be:
    A. isotonic crystalloids such as normal saline or Ringer's lactate.
    B. D5$\frac{1}{2}$NS (dextrose 5% and 0.45% NaCl).
    C. warmed to 38° C (100.4° F).
    D. A and C.
    E. None of the above.

44. What potential complications are most likely in this patient?
    A. volume overload
    B. respiratory insufficiency due to carbon monoxide poisoning
    C. respiratory compromise due to thoracic eschar formation
    D. compartment syndrome in the lower extremities
    E. A and C

45. The most appropriate pain relief agents for burn patients requiring high-concentration oxygen are:
    A. nitronox (50/50 nitrous oxide and oxygen mixture).
    B. opioids such as fentanyl or morphine.
    C. benzodiazepines such as midazolam.
    D. dissociative anesthetics such as ketamine.
    E. barbiturate sedatives.

46. Other than nitrous oxide, all analgesics in burn patients should be administered via which route?
    A. oral
    B. subcutaneous
    C. intravenous
    D. intramuscular
    E. transdermal

47. In general terms, dressings for burns of greater than 10% TBSA should be:
    A. impregnated with an antimicrobial agent.
    B. moistened to aid in halting the burning process.
    C. applied over a thin layer of Silvadene ointment.
    D. dry and sterile.
    E. none of the above.

48. Escharotomies should be performed only:
    A. on circumferential burns.
    B. by the surgeon at the burn center.
    C. when respiratory, hemodynamic, or neurological compromise results from the eschar formation.

D. on very deep burns.

E. none of the above.

49. A patient with carbon monoxide poisoning will always have:
    A. cherry red skin.
    B. elevated carboxyhemoglobin levels despite otherwise normal arterial blood gases.
    C. low oxygen saturation on the pulse oximeter.
    D. tachypnea.
    E. none of the above.

50. Carboxyhemoglobin levels of 5–10% may:
    A. result in obtundation and coma.
    B. be a normal finding in a heavy smoker.
    C. cause anxiety and restlessness in most patients.
    D. be fatal.
    E. be the name of a Willie Nelson song.

51. Severity of electrical burns is determined by strength of current and:
    A. duration of contact.
    B. resistance of the tissue contacted.
    C. direction of flow.
    D. all of the above.
    E. A and C.

52. What is the most confounding factor in determining severity of electrical burns?
    A. Severe pain in the patient makes assessment difficult.
    B. It may be impossible to determine the voltage and duration of exposure.
    C. Metal objects worn by the patient often result in horrific but non-life-threatening "blowout" burns.
    D. Much of the damage is internal.
    E. none of the above

53. Laboratory findings that may indicate a severe electrical burn in the patient with otherwise unimpressive external signs of injury include:
    A. radiographic studies indicating swelling of internal organs.
    B. presence of myoglobinuria.
    C. serum creatine kinase levels above 1,000 IU.
    D. all of the above.
    E. B and C.

54. Of the types of electrical current, which of the following produces the most severe injuries?
    A. low voltage direct current (DC)
    B. high voltage alternating current (AC)
    C. low voltage AC
    D. high voltage DC
    E. none of the above

55. Patients injured by arcing of electrical energy often present with:
    A. associated thermal burns resulting from ignition of their clothing.
    B. no visible signs of injury.
    C. respiratory arrest caused by tetany of the breathing muscles.
    D. blunt trauma injuries resembling those from an explosion.
    E. A and D.

56. The patient injured by exposure to household electrical current will often present with:
    A. cardiac arrest.
    B. respiratory arrest due to tetany of the breathing muscles.
    C. no visible signs of injury.
    D. all of the above.
    E. none of the above.

57. The most life-threatening injuries from a lightning strike are generally considered to be:
    A. cardiac.
    B. deep tissue burns.
    C. neurologic.
    D. tetany or paralysis of respiratory muscles.
    E. A and C.

58. Presence of rhabdomyolysis is often indicated by:
    A. high serum potassium levels.
    B. presence of port-wine colored pigments in urine.
    C. elevated creatine kinase levels on a cardiac enzyme panel.
    D. polyuria.
    E. none of the above.

59. Treatment of rhabdomyolysis usually consists of:
    A. blood transfusions to replace the lost hemochromogens.
    B. administration of sodium bicarbonate until urine pH is less than 6.0.
    C. IV fluid therapy titrated to maintain urine production of at least 75–100 mL/hr.
    D. administration of mannitol to aid in diuresis.
    E. B, C, and D.

60. Examples of acids that can potentially cause severe burns are:
    A. drain cleaners.
    B. swimming pool chemicals.
    C. disinfectants.
    D. refrigerants.
    E. three-alarm chili.

61. Examples of alkalis that can potentially cause severe burns are:
    A. baking soda.
    B. drain cleaners.
    C. wet cement.
    D. disinfectants.
    E. A and C.

62. Of the following types of chemicals, which has the potential to cause the most severe burns?
    A. alkalis
    B. acids
    C. organic compounds
    D. noble gases
    E. none of the above

63. General care of the patient with chemical burns includes all of the following EXCEPT:
    A. removal of contaminated clothing.
    B. use of other chemical agents to neutralize the burning chemical.
    C. brushing off of any dry chemicals.
    D. copious irrigation of most chemical burns.
    E. protection of medical personnel from chemical exposure.

64. Hydrofluoric acid burns are especially dangerous because:
    A. severe coagulation necrosis and protein precipitation usually result in extensive tissue damage.
    B. liquefaction necrosis and protein denaturation usually result in extensive tissue damage.
    C. hydrofluoric acid is especially toxic to the liver.
    D. high concentrations of hydrofluoric acid rapidly bind free calcium in the blood, causing life-threatening hypocalcemia.
    E. none of the above.

65. Burns from anhydrous ammonia often require:
    A. copious irrigation of affected tissues until the ammonia smell is gone.
    B. neutralization with 50% polyethylene glycol solution.

C. intubation and mechanical ventilation for inhalation cases.
D. covering of the burned area with petroleum jelly to retain moisture and slow the desiccating effects of the chemical.
E. A and C.

66. Of the following types of radiation, which poses the greatest danger?
    A. photons
    B. alpha radiation
    C. gamma radiation
    D. beta radiation
    E. ultraviolet B rays

67. Which of the following best describes a patient who should be referred to a specialized burn center?
    A. 60-year-old man with first-degree burns (sunburn) over his entire posterior body
    B. 30-year-old female with second-degree scald burns over 8% of her body and first-degree burns over 30%
    C. 20-year-old male with second-degree burns to the anterior chest (9%) and inhalation injury
    D. 12-year-old male with second-degree scald burns to the thighs and genitalia
    E. C and D

68. The deepest layer of the epidermis is termed the:
    A. stratum corneum.
    B. stratum lucidum.
    C. stratum granulosum.
    D. stratum germinativum.
    E. stratum spinosum.

69. The most superficial layer of the dermis is termed the:
    A. papillary layer.
    B. reticular layer.
    C. cortical layer.
    D. stratum lucidum.
    E. "Layla" by Derek and the Dominoes.

70. Epidermal cells in which of the following layers convert the precursor steroid into Vitamin D though ultraviolet light exposure?
    A. stratum corneum
    B. stratum lucidum
    C. stratum germinativum
    D. stratum spinosum
    E. C and D

71. Apocrine sweat glands can be found in which of the following body areas?
    A. upper lip
    B. armpit
    C. nipple area
    D. groin
    E. B, C, and D

72. Merocrine glands are most concentrated in which of the following body areas?
    A. soles
    B. groin
    C. palms
    D. A and B
    E. A and C

73. Which of the following statements about the skin and the effects of aging is false?
    A. Hair thickens and changes color.
    B. The ability to lose heat decreases.
    C. The skin becomes drier.
    D. The sensitivity of the immune system is reduced.
    E. Skin injuries and infection become more common.

74. The pigmentation in the skin is due to a substance produced by which cell type?
    A. transitional cells
    B. melanocytes
    C. plasma cells
    D. erythrocytes
    E. none of the above

75. Which of the following cell types is found in the epidermis?
    A. stratified columnar
    B. ciliated columnar
    C. stratified squamous
    D. transitional cells
    E. none of the above

CHAPTER 19
Principles of Orthopedic Care

19: PRINCIPLES OF ORTHOPEDIC CARE

DIRECTIONS Each of the questions or incomplete statements below is followed by suggested answers or completions. Select the **one answer** that is best in each case.

1. Which of the following is NOT a function of the skeletal system?
   A. support
   B. leverage
   C. protection
   D. storage
   E. white blood cell production

2. The central shaft of a long bone is called:
   A. diaphysis.
   B. epiphysis.
   C. periosteum.
   D. endosperm.
   E. none of the above.

3. The central canal of a long bone is called:
   A. Venetian canal.
   B. haversian canal.
   C. aqueduct of Sylvan.
   D. foramen magnum.
   E. canaliculi.

4. Spongy bone is called _____ bone.
   A. spongy
   B. compact
   C. compliant
   D. cancellous
   E. none of the above

5. Which of the following cells are responsible for the production of new bone?
   A. osteocytes
   B. osteoclasts
   C. osteoblasts
   D. iconoclasts
   E. none of the above

6. A type of bone development is:
   A. osteoclastic ossification.
   B. intramembranous ossification.
   C. endochondrial ossification.
   D. A and B.
   E. B and C.

7. While bone elongates, the process by which the diameter of the bone increases is called:
   A. aggregational growth.
   B. congregational growth.
   C. oppositional growth.
   D. appositional growth.
   E. none of the above.

8. During bone growth, the area that separates the bone of the shaft and the bone of each epiphysis is called:
   A. ossification center.
   B. epiphyseal plate.
   C. haversian canal.
   D. intramedullary canal.
   E. none of the above.

9. Which of the following vitamins does NOT play a major role in bone growth?
   A. vitamin B_1
   B. vitamin D_3
   C. vitamin A
   D. vitamin C
   E. none of the above

10. Which of the following hormones elevate(s) calcium levels in the body?
    A. parathyroid hormone (PTH)
    B. calcitriol
    C. calctonin
    D. A and B
    E. A and C

11. Following a fracture, cells of the endosteum lay down:
    A. internal callus.
    B. external callus.

C. fracture hematoma.
D. tophi.
E. none of the above.

12. The cribriform plate is a part of which bone?
    A. frontal
    B. sphenoid
    C. palatine
    D. nasal
    E. ethmoid

Match the following terms:

13. _____ diarthrosis
14. _____ amphiarthrosis
15. _____ synarthrosis
16. _____ enarthrosis
17. _____ ginglymus

    A. ball and socket joint
    B. nonmovable joint
    C. hinge joint
    D. slightly movable joint
    E. movable joint

Match the following terms:

18. _____ arthrodia
19. _____ trochoid
20. _____ condyloid

    A. pivot joint
    B. saddle joint
    C. gliding joint

21. Which of the following is NOT a classification of bony orthopedic injury?
    A. fractures
    B. dislocations
    C. subluxations
    D. sprains
    E. none of the above

22. A fracture where the bone is broken into multiple parts is termed:
    A. comminuted.
    B. spiral.
    C. impacted.
    D. transverse.
    E. none of the above.

23. Open fractures are often graded by which system?
    A. Salter-Harris system
    B. Tscherne system
    C. Gustilo system
    D. Sager system
    E. none of the above

24. All high-velocity gunshots causing open fractures are classified as:
    A. Gustilo Type III.
    B. Salter-Harris Type V.
    C. Tscherne Grade 1.
    D. Mobitz III.
    E. none of the above.

25. Testing of the biceps deep tendon reflex (DTR) assesses what nerve root?
    A. C1
    B. C3
    C. C5
    D. C7
    E. C8

26. A child sustains a wrist fracture where a portion of the epiphysis and metaphysis are broken off. This is what classification of fracture?
    A. Gustilo Type I
    B. Salter-Harris Type III
    C. Salter-Harris Type I
    D. Salter-Harris Type IV
    E. none of the above

Labeling

Questions 27–29 refer to Figure 19–1.

For Figure 19–1, growth plate in a child's long bone, decide what label is correct for each of the blank lines numbered 27 through 29. Select from choices A through E.

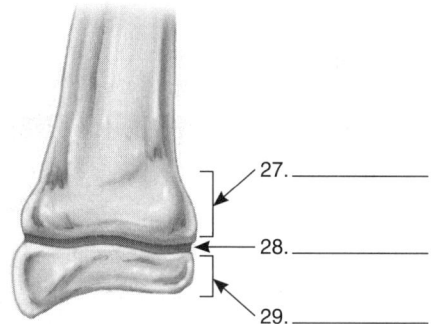

Figure 19–1

27. _____
28. _____
29. _____
   A. epiphysis
   B. physis
   C. diaphysis
   D. metaphysis
   E. suphysis

30. The act of realigning fracture segments to their normal position is called:
   A. subluxation.
   B. fixation.
   C. fabrication.
   D. osteopathic manipulation.
   E. none of the above.

31. You are called to transport a critically injured patient from a community hospital to a trauma center. The X-ray and physical exam show a pelvic fracture that is vertically stable but rotationally unstable. What Tile class pelvic fracture would this be?
   A. type A
   B. type B
   C. type C
   D. type D
   E. none of the above

32. Which of the following statements about unstable, "open-book" pelvic fractures is FALSE?
   A. They can result in life-threatening hemorrhage.
   B. They can be treated with external devices such as the SAM splint.
   C. Urinary tract injuries are common.
   D. They often require specialized trauma center care.
   E. none of the above

33. Important concerns in isolated long bone fractures include:
   A. assurance of the ABCs.
   B. fracture stabilization.
   C. provision of analgesia.
   D. peripheral pulse checks.
   E. all of the above.

34. Acceptable prehospital treatment modalities for isolated femur fractures include:
   A. MAST.
   B. Sager traction splint.
   C. REEL splint.
   D. Hare Traction splint.
   E. all of the above.

Labeling

Questions 35–38 refer to Figure 19–2.

For Figure 19–2, hip fracture types, decide what label is correct for each of the blank lines numbered 35 through 38. Select from choices A through E.

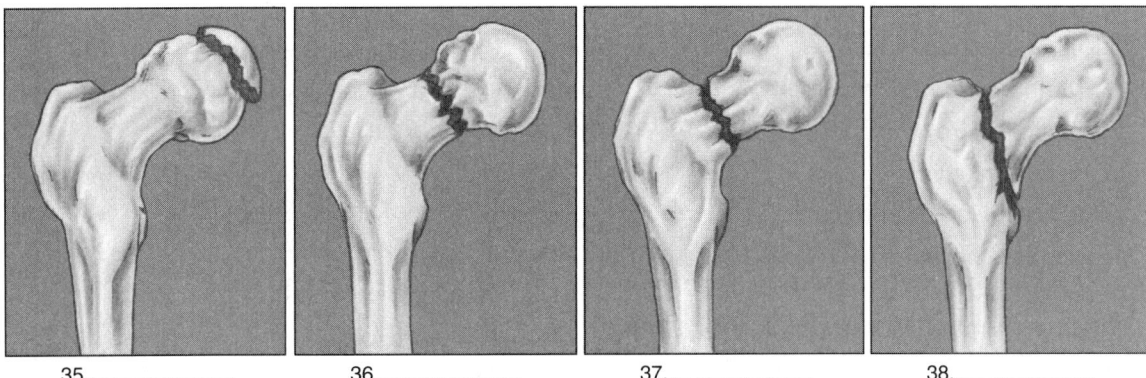

35. _____ 36. _____ 37. _____ 38. _____

Figure 19–2

35. _____
36. _____
37. _____
38. _____
   A. intertrochanteric
   B. capital
   C. subcapital
   D. basicervical
   E. transcervical

39. The most common cause of vertebral fractures is:
   A. diving.
   B. penetrating injuries.
   C. football injuries.
   D. motor vehicle collisions.
   E. none of the above.

40. Which of the following statements is **FALSE**?
   A. There are 8 pairs of cervical spinal nerves.
   B. There are 12 pairs of thoracic spinal nerves.
   C. There are 5 pairs of lumbar spinal nerves.
   D. There are 7 pairs of cervical spinal nerves.
   E. none of the above

Labeling

Questions 41–42 refer to Figure 19–3.
For Figure 19–3, hip fracture types, decide what label is correct for each of the blank lines numbered 41 and 42. Select from choices A through E.

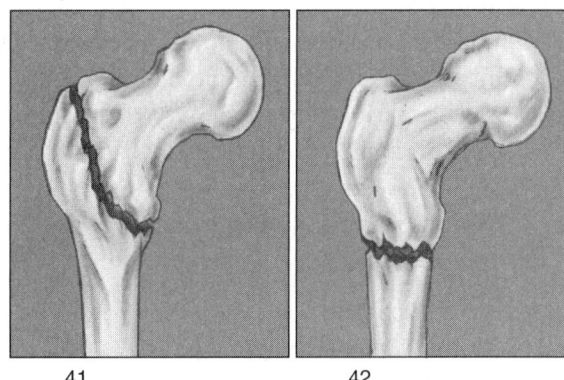

41. _____ 42. _____

Figure 19–3

41. _____
42. _____
   A. intertrochanteric
   B. capital
   C. subcapital
   D. supratrochanteric
   E. subtrochanteric

43. The Denis system is used for which of the following fracture types?
    A. lumbar vertebral fractures
    B. pediatric growth plate fractures
    C. pelvic fractures
    D. cervical vertebral fractures
    E. none of the above

44. Which of the following is **NOT** true with regard to pediatric distal humerus fractures?
    A. They are often associated with growth plate injury.
    B. They can result in permanent disability.
    C. Associated nervous and vascular injuries are uncommon.
    D. Prehospital treatment should include splinting and analgesia.
    E. none of the above

45. You have a 22-year-old male patient who was thrown from his motorcycle when he hit an armadillo crossing the road. He has a pulseless right leg secondary to a significantly angulated fracture. His vital signs are stable and he has no other injuries. Which of the following treatment steps is appropriate?
    A. analgesia
    B. returning the leg to a more natural position
    C. splinting
    D. all of the above
    E. A and C

46. The accumulation of fluid in a muscle compartment is termed:
    A. rheumatism.
    B. compartment syndrome.
    C. myofascial syndrome.
    D. orthopedic syndrome.
    E. none of the above.

47. The only injectable NSAID approved for use in the United States is:
    A. ibuprofen.
    B. naproxen sodium.
    C. ketorolac.
    D. acetaminophen.
    E. none of the above

48. Of the following treatments, which would **NOT** be an appropriate treatment for long-distance transport involving a patient with multiple open fractures?
    A. crystalloid therapy
    B. intravenous analgesia
    C. intravenous antibiotics
    D. tetanus prophylaxis
    E. none of the above

49. Which of the following statements about low-molecular-weight heparin is **FALSE**?
    A. It permits Factor IIa to function.
    B. It allows localized hemostasis.
    C. It inhibits Factor Xa.
    D. It is given intravenously.
    E. none of the above

50. Which of the following fractures is least likely to result in significant hemorrhage?
    A. pelvic fracture
    B. femur fracture
    C. rib fracture
    D. calcaneal fracture
    E. open humerus fracture

CHAPTER 20
Special Patients: Pediatric, Geriatric, and Obstetrical Trauma

DIRECTIONS

Each of the questions or incomplete statements below is followed by suggested answers or completions. Select the **one answer** that is best in each case.

1. Which is the most common type of pediatric trauma?
   A. motor vehicle accidents
   B. gunshot wounds
   C. falls
   D. burns
   E. Nintendo thumb

2. The most common cause of pediatric trauma-related deaths and permanent head injuries is:
   A. falls.
   B. abuse.
   C. bicycle accidents.
   D. motor vehicle accidents.
   E. gunshot wounds.

3. The leading cause of death in the home for children ages 14 and under is:
   A. falls.
   B. burns and smoke inhalation.
   C. firearm accidents.
   D. abuse.
   E. bathtub drownings.

4. Assessment of the injured or ill child must be done:
   A. within the context of their emotional and physiologic development.
   B. just as it is done in an adult.
   C. from head to toe.
   D. from toe to head.
   E. using as many technological assessment tools as possible.

5. Among the many fears children experience when ill or injured, fear of more pain is among the most common. Which of the following represents steps the critical care paramedic should take to minimize a child's fear and anxiety?
   A. Assure the child you are there to help and that you will do nothing to cause them more pain.
   B. Use motivational phrases such as "Big boys don't cry."
   C. Have the parents help physically restrain the child.
   D. Answer truthfully if the child asks if a procedure will hurt, and minimize lag time between informing the child and actually performing the procedure.
   E. Threaten them with a spanking if they do not cooperate.

6. The critical care paramedic is about to apply a blood pressure cuff to an anxious 3-year-old with a fractured right femur. She reacts fearfully, pulling away and asking what the medic plans to do with the cuff. The medic answers, "I'm going to wrap this funny thing around your arm and when I pump it up, it's going to give your arm a hug. Which arm would you like me to put it on?" This is an example of:
   A. an outright lie and a good way to destroy any rapport the medic has built with the child.
   B. involving the child in her own care and reducing her feelings of helplessness.

C. an attempt by the medic to obtain informed consent to auscultate a blood pressure.

D. an attempt to divert the child's attention from her broken leg.

E. gratuitous coercion.

7. Often, like the ill or injured child, parents and caregivers may feel overwhelmed by fear. All of the following are good techniques that can help alleviate these fears **EXCEPT**:

    A. Assure the parents everything will be okay and that the child will be fine.

    B. If possible, have one crew member be the point of contact with the parents to avoid giving conflicting information.

    C. Keep the parents informed about the child's condition and give them periodic updates.

    D. Allow a parent to accompany the child, provided the parent can be calm and reassuring and not heighten the child's fear and anxiety.

    E. Assure the parents that everything possible is being done for their child.

8. The APGAR scale is the most frequently used scoring system to assess newborns. In this system, APGAR stands for Appearance, Pulse, Grimace, _____ and Respirations.

    A. Agitation
    B. Airway
    C. Activity
    D. Alertness
    E. Awakeness

9. Although usually associated with a minor illness, _____ in a neonate (< 1 month of age) may be the only sign of a major illness such as meningitis.

    A. diminished interaction with the environment
    B. cyanosis of the hands and feet (acrocyanosis)
    C. fever
    D. jaundice
    E. lack of protest when separated from the parents

10. Infants in the 6- to 12-month age group should be examined:

    A. while sitting in the parent's or caregiver's lap.
    B. in a quiet, softly lit area away from the parent's view.
    C. from toe to head.
    D. from head to toe.
    E. A and C.

11. You are transferring a 3-year-old with burns to her face, chest, and forearms. She is only able to answer questions with a "yes" or "no." As you continue your assessment and treatment plan, it is important to:

    A. get all the painful and unpleasant procedures out of the way first.
    B. explain to the child any procedures you perform, because her ability to understand may surpass her ability to talk.
    C. usher the parents from the room while you work.
    D. document signs of abuse, because the child's behavior is not normal.
    E. none of the above.

12. You are examining a 16-year-old girl who is being transferred to a tertiary care center for psychiatric evaluation and further care. The patient's parents had discovered her in the act of swallowing an unknown quantity of 500 mg acetaminophen tablets and immediately drove her to the hospital. The girl seems evasive in answering history questions, and there is obvious tension between her and her mother, who stridently insists that the patient answer your questions. Of the following, which is most likely to be the most effective approach in obtaining a history from this patient?
    A. Threaten the patient with nasogastric lavage and a second large-bore IV access if she does not answer your questions.
    B. Attempt to build a rapport with your patient by telling her you know how she feels.
    C. Gently escort the mother from the room while your female partner continues questioning the patient.
    D. Ask the girl's father to step into the room to speak with the patient.
    E. Use a puppet of "Triumph the Insult Comic Dog" and make her laugh until she spills the beans.

13. An important component of the initial assessment in a pediatric patient is the:
    A. blood pressure.
    B. general appearance and mental status.
    C. lab values and diagnostic imaging.
    D. heart rate.
    E. all of the above.

14. The pediatric assessment triangle is an assessment tool that:
    A. uses the triad of technological assessment data comprised of capillary blood glucose, pulse oximetry, and EKG tracing.
    B. requires a great deal of hands-on examination.
    C. can be accomplished, for the most part, from across the room.
    D. eliminates the need for a detailed physical examination.
    E. none of the above.

15. A poor impression of the child's general appearance and mental status may indicate:
    A. obvious CNS depression.
    B. shock.
    C. respiratory failure.
    D. instability and/or decompensation of physiologic status.
    E. none of the above.

16. Measuring oxygen saturation via pulse oximetry allows for continuous monitoring of:
    A. adequacy of ventilation.
    B. adequacy of oxygenation.
    C. hemoglobin levels.
    D. alveolar oxygen concentration.
    E. oxygen delivery at the cellular level.

17. Which of the following is NOT typically a clinical sign of increased work of breathing?
    A. poor ventilatory mechanics such as retractions and "see-saw" breathing
    B. low arterial oxygen saturation
    C. nasal flaring
    D. use of accessory muscles
    E. elevated respiratory rate

18. You are transporting an eighteen-month-old child with croup from a community hospital to a PICU at the tertiary care center 40 minutes away. The child has a patent IV access, is on an EKG monitor, and is receiving beta-agonist bronchodilators and humidified oxygen during transport. Initially the child exhibited significant airway stridor, anxiousness, and tachypnea at 50 breaths per minute. During transport, your reassessment reveals the child to be quiet with a respiratory rate of 18 breaths per minute. This is:
    A. a sign of effective treatment and resolution of the bronchospasm.
    B. a sign of respiratory fatigue and impending respiratory arrest.
    C. a normal sleep pattern.
    D. an absolute indication for endotracheal intubation.
    E. none of the above.

19. In pediatric patients, bradycardia is:
    A. common.
    B. usually the first sign of primary cardiac abnormality.
    C. often a sign of critical hypoxia.
    D. almost always a sign of increased intracranial pressure.
    E. B and D.

20. An indirect measure of end-organ perfusion that may be of use to the critical care paramedic is:
    A. urinary output.
    B. rectal sphincter tone.
    C. pupillary reaction.
    D. presence or absence of hepatic congestion and ascites.
    E. none of the above.

21. The most common pathophysiological cause of pediatric death is:
    A. blunt chest/abdominal trauma.
    B. childhood respiratory illnesses.
    C. burns.
    D. head trauma.
    E. none of the above.

22. Assessing the Glasgow Coma Score in young infants:
    A. requires modification for measuring response to verbal commands and verbal responses.
    B. is of no use to the critical care paramedic because young infants cannot be accurately measured using existing criteria.
    C. is done exactly the same as in adults.
    D. should be done the same way for 5-year-olds as it is for 5-month-olds.
    E. none of the above.

23. On the pediatric Glasgow Coma Scale, an infant who opens his eyes to shouting, localizes painful stimuli, and cries appropriately would receive a score of:
    A. 15.
    B. 13.
    C. 11.
    D. 12.
    E. none of the above.

24. Children older than 1 year of age should respond like adults on all areas of the Glasgow Coma Scale EXCEPT:
    A. verbal response.
    B. motor response.
    C. eye opening.
    D. flexion.
    E. none of the above.

25. A child with a Glasgow Coma Scale score of 8 would be classified as:
    A. mild acuity.
    B. moderate acuity.
    C. severe acuity.
    D. dead.
    E. nonacute.

26. You are called to community hospital to transport a 6-year-old patient to the pediatric tertiary care center an hour away. The child was struck by a motor vehicle at low speed, sustaining a broken right arm and bruises to the chest. The Emergency Department physician tells you the child likely has a pulmonary contusion. The child's arterial oxygen saturation is only 85% despite being on high-concentration oxygen via mask. The chest X-ray taken 20 minutes ago reveals no pneumothoraces, hemothoraces, or rib fractures. Upon further examination, the child appears dusky and has diminished breath sounds on the left side and subcutaneous emphysema in the left axilla. The most likely cause of this child's respiratory distress is:
    A. pulmonary contusion.
    B. cardiac tamponade.
    C. tension pneumothorax.
    D. simple pneumothorax.
    E. none of the above.

27. The first intervention to be taken for the child in question 26 is:
    A. needle pericardiocentesis.
    B. needle thoracentesis and/or placement of a chest tube.
    C. repeat chest radiographic films to assess for a possible tension pneumothorax or cardiac tamponade.
    D. bag-valve-mask ventilation.
    E. all of the above.

28. Of the following, which is an early sign of increased intracranial pressure (ICP)?
    A. Cushing's triad
    B. anisocoria
    C. decorticate posturing
    D. decerebrate posturing
    E. sustained ICP > 20 mmHg for thirty minutes or more

29. Which of the following does NOT influence ICP?
    A. blood volume
    B. CSF volume
    C. brain volume
    D. tidal volume
    E. none of the above

30. You are transporting an 8-year-old patient with blunt chest trauma to the tertiary care center. During your ongoing assessment, you note that the patient's chest tube has stopped draining. Your first step in ensuring patency of the tube is to:
    A. clamp the tube with padded hemostats and replace the drainage unit.
    B. check patient position and reposition if necessary, checking tube for kinks or clots.
    C. check the water seal in the drainage system, making sure the chambers are filled to the proper level.
    D. disconnect the drainage system from the suction unit, checking to make sure the suction unit is operating properly.
    E. increase the vacuum pressure on the suction unit.

31. Treatment for the pediatric patient in shock usually includes:
    A. vasopressor and inotropic support.
    B. fluid boluses of 20 mL/kg of an isotonic crystalloid solution.

C. fluid boluses of 3 mL/kg of 3% NaCl solution.
D. PASG.
E. none of the above.

32. An easily accessible, non-collapsible vascular access often used for critically ill infants and children is:
    A. cannulation of the femoral vein using the Seldinger technique.
    B. a peripherally inserted central catheter (PICC) line.
    C. cannulation of the intraosseous spaces.
    D. intra-cardiac injection of resuscitation fluids and medications.
    E. extracorporeal membrane oxygenation (ECMO).

33. Common causes of acute deterioration of the intubated and mechanically ventilated pediatric patient include:
    A. tube displacement.
    B. obstruction of the endotracheal tube or ventilator circuit.
    C. pneumothorax.
    D. equipment failure.
    E. all of the above.

34. Changes to the respiratory system in elderly patients include:
    A. increase in functional reserve capacity due to trapped air.
    B. decrease in chest wall excursion and tidal volume.
    C. pulmonary hypertension increases O_2 and CO_2 exchange, thus predisposing to respiratory alkalosis.
    D. maximum oxygen uptake increases by up to 70%.
    E. none of the above.

35. Age-related decline in cardiovascular systems includes:
    A. loss of elasticity and hardening of arteries.
    B. deterioration of the cardiac conduction system, predisposing to dysrhythmias.
    C. decline in myocardial contractility.
    D. all of the above.
    E. none of the above.

36. Of the following physiologic abnormalities, which should be of particular concern to the critical care paramedic before administering medication to the elderly patient?
    A. decline in renal function impairs the elderly patient's ability to compensate for low perfusion states
    B. reduction in solute filtration contributes to electrolyte imbalances
    C. decline in renal function predisposes to drug toxicity
    D. decline in the kidneys' ability to regulate fluid reabsorption contributes to hypertension
    E. none of the above

37. Caution should be exercised in assessing the elderly fall victim because:
    A. reduction in nerve impulse velocity decreases the patient's perception of pain.
    B. declines in the elderly patient's mental status may pose challenges in obtaining patient history.
    C. shrinkage in brain size makes head injury more likely and may result in delayed appearance of symptoms.
    D. all of the above.
    E. none of the above.

38. Which of the following is NOT a consideration in treating the elderly trauma patient with osteoporosis?
    A. greater likelihood of occult fractures
    B. decreased pain perception in elderly patients makes analgesia rarely necessary
    C. immobilization techniques may need to be modified
    D. high likelihood of closed head injury
    E. none of the above

39. The most common posttraumatic condition the critical care paramedic will have to deal with in obstetrical trauma is:
    A. fetal anoxia secondary to maternal hemorrhage.
    B. musculoskeletal injury of the fetus due to deformation of the uterus.
    C. placental separation.
    D. premature rupture of membranes.
    E. none of the above.

40. You are called to transport a woman injured in an automobile crash. The patient is an expectant mother at 32 weeks gestation who has sustained blunt trauma to the abdomen. She complains of abdominal cramps and tenderness. Her vital signs are: HR = 88 beats per minute, RR = 24 breaths per minute, and BP = 128/80 mmHg. A fetal heart rate monitor shows a rate of 116 beats per minute with little variability and recurrent decelerations. Despite the absence of any clinical signs of hemorrhage in the mother, what physiologic changes of pregnancy may account for the fetal distress?
    A. Increased maternal blood volume may delay the appearance of clinical signs of shock in the mother until well after the fetus is compromised.
    B. Fetal heart rate usually closely parallels maternal heart rate.
    C. Shunting of blood away from the uterus may promote fetal distress well before clinical signs of shock develop in the mother.
    D. Relative hemodilution from administration of IV boluses in the mother results in decreased oxygen-carrying capability to the uterus and resultant hypoxia-induced bradycardia.
    E. A and C

41. For the third-trimester pregnant trauma patient exhibiting signs of fetal distress, the most appropriate course of treatment available to the critical care paramedic is:
    A. emergency cesarean section.
    B. stabilization of maternal oxygenation, ventilation, and perfusion.
    C. prophylactic administration of tocolytics.
    D. vasopressor support of the mother's blood pressure.
    E. induction of labor and delivery of the fetus.

42. Elements of the maternal history of particular concern to the critical care paramedic include:
    A. sex of the fetus.
    B. number of fetuses.
    C. complications with current or previous pregnancies.
    D. history of previous uncomplicated cesarean section.
    E. all of the above.

43. Which of the following is NOT considered a normal physiologic change of pregnancy?
    A. mild leukocytosis
    B. mild respiratory alkalosis
    C. increased systolic and diastolic blood pressure

- D. flat or inverted T waves in Leads III, V1 and V2
- E. heart rate increased by 10–15 beats per minute

44. Which of the following statements about breathing is FALSE?
    A. Breathing is good.
    B. Apnea is bad.
    C. Cellular oxygenation is dependent upon adequate breathing.
    D. The number of times a person breathes per minute is called the respiratory rate.
    E. none of the above

45. Which of the following factors is NOT associated with increased fetal mortality?
    A. sex of the mother
    B. high maternal injury severity score (ISS)
    C. maternal hemorrhage
    D. maternal alcohol usage
    E. maternal smoking history

CHAPTER 21
Pulmonary Emergencies

DIRECTIONS Each of the questions or incomplete statements below is followed by suggested answers or completions. Select the **one answer** that is best in each case.

1. The respiratory epithelium is made up of many cells, including:
   1. bronchioles.
   2. cilia.
   3. goblet cells.
   4. lamina propria.
   5. alveoli.

   A. 1 and 2
   B. 2 and 3
   C. 1, 2, and 3
   D. 2, 3, and 4
   E. 1, 2, 3, 4, and 5

2. It is an accepted clinical point of reference that a blockage or obstruction between the _____ and _____ will result in a fatal event if not corrected.
   A. epiglottis, arytenoids
   B. glottic opening, inferior carina
   C. epiglottis, superior carina
   D. glottic opening, arytenoids
   E. none of the above

3. The trachea begins at the level of _____ and extends inferiorly for approximately 11 cm, terminating at the _____.
   A. C-2/C-3, carina
   B. C-3/C-4, 6th tracheal ring
   C. C-4/C-5, 7th tracheal ring
   D. C-5/C-6, carina
   E. C-6/C-7, carina

4. The collection of structures held in place by the roots at the level of T-5 and T-6 are:
   1. trachea
   2. primary bronchi
   3. pulmonary vessels
   4. pulmonary nerves
   5. hilum

   A. 1 and 2
   B. 1, 2, and 3
   C. 1, 2, 3, and 4
   D. 1, 2, 3, 4, and 5
   E. 1, 3, and 5

5. Gas exchange in the lungs takes place predominantly in the:
   A. bronchioles.
   B. alveoli.
   C. terminal bronchioles.
   D. respiratory bronchioles.
   E. alveolar sacs.

6. Factors that decrease the efficiency of gas exchange between the cardiovascular and respiratory systems can include:
   A. increased width of the interstitial space.
   B. interruption of the alveolar epithelial membrane.
   C. lack of perfusion of the pulmonary capillaries.
   D. all of the above.
   E. A and B.

7. Small holes in alveolar walls, called the _____, allow for limited interalveolar communication; likewise, the _____ allow for collateral air distribution between the bronchioles.
   A. pores of Kohn, canals of Lambert
   B. pores of Lambert, canals of Kohn
   C. pores of Cohn, canals of Lampert
   D. pores of Lampert, canals of Cohn
   E. none of the above

8. A combination of phospholipids that helps decrease the surface tension of water in the alveoli, preventing collapse or atalectasis, is known as:
   A. pulmonary surfactoids.
   B. pulmonic surfactants.
   C. pulmonary surfactants.
   D. all of the above.
   E. none of the above.

9. There are three types of cells present in the alveoli. Match the name of each type with its function.
   1. type I pneumocytes
   2. type II pneumocytes
   3. alveolar macrophages

   a. surfactant producers
   b. debris cleaners
   c. assist gas exchange

   A. 1–a, 2–b, 3–c
   B. 1–b, 2–a, 3–c
   C. 1–a, 2–c, 3–b
   D. 1–c, 2–a, 3–b
   E. 1–b, 2–c, 3–a

10. Alveolar macrophages are a type of _____ cell.
    A. lymphocytic
    B. phagocytic
    C. macrophagic
    D. lamanictic
    E. none of the above

11. The _____ pleura covers the lungs and the _____ pleura attaches to the chest wall.
    A. visceral, parietal
    B. parietal, visceral
    C. pulmonary, parietal
    D. visceral, pulmonary
    E. parietal, visceral

12. In addition to their role in gas exchange, the _____ are the site of production of angiotensin-converting enzyme.
    A. alveolar capillaries
    B. pulmonary capillaries
    C. alveolar bronchioles
    D. all of the above
    E. none of the above

13. Acute respiratory failure can be defined as a state of:
    A. chronic respiratory insufficiency.
    B. hypercarbia.
    C. inadequate gas exchange.
    D. hypocarbia.
    E. all of the above.

14. The generally accepted oxygenation failure syndromes include cardiogenic shock, low FiO_2, and which of the following?
    1. hyperventilation
    2. ventilation/perfusion mismatch
    3. diffusion defect(s)
    4. intrapulmonary shunting
    5. hypoventilation

    A. 1 and 2
    B. 1, 2, and 3
    C. 1, 3, and 5
    D. 1, 2, 3, and 4
    E. 2, 3, 4, and 5

15. Alveolar hypoventilation can result from depression of the respiratory center secondary to:
    A. drug intoxication.
    B. increased intracranial pressure.
    C. CNS sedation.
    D. all of the above.
    E. B and C.

16. You are transporting a patient with head, neck, chest and pelvic trauma to a Level I Center by ground. The patient is intubated

and sedated for transport. Five minutes into the trip, the automatic ventilator alarm begins to sound. You notice the patient's O_2 saturation is decreasing and the CO_2 level has increased precipitously. You also note the patient has now become quite pale, the VS monitor is reading 52/26 mmHg, and the monitor shows an apparent sinus tachycardia at a rate of 130 beats per minute. As you auscultate lung sounds, you suspect the patient is exhibiting signs of respiratory failure as a result of:
   A. V/O mismatch.
   B. V/P mismatch.
   C. V/Q mismatch.
   D. V/R mismatch.
   E. none of the above.

17. Nontraumatic reasons why a patient might experience ventilation/perfusion mismatch could include:
   A. right ventricular failure.
   B. pulmonary embolus.
   C. severe hypervolemia.
   D. A and B.
   E. A and C.

18. The equation:

$$\frac{QPS}{QT} = \frac{CiO_2 - CaO_2}{CiO_2 - CvO_2}$$

has to do with physiological shunting, where QPS is the shunt flow, QT is the _____ and CiO_2 is the concentration of oxygen in arterial blood flow when the _____ is ideal.
   A. venous oxygen concentration, V/Q
   B. cardiac output/minute, V/R
   C. mixed venous oxygen concentration, V/X
   D. cardiac output/minute, V/Q
   E. none of the above

19. What is the normal ventilation/perfusion (V/Q) ratio in a healthy adult?
   A. 4/5 or 0.8
   B. 4/6 or 0.6
   C. 4/7 or 0.57
   D. 4/8 or 0.5
   E. 5/4 or 1.25

20. In a case of a V/Q ratio less than 0.8, where an area of lung is not properly ventilated and perfusion remains normal, the PaO_2 will shunt:
   A. up and down.
   B. left to right.
   C. right to left.
   D. A and C.
   E. none of the above.

21. Normal oxygen transport within the human body can be represented in a formula as:
   O_2 transport = _____.
   A. $CaO_2 \times CO \times 10$
   B. $CaO_2 \times PCO_2 \times 10$
   C. $PCO_2 \times CaO_2 \times 5$
   D. $CaO_2 \times CO_2 \times 5$
   E. $PCO_2 \times CO_2 \times 10$

22. Disturbances to the relationship between the pulmonary capillaries and alveoli affecting O_2 and CO_2 diffusion can occur as a result of:
   A. interstitial edema.
   B. pulmonary hypertension.
   C. fibrotic changes.
   D. heart failure.
   E. all of the above.

23. In a diffusion deficit abnormality, _____ diffuses less readily than _____ and hypoxemia often results before signs of _____ are seen.
   A. CO_2, O_2, hypocapnia
   B. CO_2, O_2, hypercarbia
   C. O_2, CO_2, hypocapnia
   D. O_2, CO_2, hypercarbia
   E. O_2, CO_2, hypercapnia

24. A V/Q mismatch can occur in an area of a lung where ventilation is greater than the blood flow to that area, resulting in:
   A. hypocarbia.
   B. hypocapnia.
   C. hypercarbia.
   D. hypercapnia.
   E. hypoxycarbia.

25. Ventilation failures resulting in hypercapnia can be measured by evaluating the _____ via arterial blood gas (ABG) analysis.
   A. PAO$_2$
   B. PCO$_2$
   C. PaCO
   D. PaO$_2$
   E. PaCO$_2$

26. While inspecting a patient's chest, you place your hands on the lower costal border with your thumbs at the xyphoid process. When the patient inhales, your thumbs separate approximately 0.5 inches. You know that this expansion distance is indicative of:
   A. minimal excursion.
   B. normal excursion.
   C. maximum excursion.
   D. labored excursion.
   E. none of the above.

27. As you assess the contour of a patient's chest, you decide it has a "barrel" conformation based upon the 2:2 ratio of the AP and lateral aspects of the patient's thorax. The normal ratio is _____.
   A. 1:2
   B. 1:3
   C. 2:1
   D. 3:1
   E. none of the above

28. Chest contour variations can include:
   A. kyphosis and scoliosis.
   B. pigeon breast and funnel chest.
   C. barrel and concave chest.
   D. all of the above.
   E. B and C.

29. The purpose of the Heimlich valve is to prevent:
   A. leakage of fluids from a chest tube.
   B. loss of vacuum seal around a chest drainage jar.
   C. loss of chest tube placement during movement.
   D. accidental entrainment of air into the pleural cavity.
   E. all of the above.

30. One purpose of chest palpation is to assess for:
   A. subcutaneous emphysema.
   B. pain and tenderness.
   C. symmetry.
   D. all of the above.
   E. B and C.

31. Conditions that may result in deviation of the trachea toward the affected side are:
   1. tension pneumothorax.
   2. atelectasis.
   3. pleural effusion.
   4. phrenic nerve paralysis.
   5. fibrosis.

   A. 1 and 2
   B. 2 and 3
   C. 2, 3, and 4
   D. 1, 3, and 5
   E. 2, 4, and 5

32. Tactile fremitus is _____ over areas of lung consolidation and _____ over bronchial obstructions.
   A. not heard, always heard
   B. increased, diminished
   C. diminished, increased
   D. always heard, not heard
   E. quiet, loud

33. Sounds produced by percussion are described as:
    1. resonant.
    2. hyperresonant.
    3. tympanic.
    4. dull.
    5. flat.

    A. all of the above
    B. 1, 2, and 3
    C. 2, 3, and 4
    D. 1, 3, and 5
    E. none of the above

34. Percussive sounds are generally described in terms of their:
    1. pitch.
    2. tenor.
    3. intensity.
    4. quality.
    5. duration.

    A. 1 and 3
    B. 2 and 4
    C. 1, 3, and 5
    D. 2, 3, and 4
    E. 1, 2, 3, 4, and 5

35. During auscultation of a 24-year-old AIDS patient's lung sounds, you ask her to continuously speak the letter "E." Your patient has complained of shortness of breath over the last 3 days. She denies coughing but admits to "some discomfort at times." As you percuss the chest you note a hollow intense, low pitch over the right upper lobe and flat, dull sounds over the left lower lobe. Auscultation confirms your assessment that the patient's lungs seem to be:
    A. normal in the right and upper left lobes, abnormal in the left lower lobe.
    B. normal in the left lower lobe, abnormal in the right and upper left lobes.
    C. normal in all fields; you just didn't percuss correctly across the entire surface.
    D. abnormal in all fields with serious consolidation in the left lower lobe.
    E. none of the above.

36. The four types of normal lung sounds are generally described as:
    1. bronchial.
    2. tracheovesicular.
    3. bronchovesicular.
    4. vesicular.
    5. tracheal.

    A. 1, 3, and 5
    B. 2, 4, and 5
    C. 1, 3, 4, and 5
    D. 1, 2, 3, 4, and 5
    E. 1 and 4

37. The art of assessing lung sounds involves knowing the normal findings one should expect to hear in different areas of the respiratory tree. Match the following with their appropriate sounds and characteristics.
    1. Loud, harsh, equal inspiratory and expiratory phases
    2. Loud, high, longer expiratory than inspiratory phases
    3. Medium, similar inspiratory and expiratory phases
    4. Soft, low, longer inspiratory than expiratory phases

    a. Bronchial
    b. Vesicular
    c. Bronchovesicular
    d. Tracheal

    A. 1–a, 2–b, 3–c, 4–d
    B. 1–b, 2–c, 3–d, 4–a
    C. 1–c, 2–d, 3–a, 4–b
    D. 1–d, 2–a, 3–c, 4–b
    E. 1–d, 2–a, 3–b, 4–c

38. Adventitious lung sounds are described as:
    A. crackles, rhonchi, wheezes, and friction rubs.
    B. crackles, rhonchi, whistling, and pops.
    C. rhonchi, crackles, friction rubs, and whistling.
    D. grunts, rhonchi, wheezes, and crackles.
    E. none of the above.

39. During auscultation of a 24-year-old AIDS patient's lung sounds, you ask her to continuously speak the letter "E," and as she does so you note egophony. Specifically, there is a bilateral change from the "E" you hear at the lower lobes to a flat "A" sound you hear in the mid-thoracic region. You know this change is probably indicative of:
    A. distortion of the voice.
    B. pleural effusion.
    C. pulmonary edema.
    D. all of the above.
    E. B and C.

40. Asking a patient to whisper as you auscultate lung sounds, is a type of assessment known as:
    A. bronchial egophany.
    B. whispered egophany.
    C. whispered pectoriloquy.
    D. vesicular pectoriloquy.
    E. ventriloquy.

41. Match the following terms and values for standard ABG results:
    1. SAO$_2$
    2. PaO$_2$
    3. PaCO$_2$
    4. pH
    5. HCO$_3^-$

    a. 22–26 mEq/L
    b. 7.35–7.45
    c. 35–45 mmHg
    d. 94–99%
    e. 80–100 mmHg

    A. 1–a, 2–b, 3–c, 4–d, 5–e
    B. 1–b, 2–c, 3–d, 4–e, 5–a
    C. 1–d, 2–e, 3–c, 4–b, 5–a
    D. 1–d, 2–e, 3–a, 4–c, 5–b
    E. 1–c, 2–e, 3–b, 4–e, 5–b

42. You are using a pulse oximeter to measure SpO$_2$ in the field. The reading is 90%. You know this means the PaO$_2$ is approximately:
    A. 40 mmHg.
    B. 50 mmHg.
    C. 60 mmHg.
    D. 70 mmHg.
    E. none of the above.

43. The major critical limitation of pulse oximetry is that it will report fairly accurate data of a patient's _____ status, but does not offer data concerning the patient's _____ status.
    A. ventilation, oxygenation
    B. pulmonary, ventilation
    C. oxygenation, ventilation
    D. pulmonary, oxygenation
    E. none of the above

44. End tidal capnography (ETCO$_2$) level is an approximation of PaCO$_2$, but it still allows a fairly accurate approximation of what value?
    A. bronchial respiration
    B. alveolar ventilation
    C. vesicular respiration
    D. bronchovesicular ventilation
    E. all of the above

45. The four phases of a normal capnogram include the following:
    a. completion of the inhalatory phase
    b. exhalation of CO$_2$ from the lungs

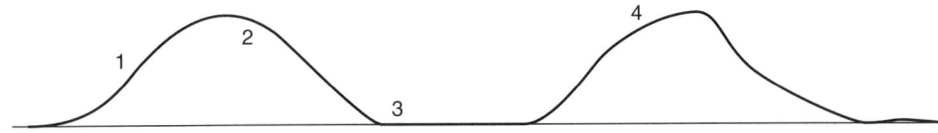

Figure 21–1

c. exhalation of CO_2 from the terminal and alveolar spaces

d. inception of the inhalatory phase

Match the letter for each phase listed above with the number (1, 2, 3, or 4) that corresponds to its waveform part as illustrated in Figure 21–1.

A. a–1, b–2, c–3, d–4
B. a–3, b–1, c–4, d–2
C. a–2, b–1, c–4, d–3
D. a–4, b–3, c–1, d–2
E. a–1, b–3, c–2, d–1

46. When presented with elevated $ETCO_2$ levels, the critical care paramedic should consider all of the following as a possible cause EXCEPT:
    A. conditions resulting in increased CO_2 production.
    B. decreased alveolar ventilations.
    C. equipment malfunction.
    D. increased alveolar ventilations.
    E. decreased minute ventilations.

47. High concentrations of _____ can present false low readings and excessive _____ can present false high readings in $ETCO_2$ monitoring.
    A. carbon dioxide, oxygen
    B. oxygen, nitrogen
    C. nitrogen, water vapor
    D. oxygen, water vapor
    E. carbon dioxide, oxygen

48. The basic goal of management in acute respiratory failure—as with all respiratory ailments—is to ensure adequate:
    A. ventilation.
    B. oxygenation.
    C. carbon dioxide elimination.
    D. all of the above.
    E. A and B.

49. The generally accepted indication for _____ is a $PaCO_2$ less than 50 mmHg, a PaO_2 less than 60 mmHg, and an arterial pH less than 7.30 on room air.
    A. ventilations using a bag-valve mask (BVM)
    B. oxygen therapy via nonrebreather mask (NRB)
    C. extubation
    D. intubation
    E. none of the above

50. You are assessing a 15-year-old male patient who cannot speak and is sitting in a tripod position. His mother tells you he was mowing the lawn when this came on suddenly. She denies any previous medical history for the patient. When you inquire about chest pain or trauma, the patient shakes his head "no." Further assessment reveals pale, cool, non-diaphoretic skin and audible wheezes but no visible urticaria. His RR is 32 and labored, HR is 130, and BP is 98/68. As you administer 100% oxygen, you begin to check off your list of differentials—a list that might include all of the following EXCEPT:
    A. acute asthma attack.
    B. acute pulmonary embolism.
    C. acute respiratory failure.
    D. organophosphate poisoning.
    E. anaphylaxis.

51. Acute asthma attacks normally follow a two-phase response. The first phase involves the inhalation of an antigen that contacts IgE antibodies and triggers mast cell degranulation. A result of this response is the release of several substances including prostaglandins and thromboxanes as well as:
    1. histamine.
    2. leukotrienes.
    3. cytokines.
    4. interleukins.
    5. eosinophil factors.

    A. 1 and 3
    B. 1, 2, and 3
    C. 1, 2, 3, and 4
    D. 1, 2, 3, 4, and 5
    E. 1, 2, and 4

52. The release of substances such as platelets, eosinophils, and leukocytes into the bronchial tract signals the _____ phase of an asthma attack.
    A. primary
    B. initial
    C. secondary
    D. tertiary
    E. restorative

53. You respond to a 52-year-old female who is complaining of shortness of breath. She is using accessory muscles, appears lethargic, and is having difficulty focusing on you or your voice. The patient has a known history of asthma, and her husband tells you she has used her albuterol inhaler several times in the last 30 minutes with no relief. You begin treatment with nebulized albuterol as you auscultate the patient's chest and your partner obtains vital signs. You note paradoxical breathing, hyperresonance upon percussion, and a "silent chest." Your next action is to:
    A. consider the use of subcutaneous epinephrine 1:1000.
    B. consider the use of inhaled ipratropium bromide.
    C. consider nasal intubation.
    D. all of the above.
    E. B and C.

54. The presence of escalating airway compromise in asthmatics can be diagnostically demonstrated with capnography and recognized by the change in the normal wave form to a _____ appearance.
    A. "porgy fin"
    B. "shark fin"
    C. "trout fin"
    D. "flounder fin"
    E. none of the above

55. In restrictive respiratory syndromes, the FVC and FEV_1 are reduced _____; in obstructive syndromes the FVC and FEV_1 are reduced _____.
    A. appropriately, inappropriately
    B. inappropriately, appropriately
    C. proportionately, disproportionately
    D. disproportionately, proportionately
    E. 40–50%, 60–80%

56. _____ agonists are most beneficial in asthma because they reduce mediator release, relax smooth muscle, and promote mucociliary release.
    A. $Alpha_1$ antagonists
    B. Mixed $alpha_2$ and $beta_1$ agonists
    C. Both $beta_1$ and $beta_2$ antagonists
    D. $Beta_2$ agonists
    E. $Beta_2$ antagonists

57. Anticholinergic drugs are used in the treatment of asthma because of their:
    A. ability to block vagal tone.
    B. bronchodilatory effects.
    C. positive effect on FEV_1 and PEFR.
    D. all of the above.
    E. A and B.

58. You are interviewing a 25-year-old male patient with a known history of asthma. He is not complaining of respiratory problems today, but he states he has been feeling "really funny" since he used his albuterol inhaler yesterday. He also says he feels nauseated and has a headache that will not go away. During assessment you note wave abnormalities in his 12-Lead ECG, although his vital signs are normal for his age and condition. He takes theophylline daily and uses an albuterol inhaler "p.r.n." (as necessary). As a part of your continued work-up you should consider the possibility of _____ toxicity.
    A. aminophylline
    B. theophylline
    C. ipatropium bromide
    D. albuterol
    E. A and B

59. Another name for CPAP (continuous positive airway pressure) is:
    A. PERP (positive-pressure endotracheal respiratory pressure).
    B. NPPV (noninvasive positive-pressure ventilation).
    C. ETPV (endotracheal positive-pressure ventilation).
    D. IPPV (intermittent positive-pressure ventilation).
    E. all of the above.

60. CPAP uses continuous positive pressure throughout the respiratory cycle, while BiPAP (bilevel continuous positive airway pressure) uses _____ positive pressure during inhalation and _____ positive pressure during exhalation.
    A. higher, lower
    B. lower, higher
    C. maximum, minimum
    D. minimal, maximal
    E. none of the above

61. There is a severe risk of barotrauma in patients receiving PPV (positive-pressure ventilation). This most often occurs when:
    A. returned volume is greater than tidal volume.
    B. tidal volume is greater than returned volume.
    C. initial PPV value is lower than end PPV.
    D. settings are too high from the beginning.
    E. settings are too low from the beginning.

62. The archetypal "blue bloater" (with chronic bronchitis) and "pink puffer" (with emphysema) have similar underlying pathologies. However, there is a hallmark difference in presentation. The chronic bronchitis patient will present with _____, while the emphysema patient will present with _____.
    A. increased sputum; a dry cough
    B. decreased sputum; a productive cough
    C. wheezing; no wheezing
    D. A and C
    E. none of the above

63. The GOLD (Global Initiative for Chronic Obstructive Lung Disease) criteria allow clinicians to diagnose and classify COPD (chronic obstructive pulmonary disease) on the basis of:
    A. severity.
    B. length of diagnosed disease.
    C. amount of sputum production.
    D. pulmonary function as determined by spirometry results.
    E. all of the above.

64. The pathogens most commonly associated with exacerbation of COPD are:
    1. *Streptococcus pneumonia.*
    2. *Haemophaellius viralis.*
    3. *Haemophilus influenza.*
    4. *Moraxella catarrhalis.*
    5. *Staphylococcus aureus.*

    A. 1 and 3
    B. 2 and 3
    C. 1, 3, and 5
    D. 1, 3, and 4
    E. 1, 2, 3, 4, and 5

65. The principle characteristic of ARDS (acute respiratory distress syndrome) is its manifestation of pulmonary edema in the absence of depressed _____ function **OR** volume overload in the presence of _____.
    A. left ventricular, trauma
    B. left atrial, infection
    C. right ventricular, infection
    D. right atrial, trauma
    E. left atrial, trauma

66. Many conditions are associated with ARDS. A list of those attributed to direct injury would include near-drowning, pneumonia, aspiration, and:
    A. pulmonary contusion.
    B. sepsis.
    C. chemical exposure.
    D. A and C.
    E. A and B.

67. Management of ARDS in the clinical setting requires the use of endotracheal intubation, FiO$_2$ of no greater than _____, and PEEP settings titrated to an SpO$_2$ of 90% or better.
    A. 30%
    B. 40%
    C. 50%
    D. 60%
    E. 70%

68. The primary goal of prehospital management of ARDS during transport is to ensure an SpO$_2$ of greater than:
    A. 60%.
    B. 70%.
    C. 80%.
    D. 90%.
    E. 95%.

69. Diuretics do not have a beneficial effect upon ARDS patients because:
    A. pulmonary edema in ARDS is a result of inflammation.
    B. pulmonary edema in ARDS is managed with corticosteroids.
    C. pulmonary edema in ARDS is managed with high levels of PEEP.
    D. all of the above.
    E. none of the above.

70. The classical signs and symptoms of pneumonia include fever, increased sputum production and cough, and:
    A. tachycardia.
    B. hypertension.
    C. pleuritic pain.
    D. dyspnea.
    E. A, C, and D.

71. The decision to hospitalize a patient with pneumonia is based on assessment and history and may also be influenced by the outcome of certain lab tests, which may include:
    A. leukopenia of less than 5K cells/mm^3.
    B. leukocytosis greater than 30K cells/mm^3.
    C. more than 50% lung surface involved.
    D. all of the above.
    E. A and C.

72. As compared to nonsmokers, smokers have a _____ relative risk of spontaneous pneumothorax.
    A. 3:1
    B. 10:1
    C. 15:1
    D. 20:1
    E. 30:1

73. You are treating an 18-year-old male who collapsed while playing basketball. On your arrival, you find him in a sitting position against the wall, complaining of pain in the upper left shoulder as well as shortness of breath. Your interview elicits a history of smoking, but the patient denies other recreational drugs. His teammates also tell you he was not involved in body contact at any time during the game. The patient's vital signs are HR = 136 per minute; RR = 26 per minute, labored and irregular; BP = 110/68 mmHg; SpO$_2$ = 92%; breath sounds = diminished in upper left lobe, clear in all others.

    You know from your exam and the history of the events that this patient is most likely suffering from:
    A. tension pneumothorax.
    B. spontaneous pneumothorax.
    C. pneumonia.
    D. bronchitis.
    E. none of the above.

74. Most secondary development of a spontaneous pneumothorax is from:
    A. smoking.
    B. pleurisy.
    C. COPD.
    D. cystic fibrosis.
    E. asthma.

75. You respond to a reported high-speed, T-bone-style motorcycle-versus-automobile collision and are directed to care for a 62-year-old female who was ejected from her motorcycle over the roof of the car. She is attended by first responders who tell you she is responsive to voice prompts and has been denying any injury or pain anywhere besides her right chest wall.

    As you conduct your visual assessment, you see no obvious life-threatening injuries. However, when palpating the right chest wall you feel crepitus and then note paradoxical movement when you remove her shirt and note diminished lung sounds on the entire right side. Your patient's mental status is decreasing and her labored breathing is audible. Among your treatment modalities, you should immediately consider:
    A. 100% oxygen via BVM.
    B. intubation.
    C. needle decompression.
    D. RSI (rapid-sequence induction).
    E. all of the above.

CHAPTER 22

Cardiovascular Emergencies

DIRECTIONS Each of the questions or incomplete statements below is followed by suggested answers or completions. Select the **one answer** that is best in each case.

1. Cells of the cardiac conduction system differ from other myocardial cells in that they:
   A. lack contractile properties.
   B. possess the ability of self-excitation, or automaticity.
   C. are multinucleated.
   D. are less dependent on aerobic metabolism.
   E. none of the above.

2. Parasympathetic innervation of the heart is primarily limited to:
   A. excitation of supraventricular pacemaker sites.
   B. inhibition of supraventricular pacemaker sites.
   C. excitation of the bundle branches and the Purkinje system.
   D. inhibition of the bundle branches and Purkinje system.
   E. none of the above.

3. The mechanism by which the cells of the SA node increase their depolarization rate in response to stimuli from atrial stretch receptors is called:
   A. the Frank-Starling mechanism.
   B. autonomic reflex tachycardia.
   C. the Bainbridge reflex.
   D. benign atrial hypertrophy.
   E. Poiseuille's Law.

4. The hormone secreted in increased levels in response to atrial stretch receptors stimulated by excessive venous return is:
   A. aldosterone.
   B. angiotensin I.
   C. norepinephrine.
   D. atrial natriuretic peptide.
   E. cardioinhibitory hormone.

5. The effects of atrial natriuretic peptide include in all of the following EXCEPT:
   A. release of epinephrine and norepinephrine.
   B. increased sodium ion and water loss in the kidneys.
   C. decreased release of aldosterone.
   D. decreased release of antidiuretic hormone.
   E. peripheral vasodilation.

6. Activation of the semilunar and atrioventricular valves occurs in response to:
   A. action potentials propagated across the AV node.
   B. changes in ventricular filling pressures.
   C. the Bainbridge reflex.
   D. a timed autonomic response occurring 150 milliseconds after SA node activation.
   E. none of the above.

7. The cardiac pacemaker with an intrinsic firing rate of 40–60 impulses per minute is the:
   A. sinoatrial node.
   B. atrioventricular node.
   C. Bachman's bundle.
   D. bundle branch.
   E. Purkinje network.

8. The lateral and posterior walls of the left ventricle are perfused by the:
   A. distal branches of the right coronary artery.
   B. left common coronary artery.
   C. left anterior descending branch of the left coronary artery.
   D. circumflex branch of the left coronary artery.
   E. coronary sinus.

9. The inferior wall of the left ventricle shares a common blood supply with the:
   A. lateral wall of the left ventricle.
   B. posterior wall of the left ventricle.
   C. right ventricle.
   D. anterior wall of the left ventricle.
   E. B and C.

10. Auscultation of apical heart sounds is best done over the:
    A. fifth intercostal space on the midclavicular line.
    B. second intercostal space to the left of the sternum.
    C. second intercostal space to the right of the sternum.
    D. fifth intercostal space to the left of the sternum.
    E. none of the above.

11. The normal S2 heart sound is produced by:
    A. closing of the semilunar valves.
    B. closing of the atrioventricular valves.
    C. opening of the semilunar valves.
    D. opening of the atrioventricular valves.
    E. none of the above.

12. How can a physiologic split S2 sound be differentiated from an S3 sound?
    A. The split S2 usually occurs only during inspiration, whereas the S3 sound can be heard during inspiration and expiration.
    B. The S3 sound usually occurs only during inspiration, whereas the split S2 sound can be heard during inspiration and expiration.
    C. The S3 sound occurs between S1 and S2.
    D. The S3 sound occurs late in the diastolic phase, often immediately preceding S1.
    E. none of the above

13. An S3 heart sound:
    A. is also referred to as ventricular gallop.
    B. is also referred to as atrial gallop.
    C. often indicates hypertrophy or dysfunction of the left ventricle in adults over 35 years of age.
    D. is a sure sign of aortic stenosis.
    E. A and C.

14. The S4 heart sound:
    A. is also referred to as an ejection murmur.
    B. is also referred to as atrial gallop.
    C. occurs late in the diastolic phase and precedes the S1 sound.
    D. often indicates systemic hypertension or aortic stenosis.
    E. all of the above.

15. The S1 heart sound can be best heard:
    A. over the apex, in the 5th intercostal space in the midclavicular line.
    B. over the aorta, in the 2nd intercostal space to the right of the sternum.
    C. over the tricuspid area, in the 5th intercostal space to the left of the sternum.
    D. over the pulmonic area, in the 2nd intercostal space to the left of the sternum.
    E. none of the above.

16. The S2 heart sound can be best heard:
    A. over the apex, in the 5th intercostal space in the midclavicular line.
    B. over the aorta, in the 2nd intercostal space to the right of the sternum.
    C. over the tricuspid area, in the 5th intercostal space to the left of the sternum.
    D. over the pulmonic area, in the 2nd intercostal space to the left of the sternum.
    E. none of the above.

17. Which of the following statements is/are true of heart murmurs?
    A. They reflect a lack of patency of AV or semilunar valves.
    B. They are longer in duration than the normal S1 and S2 sounds.
    C. They always reflect serious cardiac abnormalities.
    D. Diastolic murmurs are always considered pathologic conditions.
    E. All but C are true.

18. A prolapsed mitral valve resulting in regurgitation would produce what type of murmur?
    A. systolic murmur (between S1 and S2), best heard over the left sternal border
    B. diastolic murmur (preceding S1), best heard over the aortic area
    C. diastolic murmur (preceding S1), best heard over the 5th intercostal space on the left sternal border
    D. systolic murmur (between S1 and S2), best heard over the apex
    E. none of the above

19. Of all acute coronary events, approximately _____ present without chest pain.
    A. 50%
    B. 25%
    C. 10%
    D. 40%
    E. 100%

20. Conditions that may mimic the ST-segment elevation of an acute myocardial infarction include:
    A. early repolarization.
    B. bundle branch blocks.
    C. left ventricular hypertrophy.
    D. pericarditis.
    E. all of the above.

21. Which of the following clinical or laboratory findings best indicates an acute myocardial infarction?
    A. presence of pathologic Q waves on the 12-Lead ECG
    B. elevated CK MB level with a relative index of 1.5
    C. ST-segment elevation of greater than or equal to 1 mm in two contiguous leads
    D. presence of classic substernal chest pain
    E. B natriuretic peptide (BNP) level of greater than 500 pg/dL

Scenario

Questions 22–24 refer to the following scenario:

You are called to a community hospital Emergency Department to transport a 40-year-old male to the cardiac catheterization lab at the tertiary care center. The patient began experiencing crushing substernal chest pain (10/10) while sitting at his desk at work. Local paramedics administered 325 mg of aspirin, oxygen, and three doses of sublingual nitroglycerin without relief. En route to the community hospital, they initiated IV access and administered 4 mg morphine with subsequent reduction of the chest pain to 4/10. The Emergency Department staff administered a second dose of morphine and initiated an intravenous infusion of nitroglycerin. The patient currently rates his pain as 2/10, with nitroglycerin infusing at 20 mcg/min. His current vital signs are HR 124 per minute, BP 152/90 mmHg, and RR 18 per minute with SpO_2 of 97% on 4 liters/minute of supplemental oxygen. His 12-Lead ECG reveals a sinus tachycardia at 124 beats per minute, with 3 mm ST-segment elevation in Leads V1 – V3 and QRS width within normal limits. His cardiac enzyme panel reflects elevated levels of CK-MB and Troponin T.

22. Based on the 12-Lead ECG findings, the patient is suffering from a/an:
    A. inferior wall infarction.
    B. anteroseptal infarction.
    C. posterior infarction.
    D. lateral wall infarction.
    E. anterolateral infarction.

23. Based on your knowledge of coronary artery anatomy, where is the thrombus most likely to be located?
    A. circumflex branch of the left coronary artery
    B. proximal right coronary artery
    C. marginal branch of the right coronary artery
    D. left anterior descending branch of the left coronary artery
    E. none of the above

24. Which of the following therapies would serve to help limit infarction size in this patient?
    A. Increase oxygen flow to 15 liters/minute.
    B. Consider administration of beta blockers to reduce heart rate, blood pressure and myocardial oxygen demand.
    C. Consider increasing the nitroglycerin infusion rate, titrated to pain relief and blood pressure > 90 mmHg systolic.
    D. B and C
    E. none of the above

Scenario

Questions 25–29 refer to the following scenario:

You are called to transport a 40-year-old male patient from the community hospital to the cardiac catheterization lab at the tertiary care center 30 minutes away. Family members drove the patient to the community hospital after he suffered a syncopal episode approximately 90 minutes ago. They reported that the patient complained of a sudden onset of indigestion and nausea, and when he arose from the couch to go to the bathroom, he passed out. The Emergency Department staff performed a 12-Lead ECG, which revealed sinus bradycardia with 2 mm ST-segment elevation in Leads II, III, and AVF. Subsequent testing of cardiac enzymes revealed CK-MB and troponin levels within normal limits. Initial vital signs were BP 112/70 mmHg, HR 54 per minute, and RR 18 per minute with SpO_2 of 99% on two liters per minute of oxygen. A nitroglycerin infusion is in place, but the infusion was placed on hold after the patient's blood pressure fell to 86/50 soon after beginning the infusion. After discontinuing the nitroglycerin and a fluid bolus of 250 mL, his current blood pressure is 94/60 mmHg. A rapid physical examination reveals mild diaphoresis and pallor, clear lung sounds and jugular venous distension of approximately 4 mm above the clavicles that lessens significantly with deep inspiration. Previous medical history is remarkable only for elevated cholesterol and mild hypertension.

25. Given the 12-Lead ECG findings, you suspect:
    A. septal myocardial infarction.
    B. inferior wall myocardial infarction.
    C. anterior wall myocardial infarction.
    D. posterior wall myocardial infarction.
    E. anterolateral myocardial infarction.

26. Based on your interpretation of the 12-Lead findings, which coronary artery is most likely occluded?
    A. left common coronary artery
    B. circumflex artery
    C. left anterior descending artery
    D. right coronary artery
    E. none of the above

27. Based on the patient's orthostatic syncope, 12-Lead ECG and physical exam findings and his response to treatment, you should also suspect:
    A. congestive heart failure.
    B. dehydration.
    C. right ventricular infarction.
    D. hypersensitivity to nitroglycerin.
    E. none of the above.

28. Based on your answer to question 27, what diagnostic tests might be immediately useful in confirming your suspicions?
    A. chest X-ray and B natriuretic peptide (BNP) level
    B. basic electrolyte panel and BUN and creatinine levels
    C. right-sided 12-Lead ECG, with particular scrutiny of Lead V4R
    D. try the nitroglycerin again, this time monitoring blood pressure invasively with an arterial line
    E. serial cardiac enzymes

29. Based on your answers to questions 27 and 28, which best describes the appropriate course of therapy for this patient during your transport to the tertiary care center?
    A. strict TKO fluids and administration of loop diuretics
    B. aggressive fluid therapy titrated to urinary output of 100 mL/hr
    C. judicious fluid boluses to improve preload and central venous pressure and resumption of the nitroglycerin infusion
    D. use of the nitroglycerin for coronary artery dilation and administration of vasopressors as needed to sustain a minimum systolic blood pressure of 100 mmHg
    E. none of the above

30. Which of the following is NOT a beneficial effect of morphine in the patient with acute coronary syndrome?
    A. hypotension
    B. reduction of preload
    C. pain relief, with attendant reduction in catecholamine release
    D. reduction of afterload
    E. none of the above

31. You are transporting a patient with an anterior wall myocardial infarction (3mm ST-segment elevation Lead V1–V4) to the cardiac catheterization lab 20 minutes away. Initially the patient was pain-free at the community hospital after administration of 5 mg morphine and an infusion of nitroglycerin at 20 mcg/minute. Vital signs prior to transport were HR 92 per minute, BP 134/74 mmHg, and RR 14 per minute with SpO$_2$ of 94% on 4L/min of oxygen. During transport he becomes restless and begins complaining of chest pain and increasing dyspnea. He appears pale and diaphoretic, and his cardiac rhythm changes from sinus rhythm to a second degree type II block with fixed 2:1 conduction. His heart rate drops to 44 beats per minute and his BP falls to 94/70 mmHg. The most appropriate therapy indicated for this patient is:
    A. immediate transcutaneous pacing with appropriate sedation and analgesia.
    B. administration of 0.5–1.0 mg atropine.
    C. administration of synthetic catecholamine infusion, such as epinephrine or isoproteranol, at 2–10 mcg/minute.
    D. administration of dopamine at 5–10 mcg/kg/minute.
    E. fly a kite from the ambulance and wait for a thunderstorm.

32. You are transporting a 60-year-old male to the CCU at the tertiary care center for treatment of new-onset atrial fibrillation with rapid ventricular response. The community hospital administered diltiazem 15 mg IV that subsequently reduced the ventricular rate to 80–90 beats per minute and began a maintenance infusion at 10 mg/hr. Immediately prior to your arrival the patient converted to sinus rhythm at 80 beats per minute. You quickly assess the patient, gather all needed paperwork, and continue all interventions while packaging the patient for transport. During transport, the patient begins complaining of palpitations and dyspnea, and the ECG monitor shows a narrow-complex tachycardia at 180 beats per minute. The 12-Lead ECG reveals atrial fibrillation with a rapid ventricular rate. Which of the following medications is relatively **CONTRAINDICATED**?
    A. amiodarone
    B. metoprolol
    C. procainamide
    D. repeat boluses of diltiazem
    E. none of the above

33. When transporting the acute coronary syndrome patient receiving a fibrinolytic infusion, which of the following poses the **LEAST** manageable potential complication during transport?
    A. reperfusion dysrhythmias
    B. chest pain
    C. hypotension
    D. bleeding from the patient's tunneled subclavian central venous catheter
    E. hypoxia

34. The procedure most commonly performed in the "cath lab" for the acute coronary syndrome patient is known as:
    A. high frequency radio ablation.
    B. coronary artery bypass graft (CABG).
    C. percutaneous transluminal coronary angioplasty (PTCA).
    D. Foley catheter insertion.
    E. keyhole CABG.

35. Indications for PTCA include:
    A. acute coronary syndrome with contraindications to fibrinolytics.
    B. unstable angina with nondiagnostic ECG.
    C. post-reperfusion angina with ECG findings indicative of coronary ischemia.
    D. acute coronary syndrome with persistent hemodynamic instability.
    E. A, C, and D.

36. Aortic aneurysm differs from aortic dissection in that:
    A. aneurysms arise primarily in the abdominal aorta, whereas dissections typically arise from the aortic arch.
    B. dissections involve all three layers of the aorta, whereas aneurysms usually involve a tear in the tunica intima.
    C. aneurysms involve all three layers of the aorta, whereas dissections usually involve a tear in the tunica intima.
    D. A and C.
    E. aneurysms often result from trauma, whereas dissections usually do not.

37. Clinical findings that often indicate rupture of the abdominal aortic aneurysm include:
    A. pulsatile abdominal masses.
    B. abdominal pain.
    C. oliguria.
    D. hypotension.
    E. B and D.

38. Emergency management of the patient with ruptured aortic aneurysm includes all of the following **EXCEPT** which?
    A. careful volume resuscitation with isotonic crystalloids
    B. typing and cross-matching at least 10 units of packed red blood cells

C. vasopressor support of blood pressure

D. immediate surgical intervention

E. none of the above

39. Risk factors that predispose patients to aortic dissection include:
    A. arteriosclerosis.
    B. genetic defects of connective tissues such as Marfan's disease.
    C. arterial hypertension.
    D. syphilis.
    E. all answers but A.

40. Clinical manifestations of aortic dissection may include:
    A. pulsatile abdominal masses.
    B. a "tearing" chest pain.
    C. hypotension.
    D. pulse deficits in one upper extremity as compared to the other.
    E. B and D.

41. Which class of aortic dissection is unlikely to produce an upper extremity pulse deficit?
    A. DeBakey Class I
    B. DeBakey Class II
    C. DeBakey Class III
    D. Vaughn-Williams Class I
    E. Vaughn-Williams Class II

42. Approximately 10–20% of patients with aortic dissection present with ECG changes indicative of AMI. Of the following, which additional ECG changes may increase your suspicions of aortic dissection?
    A. reciprocal changes in inferior leads
    B. left axis deviation and voltage criteria indicating left ventricular hypertrophy
    C. extreme right axis deviation
    D. prolonged QT interval
    E. none of the above

43. Supportive therapy for aortic dissection is aimed at:
    A. keeping systolic blood pressure less than 100 mmHg.
    B. keeping diastolic blood pressure less than 100 mmHg.
    C. keeping systolic blood pressure between 100-120 mmHg.
    D. maintaining a heart rate of less than 60.
    E. none of the above.

44. The most common cause of cardiogenic shock is:
    A. myocardial contusion.
    B. cardiomyopathy.
    C. acute myocardial infarction.
    D. myocarditis.
    E. endocarditis.

45. The classic presentation of cardiogenic shock is of a patient with clinical manifestations of shock accompanied by:
    A. narrowed pulse pressure.
    B. signs of CHF, particularly pulmonary edema.
    C. muffled heart sounds.
    D. fever.
    E. none of the above.

46. Which of the following is NOT a potential cause of cardiogenic shock?
    A. deficits in myocardial contractility due to muscle damage from infarction
    B. deficits in ventricular filling, such as those seen with pericardial tamponade and tension pneumothorax
    C. deficits in ventricular emptying, such as valvular insufficiency
    D. arterial vasodilation, resulting in decreased afterload
    E. none of the above

47. Invasive monitoring of the cardiogenic shock patient includes:
    A. heart rate.
    B. blood pressure.
    C. pulse oximetry.
    D. pulmonary artery pressure.
    E. none of the above.

48. For the patient in cardiogenic shock due to right ventricular infarction, which of the following pharmacologic agents should be avoided?
    A. dopamine
    B. Inocor
    C. dobutamine
    D. furosemide
    E. A and D

49. Which of the following temporary pacing methods allows dual chamber pacing?
    A. transcutaneous pacing
    B. epicardial pacing
    C. transvenous pacing
    D. pulmonary artery catheter pacing
    E. none of the above

50. Balloon pump counterpulsation augments cardiac output in what way?
    A. Properly timed inflation of the balloon raises intra-aortic pressure during diastole and lowers intra-aortic pressure during systole, thus improving coronary artery perfusion pressure and lowering afterload and myocardial workload.
    B. Properly timed inflation of the balloon lowers intra-aortic pressure during diastole and raises intra-aortic pressure during systole, thus improving coronary artery perfusion pressure and lowering afterload and myocardial workload.
    C. Blood is diverted from the damaged ventricle to a mechanical pump, thus reducing myocardial workload and preserving adequate circulation.
    D. Inflation of the balloon during ventricular systole provides back pressure, which in turn increases preload.
    E. It physically grabs the blood and moves it forward–but only if you double clutch and shift to third.

51. Which of the following is NOT considered a potential complication of IABP therapy?
    A. limb ischemia
    B. ventricular rupture
    C. hemorrhage
    D. thrombus formation
    E. damage to the aorta

52. Management of the patient receiving IABP therapy during transport include:
    A. evaluation of the effectiveness of the device in improving hemodynamics.
    B. ensuring proper timing of the counterpulsation.
    C. monitoring for complications such as malpositioning of the balloon.
    D. choosing the appropriate triggering mode of the device.
    E. all of the above.

53. The technique by which a blood is diverted from damaged ventricles, allowing them to rest, is called:
    A. intra-aortic balloon pump (IABP).
    B. extracorporeal membrane oxygenation (ECMO).
    C. left ventricular assist device (LVAD).
    D. coronary artery bypass graft (CABG).
    E. none of the above.

54. Dilated cardiomyopathy usually:
    A. results from decrease in ejection fraction and increased end-systolic volume, resulting in enlargement of chambers.
    B. results from hypertrophic changes to the left ventricle and decreased compliance.

C. occurs in young, athletic males in their twenties or thirties.
D. involves dilation of all four chambers.
E. A and D.

55. Clinical signs of dilated cardiomyopathy include:
    A. signs of right heart failure such as JVD, hepatomegaly, ascites and peripheral edema.
    B. dyspnea on exertion, orthopnea and paroxysmal nocturnal dyspnea.
    C. summation gallop (S3 and S4 sounds) evident during cardiac auscultation.
    D. ECG voltage criteria for left ventricular hypertrophy.
    E. all but D are signs of dilated cardiomyopathy.

56. Management of the patient with dilated cardiomyopathy often includes:
    A. nitrates and other vasodilators.
    B. diuretics.
    C. all but D.
    D. dopamine.
    E. anticoagulants.

57. Diagnostic findings in CHF include:
    A. elevated pulmonary capillary wedge pressure.
    B. decreased systemic vascular resistance.
    C. cardiomegaly and pulmonary congestion evident on the chest radiograph.
    D. A and C.
    E. S4 heart sound.

58. Emerging therapies used in treatment of some CHF patients that may run counter to conventional wisdom regarding the management of CHF include:
    A. use of beta-blockers.
    B. long-term use of lisinopril.
    C. fluid therapy.
    D. A and C.
    E. continuous positive airway pressure (CPAP).

59. Which of the following pharmacologic agents is NOT commonly used in the management of CHF?
    A. dobutamine
    B. furosemide
    C. Neo-Synephrine
    D. nitroglycerin
    E. morphine sulfate

60. Clinical findings indicating a hypertensive emergency include all of the following but which?
    A. acute left ventricular failure
    B. systolic blood pressure greater than 110 mmHg
    C. acute renal failure
    D. papilledema
    E. hypertensive encephalopathy

61. Hypertensive crisis with a blood pressure of greater than 160/110 mmHg during pregnancy is most often a sign of:
    A. impending eclampsia.
    B. fetal/maternal Rh incompatibility.
    C. hypertension of pregnancy.
    D. diabetes insipidus.
    E. none of the above.

62. Malignant hypertension is best described as:
    A. consistently elevated blood pressure greater than 150 systolic or 90 diastolic.
    B. chronic hypertension resulting in end-organ damage.
    C. hypertension manifested in frequent transient ischemic attacks.
    D. hypertension unable to be controlled by diet alone.
    E. none of the above.

63. Early diagnostic aids in distinguishing between aortic dissection and myocardial infarction in the hypertensive patient with chest pain include:
    A. 12-Lead ECG.
    B. laboratory testing of cardiac enzymes.
    C. transesophageal ultrasound or CT.
    D. flat and erect abdominal radiographs.
    E. none of the above.

64. Clinical signs of pericarditis may include:
    A. ST-segment elevation in all leads but AVR and V1.
    B. substernal pleuritic chest pain that worsens when leaning forward.
    C. substernal pleuritic chest pain that eases when leaning forward.
    D. A and C.
    E. A and B.

65. Cardiac auscultation in the patient with pericarditis often reveals:
    A. summation gallop.
    B. diastolic murmur.
    C. friction rub.
    D. systolic ejection murmur.
    E. all of the above.

66. The typical clinical presentation of cardiac tamponade is known as:
    A. Beck's triad.
    B. Cushing's triad.
    C. Kussmaul's sign.
    D. DeBakey syndrome.
    E. none of the above.

67. Supportive care of the patient with symptomatic aortic stenosis may include:
    A. nitrates.
    B. inotropes.
    C. diuresis.
    D. digitalis.
    E. all of the above.

68. Clinical and diagnostic findings of aortic stenosis may include:
    A. exertional syncope.
    B. extreme right axis deviation.
    C. calcification of the aorta as evident on a chest radiograph.
    D. all answers but B.
    E. left ventricular hypertrophy.

69. Mitral stenosis in adult patients is most often caused by:
    A. cardiac tumors.
    B. rheumatic fever in childhood.
    C. congenital defects.
    D. calcification.
    E. systemic lupus.

70. Management of mitral stenosis is directed at:
    A. treatment of CHF if present.
    B. rate control of atrial fibrillation.
    C. anticoagulation.
    D. surgical replacement of severely stenosed valves.
    E. all of the above.

71. Cardiac auscultation of the patient with chronic mitral regurgitation often reveals:
    A. crescendo-decrescendo murmur.
    B. S3 and S4 sounds.
    C. holosystolic murmur and split S2.
    D. A and B.
    E. none of the above.

72. Before cannulation of the radial artery, the critical care paramedic should:
    A. immobilize the hand in the position of function.
    B. occlude the brachial artery.
    C. test for adequate collateral circulation in the hand.
    D. sing American Pie.
    E. none of the above.

73. Which of the following is NOT an indication for radial arterial line placement?
    A. frequent blood gas sampling
    B. profound hypotension
    C. arterial hypertension requiring vasodilator therapy
    D. acute myocardial infarction patients receiving fibrinolytics
    E. inotropic therapy

74. Which of the following is NOT necessary for arterial cannulation?
    A. Seldinger guide wire kit
    B. constant flush device
    C. 4–0 suture material
    D. transducer and waveform pressure monitor
    E. B and C

75. After cannulation of the radial artery, the critical care paramedic should:
    A. zero the transducer and observe the waveform.
    B. immobilize the hand in 45 degrees of dorsiflexion.
    C. remove the guide wire.
    D. infiltrate 0.5 mL lidocaine on either side of the insertion site using a 25-gauge needle.
    E. none of the above.

76. Which of the following is an indication for central IV cannulation of the subclavian vein?
    A. infusion of hypotonic solutions
    B. large volume requirement requiring high flow rates
    C. transvenous pacemaker insertion
    D. IV access in patients with collapsed peripheral veins
    E. C and D

77. Which of the following is a contraindication for cannulation of the subclavian vein?
    A. conscious patient
    B. hemodynamically stable patient
    C. deformity of the chest wall
    D. hypotensive patient
    E. patient with recent pneumothorax

78. When cannulating a central vein using the Seldinger technique, one must always:
    A. maintain control of the guide wire at all times.
    B. obtain a chest radiograph as soon as possible after cannulation.
    C. insert the needle at a 90-degree angle until blood can be aspirated, then advance the catheter at a 45-degree angle.
    D. administer a local anesthetic.
    E. none of the above.

79. When performing central venous cannulation, the technique of aligning the bevel of the needle with the markings on the syringe allows the critical care paramedic:
    A. a convenient outlet for obsessive-compulsive behavior.
    B. to constantly monitor the orientation of the bevel of the needle.
    C. a better means of securing the needle than a Luer Lock.
    D. all of the above.
    E. none of the above.

80. Which of the following best describes the need for chest radiography following central venous cannulation?
    A. It is only required when internal jugular or subclavian sites are used.
    B. It should only be performed when the patient suffers post-cannulation dyspnea.
    C. It should only be performed when a hematoma occurs.
    D. It should only be performed when the initial attempt is unsuccessful.
    E. It is only done to confirm proper placement of the catheter.

81. Before utilizing a patient's peripherally inserted central catheter (PICC) or other vascular access device, the critical care paramedic should:
    A. assess the patient to determine if peripheral vascular access can be easily obtained.
    B. obtain permission to use the device from the patient or family members.
    C. cleanse the injection port with an antiseptic wipe.
    D. identify the proper injection port.
    E. all of the above.

82. Timing of IABP counterpulsation should be checked:
    A. every fifteen minutes.
    B. with the pump set to 1:2 assist ratio, if the patient can tolerate the temporary reduction in counterpulsation.
    C. only with the pump set in whatever counterpulsation ratio will be used during transport.
    D. whenever triggering modes are changed.
    E. B and D.

83. Blood in the IABP connecting tubing almost always indicates:
    A. life-threatening hemorrhage.
    B. balloon rupture.
    C. blood in the tubing is a normal finding.
    D. aortic rupture.
    E. none of the above.

84. If the critical care paramedic should find blood in the IABP connecting tubing, he should:
    A. immediately remove the catheter and apply direct pressure to the insertion site to control bleeding.
    B. immediately suspend counterpulsation to prevent helium embolus.
    C. advance the IABP catheter until the balloon tamponades the hemorrhage site.
    D. contact the base physician for orders.
    E. none of the above.

85. Even when properly performed, complications of needle pericardiocentesis include all of the following but which?
    A. pneumothorax
    B. coronary artery laceration
    C. iatrogenic pericardial tamponade
    D. air embolus
    E. all of the above

CHAPTER 23
Neurologic Emergencies

DIRECTIONS: Each of the questions or incomplete statements below is followed by suggested answers or completions. Select the **one answer** that is best in each case.

1. The cerebrum has two types of tissues: the white matter, comprised of neuronal axons, and the cortex, which forms the epicenter of:
   A. vegetative function.
   B. consciousness.
   C. thought.
   D. all of the above.
   E. B and C.

2. The cerebrum is divided laterally into left and right hemispheres and its surface area is creased by deep valleys called _____ and ridges knows as _____.
   A. gyri, sulci
   B. lobes, gyri
   C. sulci, gyri
   D. lobes, sulci
   E. none of the above

3. The generally accepted terms for the functionally diverse areas of the brain are:
   1. frontal.
   2. parietal.
   3. ocular.
   4. temporal.
   5. occipital.
   6. maxillary.

   A. 1 and 3
   B. 2 and 4
   C. 1, 2, and 3
   D. 1, 2, 4, and 5
   E. 1, 2, 4, and 6

4. The area of the brain responsible for coordination and stabilization of fine motor skills and complex movement as well as ability to judge spatial relationships is called the:
   A. thalamus.
   B. cerebellum.
   C. diencephalon.
   D. hypothalamus.
   E. medulla.

5. The area of the brain that is composed of the thalamus, epithalamus, and hypothalamus is called the:
   A. midbrain.
   B. pons.
   C. diencephalon.
   D. medulla.
   E. oblongata.

6. The medulla is the most inferior structure in the brain and merges with the spinal cord at the:
   A. foramen magnum.
   B. pneumotaxic center.
   C. midbrain.
   D. pons.
   E. cerebellum.

7. An important structure within the brain, the choroid plexus, is responsible for:
   A. production of pineal hormones.
   B. production of cerebrospinal fluid.
   C. conduction of nerve signals between the pons and the medulla.
   D. all of the above.
   E. none of the above.

8. The part of the brain that is home to the majority of cranial nerve nuclei is the:
   A. cerebrum.
   B. cerebellum.
   C. brainstem.
   D. apneustic center.
   E. pneumotaxic center.

9. The midbrain houses the _____ that form(s) the pyramidal motor tracts as well as the third and fourth ventricles.
   A. choroid plexus
   B. cerebral peduncles
   C. X and VI cranial nerves
   D. pneumotaxic center
   E. none of the above

10. The two lateral ventricles are located deep in the cerebrum, and the _____ acts as a cerebrospinal fluid (CSF) drainage point into the third ventricle.
    A. foramen magnum
    B. intraventricular foramina
    C. aqueduct of Sylvius
    D. foramina of Luschka
    E. arachnoid villi

11. The openings that allow CSF to drain from the ventricular system into the subarachnoid space are the:
    1. foramina of Luschka.
    2. arachnoid villi.
    3. intraventricular foramina.
    4. foramen of Magendie.
    5. aqueduct of Sylvius.

    A. 1 and 4
    B. 1 and 5
    C. 1, 3, and 5
    D. 2, 3, and 4
    E. 3, 4, and 5

12. In order, from the brain tissue to the skull, the meninges are:
    A. pia mater, sub-arachnoid, dura mater.
    B. arachnoid, pia mater, dura mater.
    C. dura mater, arachnoid, pia mater.
    D. sub-arachnoid, pia mater, dura mater.
    E. none of the above.

13. The _____ is contiguous with the _____.
    A. pia mater, periosteum
    B. dura mater, arachnoid
    C. pia mater, arachnoid
    D. dura mater, periosteum
    E. arachnoid, periosteum

14. When looking at a cross section of the spinal cord, one would see the _____ matter in the center, surrounded by the _____ matter.
    A. white, gray
    B. gray, light
    C. light, white
    D. gray, white
    E. none of the above

15. The spinal cord is divided into the posterior and anterior median fissures, and each half of the white matter is divided into the _____, _____, and _____ funiculi.
    1. posterior
    2. inferior
    3. anterior
    4. superior
    5. lateral

    A. 1, 2, and 4
    B. 2, 3, and 5
    C. 1, 3, and 5
    D. 2, 3, and 4
    E. 2, 3, 4, and 5

16. The cell bodies of the gray matter are divided into three lobes, known as the posterior, anterior, and lateral _____, that are joined by the gray commissure.
    A. funiculi
    B. horns
    C. sulcus
    D. foramina
    E. none of the above

17. The spinal cord divides into three major nerve roots: the _____ root that projects laterally and merges with the _____ root, forming a third spinal nerve, eventually branching into the _____ nerves.
    A. ventral, dorsal, peripheral
    B. spinal, dorsal, peripheral
    C. dorsal, lateral, lateral
    D. peripheral, dorsal, ventral
    E. lateral, ventral, dorsal

18. Which of the following carries afferent (descending) sensory information?
    A. ventral root
    B. dorsal root
    C. spinal root
    D. peripheral root
    E. lateral root

19. Which of the following carries efferent (ascending) sensory information?
    A. spinal root
    B. dorsal root
    C. lateral root
    D. ventral root
    E. primary root

20. The maintenance of consistent perfusion to the brain is accomplished through autoregulation of a phenomenon that can best be characterized in the formula $X = Y - Z$. These values can best be described as:
    A. X=CPP, Y=MCP, Z=ICP
    B. X=MAP, Y=ICP, Z=ACP
    C. X=CPP, Y=MAP, Z=ICP
    D. X=ICP, Y=MRP, Z=CAP
    E. X=MCC, Y=ICP, Z=MAP

21. The series of constituent cerebral arteries that forms the foundation for the system that perfuses the brain and is located at the midline/anterior portion is called the:
    A. circle of Wilton.
    B. circle of Willis.
    C. circle of Wilson.
    D. circle of Wallace.
    E. none of the above.

22. The basilar arteries, posterior communicating arteries, middle cerebral arteries, and anterior cerebral arteries, along with the posterior and anterior communicating arteries, all combine to form the:
    A. circle of Wilton.
    B. circle of Wilson.
    C. circle of Willis.
    D. circle of Wallace.
    E. none of the above.

23. The function of the middle cerebral arteries (MCAs) is to perfuse the:
    A. midline cerebral hemispheres.
    B. inferior cerebral hemispheres.
    C. lateral cerebral hemispheres.
    D. anterior cerebral hemispheres.
    E. posterior cerebral hemispheres.

24. The cerebral veins eventually merge to form collecting veins known as the sinuses, which drain into the internal jugular vein. The exceptions to this are the occipital vein, which drains into the _____, and the vertebral vein, which drains into the _____.
    A. brachiocephalic, labyrinthine
    B. external jugular, brachiocephalic
    C. internal cephalic, external jugular
    D. vertebral jugular, basilar sinus
    E. none of the above

25. The _____, _____, and _____ are the major venous sinuses.
    A. sagittal, labyrinthine, cavernous
    B. transverse, sagittal, basilar

C. cavernous, labyrinthine, basilar
D. sagittal, transverse, cavernous
E. basilar, cavernous, transverse

26. In Figure 23–1, label the indicated circulatory landmarks of the brain, clockwise from the 6 o'clock position, using the following vocabulary list:

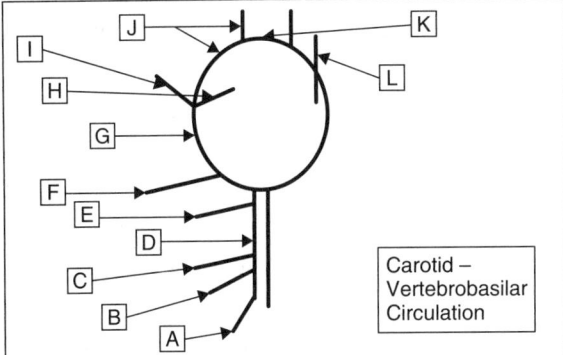

Figure 23–1

a. _____   A. anterior cerebral artery
b. _____   B. middle cerebral artery
c. _____   C. vertebral artery
d. _____   D. posterior inferior cerebellar artery
e. _____   E. internal carotid artery
f. _____   F. anterior communicating artery
g. _____   G. posterior cerebral artery
h. _____   H. superior cerebellar artery
i. _____   I. basilar artery
j. _____   J. labyrinthine artery
k. _____   K. posterior communicating artery
l. _____   L. ophthalmic artery

27. Voluntary motor control of the central nervous system resides in the:
    A. corticospinal motor system.
    B. extrapyramidal motor system.
    C. sympathetic nervous system.
    D. reptilian mid-brain.
    E. computer named HAL.

28. The corticospinal motor system, or the _____ motor system, is the primary motor control of the entire body.
    A. extrapyramidal
    B. sagittal
    C. pyramidal
    D. transverse
    E. central

29. Your 80-year-old patient is conscious, able to follow commands, and shows no obvious signs of peripheral motor function deficit during your assessment of the cranial nerves. However, it has been difficult to interview the patient because she is exhibiting symptoms of expressive aphasia and is having difficulty following your pen with her eyes. Based on these observations, you realize the patient may have damage to Broca's area, a part of the brain located in the:
    A. sulcus.
    B. frontal cortex.
    C. posterior cortex.
    D. corticobulbar tract.
    E. none of the above.

30. During clinical observation at the local stroke center, you are asked to spend some time in recreational rehabilitation working with a patient who has difficulty with voluntary movements and repetitive motor skills. Based on this reported history you know the patient has damage to the:
    A. internal capsule.
    B. extrapyramidal tract.
    C. premotor cortex.
    D. pons.
    E. cerebellum.

31. The crossing over, or _____ of most pyramidal neuron bundles, takes place at the pyramids of the medulla, contributing to contralateral motor control.
    A. decerebration
    B. decussation
    C. decclination
    D. deculcation
    E. none of the above

32. The extrapyramidal system provides involuntary control of musculature and is regulated indirectly by the:
    A. medulla.
    B. pons.
    C. cerebellum.
    D. cerebrum.
    E. all of the above.

33. Insults to the nuclei and/or axonal tracts of the extrapyramidal motor system can result in various neurologic deficits, such as:
    A. athetosis.
    B. tardive dyskinesia.
    C. tremors.
    D. ataxia.
    E. all of the above.

34. Of the six proprioceptive nerve tracts in the white matter of the spinal cord, only four are capable of delivering specific or generalized sensations. These nerve tracts terminate in the:
    A. parietal lobe.
    B. cerebellum.
    C. thalamus.
    D. all of the above.
    E. A and C.

35. The parietal lobe is the location of the _____ and is responsible for the analysis and extrapolation of information and data that helps to define sensation and the memory of those sensations.
    A. precentral gyrus
    B. postcentral gyrus
    C. subthalamic nucleus
    D. somatosensory association area
    E. lentiform nucleus

36. Place the following terms in order to trace the connection of the second cranial nerve to the occipital lobe.
    1. Thalamus relays information to the occipital lobe.
    2. Optic nerves travel to the optic chiasma.
    3. Second cranial nerve leaves retina.
    4. Partial decussation occurs prior to Circle of Willis.
    5. Visual cortex in the occipital lobe interprets images.
    6. Post decussation, optic nerve synapses in the thalamus.

    A. 5, 3, 4, 2, 6, 1
    B. 3, 2, 4, 6, 1, 5
    C. 1, 6, 2, 4, 5, 3
    D. 3, 4, 2, 6, 5, 1
    E. none of the above

37. The vestibulocochlear nerve, CN VIII, conducts auditory information to what area of the brain?
    A. parietal
    B. temporal
    C. occipital
    D. frontal
    E. medulla

38. The hypothalamus is the primary controller of the autonomic nervous system (ANS) and regulates body-core temperature, thirst, and sleep-wake cycles. It also regulates:
    1. certain emotions.
    2. heart and respiratory rate.
    3. endocrine activity.

4. reticular formation.
  5. vascular tone.
  6. end-organ response.

  A. 1, 2, and 3
  B. 4, 5, and 6
  C. 1, 3, 5, and 6
  D. 1, 2, 3, 4, and 6
  E. 1, 2, 3, 5, and 6

39. The cortical areas involved with the process of taste and smell are located in the _____ lobe.
  A. parietal
  B. occipital
  C. temporal
  D. medulla
  E. frontal

40. Preganglionic fibers are mediated by _____ and post-ganglionic fibers secrete _____.
  A. adrenaline, parathyroid hormone
  B. acetylcholine, adrenaline
  C. norepinephrine, adrenaline
  D. acetylcholine, norepinephrine
  E. none of the above

41. The sympathetic autonomic system's primary receptors are adrenergic and separated into two classes. They are:
  A. alpha.
  B. beta.
  C. theta.
  D. all of the above.
  E. A and B.

42. The nerve with the greatest overall parasympathetic control of the body is generally considered to be the _____th cranial nerve.
  A. VIII
  B. XI
  C. IX
  D. X
  E. IV

43. The prefrontal cortex is responsible for the majority of:
  A. autonomic muscle tone.
  B. repetitive memory.
  C. intellectual processes.
  D. organ response.
  E. none of the above.

44. Your 14-year-old patient is currently singing for you at the top of his lungs. You are there because he injured himself by jumping off the roof of the garage (about 8 feet from the ground) in an attempt to show off for his girlfriend. The patient's vital signs are stable, and the physical exam is unremarkable, except for the obvious fracture to his left wrist.

    As you package the patient for transport, the girlfriend tells you he is not usually so "silly and irresponsible" and was acting "kind of goofy" prior to the incident. His buddies tell you the patient has ingested approximately "two six-packs of beer" in the past hour. Based on this information, you know the patient's judgment has been impaired by the toxic assault on his _____.
  A. reticular activating system.
  B. limbic system.
  C. corticospinal system.
  D. all of the above.
  E. none of the above.

45. With any of the various stroke assessment tools, hand and arm drift are included as factors. When looking at this piece of the assessment, one is judging _____, and the status of the cerebellum.
  A. aphasia
  B. dysphasia
  C. pronator drift
  D. diplopia
  E. nystagmus

46. You are transporting a 54-year-old female stroke patient who appears to understand your directions and is able to follow motor commands without difficulty. However, when asked her name she answers "Green," and when asked how old she is she answers "Dog." During the interview all her other verbal responses display a similar lack of appropriate content. Based on this finding, you believe the patient is suffering from _____.

    A. reactive aphasia
    B. expressive aphasia
    C. global aphasia
    D. receptive aphasia
    E. conductive aphasia

47. You are asking your nonambulatory patient to alternate touching his finger to his nose and touching it to the index finger on your hand. Additionally, you move your hand to various locations in front of the patient as he attempts to follow your finger and touch it. This process is intended to assess:

    A. medullary dysphagia.
    B. cognitive response.
    C. cerebellar ataxia.
    D. occipital reflexia.
    E. none of the above

48. In the absence of contraindicating injuries, you are holding your unconscious patient's plantar foot surface and rapidly dorsiflexing the ankle. You are testing for _____ and know that the involuntary rhythmic jerking you observe is a(n) _____ response.

    A. cronis, normal
    B. clonus, abnormal
    C. cronus, normal
    D. clonius, abnormal
    E. none of the above

49. In the unconscious patient, repetitive eye movement, or "roving" eye, may be an indication of seizures. Other occulomotor functions you can assess in this patient might include:

    A. "doll's eyes."
    B. disconjugate gaze.
    C. unequal pupils.
    D. all of the above.
    E. A and B.

50. The most common types of diagnostic imaging you may encounter as a critical care paramedic are:

    1. magnetic resonance imaging (MRI).
    2. myelography.
    3. cerebral angiography.
    4. evoked electrical potential.
    5. transcranial Doppler ultrasound.
    6. electroencephalogram (EEG).
    7. lumbar puncture.
    8. PET scan.
    9. computed tomography scan (CT scan).

    A. 1, 3, 5, 7, and 9
    B. 1, 2, 3, 5, 7, and 9
    C. 1, 3, 5, 6, and 9
    D. 1, 2, 3, 4, 5, and 6
    E. 4, 5, 6, and 8

51. With regard to ischemic stroke, the _____ describes an area of brain tissue distal to an occluded vessel and without collateral circulation.

    A. penumbra
    B. hypercoagulated zone
    C. zone of infarction
    D. thromboembolic zone
    E. polycythemic zone

52. Cellular ischemia causes a transition to anaerobic metabolism, producing damaging byproducts, such as:

    A. lactate.
    B. myohemoglobenemia.
    C. glycol.

D. adenosine triphosphate.
E. all of the above.

53. With regard to ischemia, an area of tissue that becomes necrotic after an infarct occurs and perfusion is not restored is called the:
   A. penumbra.
   B. hypercoagulated zone.
   C. zone of infarction.
   D. thromboembolic zone.
   E. polycythemic zone.

54. Match the terms listed at left with the sequence of steps in the pathogenesis of stroke.

   A. acidosis   1. _____
   B. depolarization   2. _____
   C. imbalance of ions 3. _____
   D. ischemia   4. _____
   E. cell injury/death 5. _____
   F. energy failure   6. _____
   G. intracellular   7. _____
      calcium
   H. cell membrane/   8. _____
      protein
      degradation
   I. glutamate   9. _____

55. An infarct of the middle cerebral artery (MCA) can result in significant disabilities that may present as:
   1. dysphasia.
   2. aphagia.
   3. ipsilateral gaze.
   4. contralateral hemiplegia.
   5. contralateral hemisensory loss.
   6. homonymous hemianopsia.

   A. 1, 3, and 5
   B. 1, 2, 3, and 4
   C. 1, 2, 3, 4, 5, and 6
   D. 1, 3, 4, 5, and 6
   E. 2, 3, 4, and 5

56. Contralateral lower extremity weakness and intellectual or behavioral changes may be indicative of ischemic damage secondary to aneurysm or thrombus in the:
   A. vertebral artery.
   B. basilar artery.
   C. middle cerebral artery.
   D. posterior cerebral artery.
   E. anterior cerebral artery.

57. You are reading the history of a patient who has been diagnosed with cortical blindness and is in denial of the fact that she has lost all ability to see. You know this syndrome is a result of:
   A. hemorrhage of the MCA.
   B. bilateral occlusion of the PCA.
   C. basilar occlusion of the PCA.
   D. A and C.
   E. B and C.

58. Your patient is experiencing an inability to move his extremities as well as an inability to speak. He has no sensory loss and appears oriented in all other aspects, but he is only able to move or blink his eyes at your request. There is a concern that an apparent stroke has resulted in a rare phenomenon known as "locked-in syndrome," a condition resulting from:
   A. damage to the medulla.
   B. complete infarct of the pons.
   C. hemorrhage of the cerebellum.
   D. occlusion of the ACA.
   E. hemorrhage of the MCA.

59. Transient ischemic attacks (TIAs) are sometimes associated with unilateral ataxia, facial paresis, and dysarthria ("clumsy hand") syndrome. When a TIA is suspected in conjunction with these signs and symptoms, there is concern for which neurologic syndrome?
   A. watershed infarction
   B. contralateral hemiplegia
   C. homonymous hemianopsia
   D. lacunar infarction
   E. none of the above

60. Of the generally accepted stroke deficit assessments, the two most common are the _____, which evaluates level of consciousness, cognition, and motor/sensory function, as well as the _____, which specifically evaluates facial droop, arm drift, and clarity of speech.
    A. Cincinnati Stroke Scale (CSS), National Institute of Health Stroke Scale (NIHSS)
    B. NIHSS, CSS
    C. Both assessment tools evaluate the same things.
    D. Only NIHSS evaluates for all the indicated factors.
    E. Only CSS evaluates for all the indicated factors.

61. In order to qualify for fibrinolytic therapy the patient must have a clinical diagnosis of stroke within three hours of symptoms and:
    A. be between 18 and 75 years of age.
    B. have significant neurologic compromise to warrant therapy.
    C. have had a CT scan that ruled out intracranial hemorrhage.
    D. all of the above.
    E. both B and C.

62. Additional exclusion criteria for fibrinolytic therapy are extensive and include many items that deal specifically with history of recent:
    A. pregnancy, drug abuse, metabolic disorder.
    B. bleeding disorders, surgery, and/or major trauma.
    C. illnesses affecting the blood, brain, heart, or MAP.
    D. B and C.
    E. A, B and C.

63. Patients excluded from fibrinolytic therapy are normally treated with:
    A. antibiotic therapy.
    B. antiplatelet therapy.
    C. tincture of time.
    D. intra-arterial tPA.
    E. B and D.

64. Cerebral aneurysms and arteriovenous malformations that rupture are hallmarked by subarachnoid hemorrhage and three specific injury cascades. These are:
    1. mass effect of the blood, itself.
    2. cerebral vasospasm.
    3. cerebral vasodilation.
    4. intraventricular hemorrhage.
    5. extraventricular hemorrhage.

    A. 1, 2, and 3
    B. 2, 3, and 4
    C. 3, 4, and 5
    D. 1, 2, and 4
    E. 2, 3, and 5

65. The Fisher scale and the Hunt and Hess scale are indicators of blood pattern distribution and prognosis involving what type of event?
    A. subarachnoid hemorrhage
    B. level VI hemorrhage
    C. epidural hemorrhage
    D. subdural hemorrhage
    E. level X hemorrhage

66. You are triaging a 50-year-old female at the Walk-In Clinic who is complaining of a sudden, severe headache and photophobia. As you interview the patient, she tells you that this is the "worst headache of my life" and it felt like a "thunderclap" in her head. She denies a history of migraines or other headache syndromes as well as recent illness. As you speak with her, she begins to complain of nausea and asks to lie down. You also note the patient's mentation is deteriorating during the interview and she is becoming quiet and lethargic. As you begin checking vital signs, you contact the physician on duty. Based on the patient's chief complaints and declining mentation, you

tell her you suspect the patient may be suffering from:
A. level VI hemorrhage.
B. subarachnoid hemorrhage.
C. subdural hemorrhage.
D. level X hemorrhage.
E. epidural hemorrhage.

67. Transcranial Doppler studies or the Lindegaard ratio can help gauge the severity of vasospasm in a suspected arterial cranial hemorrhage by extrapolating the ratio of the velocity of blood traveling through the _____ to that traveling through the _____ artery.
A. PCA, spinal
B. MCA, vertebral
C. ACA, vertebral
D. PCA, vertebral
E. MCA, spinal

68. Patients suffering vasospasms secondary to a subarachnoid hemorrhage may be treated with a type of therapy known as "Triple-H." The point of this therapy is to:
1. hypotense.
2. hypervolumize.
3. hemodilute.
4. hypertense.
5. hypovolumize.
6. hemoperfuse.

A. 1, 2, and 3
B. 2, 3, and 4
C. 3, 4, and 5
D. 4, 5, and 6
E. none of the above

69. One of the possible reasons for a patient to develop an intracranial hemorrhage is a vascular disorder caused by deposits of _____ that can weaken the walls of the cerebral vasculature.
A. calcium
B. potassium
C. amyloid
D. cortisol
E. none of the above

70. Patients who are unable to maintain the integrity of the protection offered by the bone and meninges around their brain are at risk for developing:
A. meningitis.
B. subarachnoid hemorrhage.
C. ventriculitis.
D. all of the above.
E. A and C.

71. The bacteria associated with meningococcal meningitis are:
A. *Neisseria meningitides*.
B. *Streptococcus pneumonia*.
C. *Haemophilius influenza*.
D. *Klebsiella pneumonia*.
E. all of the above.

72. Syphilis, Lyme disease and *Leptospira interrogans,* as well as _____ and _____, may cause meningitis.
A. malaria, encephalitis
B. hemophilia, toxoplasmosis
C. toxoplasmosis, malaria
D. all of the above
E. none of the above

73. Viral infections and syndromes associated with meningitis can include:
1. West Nile.
2. measles.
3. herpes.
4. Guillian-Barré.
5. Epstein-Barr.
6. eastern equine encephalitis.

A. 1, 3, and 5
B. 2, 3, and 4
C. 1, 3, and 5
D. 2, 3, and 6
E. 1, 2, 3, 5, and 6

74. Several diagnostic tests can be used to rule out other differentials from meningitis. Among them might be:
    1. CT scan.
    2. MRI.
    3. Lumbar puncture.
    4. Blood cultures.
    5. X-ray.

    A. 1, 3, and 4
    B. 2, 3, and 4
    C. 1, 3, and 5
    D. 2, 3, and 5
    E. 1, 2, 3, and 4

75. Your 32-year-old male AIDS patient presents with an altered mental status and has developed a high fever. Lab tests show the patient is suffering from an infection in the brain. The most likely suspects are:
    A. toxoplasmosis.
    B. cytomegalovirus.
    C. crytococcal encephalitis.
    D. all of the above.
    E. A and B.

76. The term "encephalitis" describes inflammation of the brain _____ as the result of viral exposure to an agent contributing to this etiology.
    A. vasculature
    B. parenchyma
    C. sulcus
    D. ventricles
    E. meninges

77. You are transporting a 24-year-old male from a small rural hospital to a specialized facility for a neurologic consult and CT scan. The patient presented earlier today with a severe headache, nausea, visual deficits, and ataxia. The written history accompanying the patient state these signs and symptoms have been increasing in frequency and severity over several months. The patient came to the ED today because he had lost his peripheral vision and was having difficulty walking. Based on this information you know that the patient may have a brain lesion that is most likely in or near the:
    A. occipital lobe.
    B. medulla.
    C. pons.
    D. frontal lobe.
    E. temporal lobe.

78. Cells within the brain that comprise the supportive structure around neurons are called:
    A. gillial cells.
    B. neuroglia cells.
    C. neuralgia cells.
    D. neurologic cells.
    E. none of the above.

79. Gliomas of the brain can include:
    1. astrocytomas.
    2. oligodendrogliomas.
    3. blastomas.
    4. ependymomas.
    5. schwannomas.

    A. 1, 3, and 5
    B. 2, 4, and 5
    C. 1, 2, and 4
    D. 2, 3, and 5
    E. 1, 2, 3, 4, and 5

80. Types of brain tumors that have been identified can include:
    A. neuroblastomas.
    B. schwannomas.
    C. meningiomas.
    D. astrocytomas.
    E. all of the above.

81. Recurring localized back pain, intermittent parasthesias, and unexplained incontinence, along with autonomic system dysfunction may be signs of:
    A. meningitis.
    B. dyskinesia.
    C. chordoma.

D. dementia.
E. all of the above.

82. The major known causes of encephalopathy include:
    1. hypoxia.
    2. hypoperfusion.
    3. hyperperfusion.
    4. metabolic disorders.
    5. viral infection.
    6. toxoplasmosis.

    A. 1, 3, and 5
    B. 2, 4, and 6
    C. 1, 2, 3, and 4
    D. 3, 4, 5, and 6
    E. 1, 2, 3, 4, 5, and 6

83. An encephalopathy associated with Vitamin B1 deficiency, alcoholism, and Korsakoff's syndrome is:
    A. hepatic.
    B. AIDS.
    C. Wernicke's.
    D. chronic.
    E. none of the above.

84. Local EMS has delivered a patient to your ED who appears to be intoxicated and has a diminished sense of self. Vital signs are within acceptable limits for his age and emaciated condition and you decide to let him sleep it off. When the previously ordered tests are completed, they are negative for blood alcohol, narcotics, and other toxins. Additionally, the blood glucose level is 72, not nearly low enough to account for the symptoms. You wake the patient up and, while attempting to elicit a more detailed history, you notice the patient has mild jaundice and exhibits a flapping motion of his hands when they are raised in front of him. Based on these signs and symptoms, you suspect the patient may suffer from:
    A. hepatic encephalopathy.
    B. Wernicke's encephalopathy.
    C. Korsakoff's syndrome.
    D. diabetes mellitus.
    E. agranulocytosis.

85. Acute and chronic encephalopathic syndromes may be caused by exposure to various drugs and chemicals. Examples of such exposures might include:
    1. huffing.
    2. smoking.
    3. IV drug abuse.
    4. glue sniffing.
    5. ink making.
    6. organophosphate production.

    A. 1, 2, and 3
    B. 2, 3, and 4
    C. 1, 3, 4, and 5
    D. 1, 3, 4, and 6
    E. 1, 2, 3, 4, 5, and 6

86. Your patient is experiencing what appear to be tonic-clonic seizures, reported to have been ongoing for over 15 minutes. You begin ventilations via bag-valve mask with 100% O_2, gain IV access, and administer a benzodiazepine that appears to have no effect 2 minutes later. En route to the hospital you realize the patient is at risk for multiple sequelae that minimally include:
    1. hypoxia.
    2. hypothermia.
    3. rhabdomyolosis.
    4. cardiac dysrhythmias.
    5. intracranial hypotension.
    6. electrolyte imbalance.

    A. 1, 2, and 3
    B. 2, 3, and 4
    C. 1, 3, 4, 5, and 6
    D. 2, 3, 4, 5, and 6
    E. none of the above

87. For the patient in question 86, further drug treatment modalities are available to you. Among them are:
    A. narcotics.
    B. barbiturates.
    C. antibiotics.
    D. vitamins.
    E. none of the above.

88. Many acute and chronic neurologic disorders have systemic signs and symptoms. Regardless of the etiology, the critical care paramedic should be prepared to deal with concomitant compromise of the _____ system, as well as _____ care.
    A. cardiorespiratory, end-of-life
    B. cardiovascular, end-of-shift
    C. endocrine, end-of-breathing
    D. limbic, end-of-disease
    E. cardiorespiratory, end-of-shift

89. _____ is described as a primary dementia caused by hippocampal degeneration, neurofibrillary tangles, and senile plaques.
    A. Multiple sclerosis
    B. Alzheimer's disease
    C. Muscular dystrophy
    D. Poliomyelitis
    E. Parkinson's disease

90. Aside from the known memory and informational deficits, it is important for the critical care paramedic to recognize that Alzheimer's patients are vulnerable to and at high risk for:
    1. physical debilitation.
    2. infection.
    3. accidental Injury.
    4. exposure.
    5. violent behavior.
    A. 1, 3, and 5
    B. 1, 2, and 4
    C. 1, 2, 3, and 4
    D. 2, 3, 4, and 5
    E. 1, 2, 3, 4, and 5

91. You have been called to transport a recovering motor vehicle trauma victim, who has been hospitalized in your locale while on vacation, back home to Florida by fixed-wing transport. The patient also suffers from an apparent dementia diagnosed as end-stage Alzheimer's. During the flight your patient begins to have short runs of bradycardia as well as hypotension. Post assessment, you are convinced this is normal for the patient and not a result of the trauma. You decide to monitor him awhile longer before making any adjustments to the ordered in-flight treatment. Why?
    A. You know the patient is OK because you are taking him home.
    B. You know the signs are normal for a person in anxiety.
    C. You know the signs are likely caused by his Alzheimer's medications.
    D. You know that the altitude is affecting your equipment and the patient is fine
    E. You are only 2 minutes from touchdown and will deal with it in then.

92. Match the following common, or primary, signs and symptoms with the disease processes listed below:
    1. _____ Parkinson's disease
    2. _____ Alzheimer's disease
    3. _____ multiple sclerosis
    4. _____ amyotrophic lateral sclerosis
    5. _____ Guillain-Barré syndrome
    6. _____ myasthenia gravis
    7. _____ neuroleptic malignant syndrome
    8. _____ malignant hypertension syndrome
    9. _____ Creutzfeldt-Jakob disease
    10. _____ bovine spongiform encephalopathy

A. familial encephalopathy
B. severe hyperthermia/muscle rigidity
C. zoonose encephalopathy
D. muscle weakness with re-stimulation
E. distal, ascending motor weakness
F. atrophy of innervated muscle
G. short-term/progressive memory loss
H. sustained muscular contractions
I. persistent tremor at 3 to 5 Hertz
J. sensory/visual alterations, fatigue

93. The patient is presenting to you with a chronic history of increased fatigue, visual disturbances, loss of sphincter control, spasticity, and cognitive dysfunction. You know this combination of factors is consistent with neurologic dysfunction. Your differential rule-outs should include organic brain syndrome (OBS), trauma, stroke, and:
    A. Parkinson's disease.
    B. amyotrophic lateral sclerosis.
    C. multiple sclerosis.
    D. muscular dystrophy.
    E. bovine spongiform encephalopathy.

94. Your 44-year-old male patient presents with increasing loss of muscle control, tone, and coordination, in spite of his active sports life. He also complains of increased respiratory difficulty and problems with swallowing that involve episodes of choking and near aspiration. Among your lab tests and other examinations, the critical care paramedic should consider the possibility that the patient is in the beginning stages of:
    A. Parkinson's disease.
    B. amyotrophic lateral sclerosis.
    C. multiple sclerosis.
    D. muscular dystrophy.
    E. bovine spongiform encephalopathy.

95. You are called to the home of a 35-year-old female complaining of severe headache and increasing lethargy accompanied by visual "blurriness." The patient's husband tells you she seemed "not herself" when she arrived home after an extended business trip in the British Isles and has gotten worse in the past two days. She denies chest pain, discomfort, and/or palpitations as well any notable respiratory difficulty. She is slightly hypertensive and bradycardic as well as nauseous "from the headache." Among your differentials, you might wish to include testing for:
    A. Parkinson's disease.
    B. amyotrophic lateral sclerosis.
    C. multiple sclerosis.
    D. muscular dystrophy.
    E. bovine spongiform encephalopathy.

96. Organophosphates, spider and snake venom, plants, and heavy metals are among items believed to contribute to symptoms and syndromes of:
    A. malignant hypertensive syndrome.
    B. Creutzfeldt-Jakob disease.
    C. Alzheimer's disease.
    D. neurotoxic disorders.
    E. none of the above.

97. The spinal cord is subject to many of the same pathophysiological insults that may occur in the brain. Among these are infarction, inflammation, and neoplastic growth. Deficits caused by any insult will depend on:
    A. the size of the lesion.
    B. the location of the injury.
    C. the malformation caused.
    D. the loss of structural integrity.
    E. all of the above.

98. Another name for "spina bifida" is:
    A. myelomeningicoccus.
    B. myelomeningocele.
    C. myelohyperplasia.
    D. all of the above.
    E. none of the above.

99. Match the following terms with their presenting malformation:
    a. _____ spina bifida occulta
    b. _____ meningomyelocele
    c. _____ memingocele
    d. _____ myelocele

    A. disorganized, open-nerve spinal tissue
    B. CSF filled cord extrusion
    C. CSF/nerve bundle filled cord extrusion
    D. vertebral cleft, dimpling, hairy indent

100. Of concern to the critical care paramedic is the likelihood that a spina bifida patient:
    A. is normally blind.
    B. may be too ill to live.
    C. is likely to have developed allergies, including to latex.
    D. is more susceptible to sunlight than other children.
    E. none of the above.

CHAPTER 24
Gastrointestinal Emergencies

DIRECTIONS
Each of the questions or incomplete statements below is followed by suggested answers or completions. Select the **one answer** that is best in each case.

1. Approximately 80% of peptic ulcers are caused by:
   A. stress.
   B. spicy foods.
   C. bacterial infection with *Helicobacter pylori*.
   D. chronic use of nonsteroidal anti-inflammatory drugs (NSAIDs).
   E. none of the above.

2. Most antiemetic medications work by blocking _____ receptors in the _____ within the brain.
   A. dopaminergic, substantia nigra
   B. serotonin, chemoreceptor trigger zone
   C. acetylcholine, cholinergic synapses
   D. gastric inhibitory peptide, posterior pituitary
   E. none of the above

3. Acute pancreatitis is caused by damage to the _____, resulting in leakage of enzymes into the surrounding tissues, subsequent activation of those enzymes, and autodigestion of pancreatic tissue.
   A. pancreatic acini
   B. islets of Langerhans
   C. common bile duct
   D. cystic duct
   E. none of the above

4. The pain associated with diverticulitis most often presents in the:
   A. transverse colon in the epigastrium.
   B. ascending colon on the right side of the abdomen.
   C. sigmoid colon, below the umbilicus.
   D. descending colon, on the left side of the abdomen.
   E. none of the above.

5. Acute cholecystitis often presents with tenderness under the right costal margin, a condition known as:
   A. referred pain.
   B. costochondritis.
   C. Murphy's sign.
   D. McBurney's point.
   E. Cullen's sign.

6. The intestinal submucosa contains sensory nerves, sympathetic postganglionic fibers and parasympathetic ganglionic neurons collectively known as:
   A. gastric nerves.
   B. mesenteric innervations.
   C. Meissner's plexus.
   D. pyloric plexus.
   E. none of the above.

7. The intestinal mucosa is a layer of epithelium organized in longitudinal and horizontal folds called:
   A. plicae.
   B. rugae.
   C. strata.
   D. columns.
   E. none of the above.

8. The veins that drain the inferior esophagus empty into the:
   A. inferior vena cava.
   B. superior vena cava.
   C. internal jugular veins.
   D. hepatic portal vein.
   E. none of the above.

9. The vermiform appendix is attached to what structure?
   A. ileum of the small intestine
   B. cecum of the large intestine

C. sigmoid colon
D. ascending colon
E. none of the above

10. Upper GI bleeds are defined as those that occur:
    A. proximal to the ligament of Trietz.
    B. proximal to the pyloric sphincter.
    C. proximal to the cardiac sphincter.
    D. between the cardiac sphincter and pylorus.
    E. none of the above.

11. Peptic ulcer disease accounts for approximately _____ of upper GI bleeds.
    A. 25%
    B. 75%
    C. 10%
    D. 50%
    E. 0.25%

12. Stress-related erosive syndrome (SRES), a phenomenon in which ulcers appear in the stomach and duodenum of some critically ill patients, is usually linked to what risk factors?
    A. use of nonsteroidal anti-inflammatory drugs (NSAIDs)
    B. long-term ventilatory support
    C. renal failure
    D. coagulopathy
    E. B and D

13. The precursor to peptic ulcer disease is often:
    A. gastritis.
    B. esophagitis.
    C. duodenitis.
    D. salmonella poisoning.
    E. none of the above.

14. Causes of gastritis include all of the following EXCEPT:
    A. radiation.
    B. chemical gastritis from NSAID or salicylate use.
    C. autoimmune disorder.
    D. *Escherichia coli.*
    E. *H. pylori* infection.

15. Liver cirrhosis often results in fibrosis and increased resistance to blood flow in the liver, which in turn leads to:
    A. congestive heart failure.
    B. hepatic portal hypertension.
    C. hepatitis.
    D. hematemesis.
    E. all of the above.

16. A venous pressure of greater than 10 mmHg will result in the formation of:
    A. ascites.
    B. varices.
    C. hepatomegaly.
    D. liver failure.
    E. splenomegaly.

17. The engorgement of esophageal and gastric veins as a result of hepatic portal hypertension is known as:
    A. upper gastrointestinal (GI) bleeding.
    B. melena.
    C. varices.
    D. ascites.
    E. hepatic hypertensive syndrome.

18. Approximately _____ of all patients with chronic liver disease will develop varices.
    A. One half
    B. 75%
    C. 90%
    D. 60%
    E. 25%

19. Although esophageal varices account for only 10% of all upper GI bleeds, approximately _____ of those cases where patients experience rebleeding will prove fatal.
    A. 10%
    B. 50%
    C. 33%
    D. 90%
    E. 20%

20. Upper GI bleeding resulting from retching, vomiting, or forceful coughing, and often associated with long-term NSAID or salicylate use, is known as:
    A. perforated peptic ulcer.
    B. bleeding esophageal varices.
    C. Mallory-Weiss syndrome.
    D. gastroesophageal reflux disease (GERD).
    E. none of the above.

21. Approximately _____ of patients with a Mallory-Weiss tear will experience hemodynamic instability and shock.
    A. 10%
    B. 25%
    C. 90%
    D. 50%
    E. 100%

22. The most common cause of lower GI bleeding is:
    A. peptic ulcers.
    B. diverticular disease.
    C. colon cancer.
    D. hemorrhoids.
    E. irritable bowel syndrome.

23. Outpouchings of the colonic mucosa, thought to be a result of increased intraluminal pressure within the colon, are known as:
    A. hemorrhoids.
    B. perforated ulcers.
    C. polyps.
    D. diverticula.
    E. none of the above.

24. The pain of diverticular disease is sometimes referred to as:
    A. indigestion.
    B. referred pain.
    C. left-sided appendicitis.
    D. heartburn.
    E. none of the above.

25. Patients with gastrointestinal hemorrhage will often present with all of the following but which?
    A. weakness and dizziness
    B. orthostatic or exertional syncope
    C. hypotension
    D. tachycardia
    E. Grey Turner's sign

26. Black, tarry stools formed by bleeding in the GI tract are known as:
    A. coffee ground stools.
    B. hematochezia.
    C. melena.
    D. tarry stool syndrome.
    E. none of the above.

27. Red or maroon stools formed by bleeding in the GI tract are known as:
    A. coffee ground stools.
    B. hematochezia.
    C. melena.
    D. bloody stool syndrome.
    E. none of the above.

28. In most cases, a lower GI bleed must produce at least _____ of blood to produce melena.
    A. 500 mL
    B. 60 mL
    C. 200 mL
    D. 100 mL
    E. 1000 mL

29. Hematocrit and hemoglobin levels in the patient with a gastrointestinal bleed:
    A. should be lowered in any significant acute hemorrhage.
    B. may not drop until 3–4 hours after bleeding starts.
    C. are unaltered by volume resuscitation using crystalloid solutions.
    D. are among the most useful lab values in the patient with gastrointestinal bleeding.
    E. B and D.

30. Blood urea nitrogen (BUN) can increase due to decreased hepatic perfusion with digestion of and subsequent absorption of hemoglobin. In patients with a suspected GI bleed, a BUN level of greater than _____ is suggestive of substantial hemorrhage.
    A. 7–20 mg/dL
    B. greater than 20 mg/dL
    C. greater than 30 mg/dL
    D. greater than 40 mg/dL
    E. greater than 80 mg/dL

31. For the patient with cirrhotic liver disease and bleeding esophageal varices, which of the following laboratory studies may be particularly useful in evaluating liver function?
    A. CBC, particularly hematocrit and hemoglobin levels
    B. BUN level
    C. coagulation studies
    D. B and C
    E. electrolyte panel

32. The process in which the patient is injected with radiolabeled potassium and then X-rayed to identify the source of extravasation of blood in the GI tract is called:
    A. intravenous pyelogram.
    B. scintigraphy.
    C. angiography.
    D. endoscopy.
    E. colonoscopy.

33. A diagnostic imaging study of particular usefulness in identifying the source of a brisk (0.5–2.0 mL/min) lower GI bleed is:
    A. scintigraphy.
    B. angiography.
    C. colonoscopy.
    D. endoscopy.
    E. barium swallow X-ray.

34. Which of the following is NOT a reliable clinical indicator of the need for a blood transfusion?
    A. low hemoglobin levels
    B. BUN greater than 40 mg/dL
    C. persistent clinical signs of shock despite administration of two liters or greater of isotonic crystalloids
    D. altered hematocrit level
    E. All are reliable indicators for the need for blood transfusion.

35. In treating the patient with bleeding esophageal varices, the critical care paramedic may consider administration of _____ to produce splanchnic vasoconstriction, thereby reducing hepatic portal hypertension.
    A. Protonix
    B. vasopressin
    C. famotidine
    D. promethazine
    E. none of the above

36. The critical care paramedic may use a _____ inserted through the nare into the stomach to tamponade bleeding varices.
    A. nasogastric tube
    B. endoscope
    C. Sengstaken-Blakemore tube
    D. Ewald tube
    E. endotracheal tube

37. Treatment of peptic ulcers includes all of the following EXCEPT:
    A. sorbitol.
    B. H₂ receptor antagonists such as famotidine.
    C. proton pump inhibitors.
    D. antacids.
    E. sucralfate.

38. Causes of obstructive pancreatitis include:
    A. *Mycoplasma* infection.
    B. organophosphate poisoning.
    C. gallstones.
    D. hepatitis.
    E. trauma.

39. The most common presenting complaint with acute pancreatitis is:
    A. nausea and vomiting.
    B. midepigastric or upper left quadrant pain.
    C. periumbilical pain.
    D. hyperglycemia.
    E. hypoglycemia.

40. The presence of Grey Turner's sign in the patient with acute pancreatitis indicates:
    A. significant hemorrhage.
    B. gallstones as the cause of the pancreatitis.
    C. associated renal failure.
    D. associated sepsis.
    E. none of the above.

41. The most specific serum marker for acute pancreatitis is:
    A. amylase.
    B. lipase.
    C. calcium.
    D. lactate dehydrogenase.
    E. none of the above.

42. When evaluating laboratory results while making a diagnosis of acute pancreatitis, it is important to remember that:
    A. elevated serum amylase always indicates pancreatitis.
    B. elevated serum lipase always indicates pancreatitis.
    C. laboratory data lacks the sensitivity and specificity to be the sole indicator for pancreatitis, and thus should be used in the context of other clinical symptoms.
    D. decreased serum amylase always indicates pancreatitis.
    E. decreased serum lipase always indicates pancreatitis.

43. The diagnostic imaging study most useful in the identification of obstructive pancreatitis secondary to biliary obstruction is:
    A. positron emission tomography (PET) scan.
    B. computed tomography (CT) scan.
    C. abdominal radiographs.
    D. ultrasound.
    E. fluoroscopy.

44. The most specific diagnostic imaging study for the identification of obstructive pancreatitis from biliary obstruction is:
    A. positron emission tomography (PET) scan.
    B. computed tomography (CT) scan.
    C. abdominal radiographs.
    D. ultrasound.
    E. fluoroscopy.

45. Treatment for severe pancreatitis includes all of the following EXCEPT:
    A. strict NPO precautions.
    B. proton pump inhibitors.
    C. IV antibiotics such as quinolone and metronidazole.
    D. hydration with IV fluids.
    E. Foley catheter to monitor urine output.

46. Inflammation of the Kupffer's cells, bile ducts, and blood vessels is called:
    A. hepatitis.
    B. hepatomegaly.
    C. portal hypertension.
    D. cirrhosis.
    E. none of the above.

47. Fibrosis of liver tissue from chronic damage that results in disruption of liver function is described as:
    A. hepatitis.
    B. cirrhosis.
    C. hepatic fibrosis syndrome.
    D. hepatomegaly.
    E. none of the above.

48. Acute liver failure associated with hepatic encephalopathy is known as:
    A. hepatitis.
    B. cirrhosis.
    C. fulminant hepatic failure.
    D. hepatomegaly.
    E. none of the above.

49. Which of the following is a sign NOT typically seen with of liver disease?
    A. dark urine and clay colored stools
    B. jaundice
    C. ascites
    D. lower GI bleeding
    E. nausea and vomiting

50. Laboratory data strongly suggestive of significant liver failure include:
    A. elevated liver enzymes (ALT and AST).
    B. prolonged prothrombin (PT) time.
    C. decreased serum albumin.
    D. elevated serum ammonia.
    E. all answers but A.

51. Hypoalbuminemia secondary to liver failure may result in:
    A. fluid shift out of the vascular spaces, requiring volume support.
    B. increased serum osmolarity and intravascular fluid shift, requiring the administration of diuretics.
    C. coagulopathy.
    D. ascites.
    E. none of the above.

52. Advantages of the Salem sump nasogastric tube over the single-lumen Levine tube include the following:
    A. the Salem sump is more easily inserted.
    B. the Salem sump is of a smaller diameter and thus causes less nasal irritation during insertion.
    C. the Salem sump allows continuous low-pressure suction without risk of damage to the gastric mucosa, whereas the Levine tube can only provide intermittent suction.
    D. the Salem sump is of a larger diameter, thus allowing for suctioning of particulate matter as well as fluids.
    E. none of the above.

53. The presence of CO_2 in the nasogastric tube following insertion most likely indicates:
    A. recent ingestion of carbonated beverages.
    B. tracheoesophageal fistula.
    C. recent use of antacids.
    D. accidental insertion of the nasogastric tube into the trachea.
    E. none of the above.

54. Nasointestinal tubes differ from nasogastric tubes in that:
    A. nasointestinal tubes are usually of smaller diameter.
    B. nasointestinal tubes have a fluid-filled distal cuff to keep them in proper position.
    C. nasointestinal tubes are usually inserted beyond the pyloric sphincter.
    D. nasointestinal tubes are less likely to clog or dislodge.
    E. A and C.

55. The procedure in which a feeding tube is inserted endoscopically along a guide wire passed through the abdominal wall is called:
    A. gastrostomy.
    B. colostomy.
    C. percutaneous endoscopic gastrostomy (PEG).
    D. Seldinger nasogastrostomy.
    E. none of the above.

56. In percutaneous endoscopic jejunostomy (PEJ), a PEG tube is first placed, and then a smaller diameter feeding tube is inserted through it. The tube is directed into the jejunum via:
    A. direct endoscopy.
    B. fluoroscopic visualization.
    C. guide wire.
    D. peristaltic contractions of the duodenum.
    E. none of the above.

57. An Anderson tube is a long _____ used to treat small bowel obstruction in patients who are high-risk surgery candidates.
    A. single-lumen, mercury-weighted
    B. double-lumen, tungsten-weighted
    C. double-lumen, mercury-weighted
    D. single-lumen, tungsten-weighted
    E. quadruple lumen, lead-weighted

58. A(n) _____ is typically used to drain bile from the gallbladder following liver, gallbladder, or common bile duct surgery.
    A. T-tube
    B. PEG tube
    C. J-tube
    D. NG tube
    E. Levine tube

59. When transporting a patient with a T-tube, care should be taken to:
    A. ensure that the tube is patent and adequately secured.
    B. empty the collection bag prior to transport.
    C. ensure that bile does not come in contact with the patient's skin.
    D. inspect the insertion site for infection or drainage.
    E. all of the above.

60. When transporting patients with a Sengstaken-Blakemore tube, care should be taken to:
    A. protect the patient's airway from aspiration.
    B. insert a Salem sump nasogastric tube above the esophageal balloon.
    C. apply gentle traction to the proximal end of the tube to hold the tube in place.
    D. apply continuous suction.
    E. all answers but D.

61. Advantages of the Minnesota tube over the Sengstaken-Blakemore tube include the following:
    A. the Minnesota tube is more easily inserted.
    B. the Minnesota tube is easier to spell.
    C. the Minnesota tube has an additional esophageal aspiration lumen, thus eliminating the need to insert another tube to remove esophageal secretions.

D. the Minnesota tube can be left in for longer periods without fear of pressure necrosis to the esophagus.

E. none of the above.

62. Prior to helicopter transport of the patient with a colostomy, the critical care paramedic should take care to:
    A. empty the collection bag prior to loading the patient in the aircraft.
    B. thoroughly flush the ostomy with sterile saline solution.
    C. ensure that the attached collection bag allows for venting of any gaseous buildup that may occur with changes in altitude.
    D. A and C.
    E. all of the above.

63. When transporting the patient with a recently placed rectal catheter, which of the following is NOT routinely necessary?
    A. Assess for potential tube obstruction.
    B. Assess for signs of rectal perforation and hemorrhage.
    C. Empty the collection chamber prior to transport.
    D. Clamp off the tube during transport.
    E. none of the above

64. When transporting the patient with a Penrose drain, Jackson-Pratt tube, or Hemovac tube, care should be taken to:
    A. remove any surgical drains prior to transport and cover the drain site with an occlusive dressing.
    B. record the amount of any discarded drainage.
    C. avoid dislodgement of the tube, as most are held in place only by absorbent dressings.
    D. flush the tube with sterile saline solution prior to transport.
    E. B and C.

65. Which of the following statements about peritoneal dialysis catheters is FALSE?
    A. The tube should be uncapped when not in use.
    B. The patient with a newly placed catheter should be frequently assessed for signs of bleeding.
    C. Dialysate solution in the abdomen may appear to make the abdomen look distended.
    D. Draining the dialysate after the appropriate dwell time is accomplished by placing the collection bag lower than the catheter.
    E. The peritoneum serves as the dialysis membrane.

CHAPTER 25

Renal and Acid-Base Emergencies

DIRECTIONS Each of the questions or incomplete statements below is followed by suggested answers or completions. Select the **one answer** that is best in each case.

1. Approximately _____ of cardiac output flows through the kidneys.
   A. 10%
   B. 20%
   C. 25%
   D. 40%
   E. 100%

2. Which of the following is an anatomical structure of the kidney?
   A. renal pelvis
   B. renal cortex
   C. renal medulla
   D. renal capsule
   E. all of the above

3. Renal filtration occurs in which of the following structures?
   A. descending loop of Henle
   B. ascending loop of Henle
   C. Bowman's capsule
   D. proximal convoluted tubule
   E. none of the above

4. Circulatory blood volume is filtered _____ times a day.
   A. 2–3
   B. 10–12
   C. 20–25
   D. 40–50
   E. 120

5. Specialized proteins on the membranes of various cells in the nephron that transport glucose, amino acids, and ions are called:
   A. transporters.
   B. nephritic countercurrent exchangers.
   C. sodium-potassium pump.
   D. ureteral stumps.
   E. none of the above.

6. Antidiuretic hormone (ADH) is secreted from which of the following structures?
   A. renal cortex
   B. adrenal cortex
   C. anterior pituitary
   D. posterior pituitary
   E. none of the above

7. Antidiuretic hormone acts on which if the following structures?
   A. distal convoluted tubule
   B. descending loop of Henle
   C. collecting duct
   D. A and B
   E. A and C

8. Renal failure secondary to cardiogenic shock would be considered:
   A. prerenal failure.
   B. intrarenal failure.
   C. post-renal failure.
   D. A and B.
   E. A and C.

9. Which of the following is NOT a major metabolic waste product found in urine?
   A. uric acid
   B. tryptophan
   C. creatinine
   D. urea
   E. none of the above

10. Which of the following is NOT an effect of angiotensin II?
    A. vasodilation
    B. elevation of glomerular pressures
    C. triggering the release of ADH
    D. stimulating secretion of aldosterone
    E. none of the above

11. Which of the following statements about aldosterone is true?
    A. It promotes the reabsorption of potassium.
    B. It is released as a result of a fall in potassium ion concentration.
    C. It is inhibited by angiotensin II.
    D. It stimulates the reabsorption of sodium ions.
    E. none of the above

12. Which enzyme converts angiotensinogen to angiotensin I?
    A. aldosterone
    B. renin
    C. fibrin
    D. fibrinogen
    E. none of the above

13. What is the most important factor affecting pH in body tissues?
    A. carbon dioxide
    B. hydrogen ions
    C. carbonic anhydrase
    D. lactic acid
    E. none of the above

14. Which of the following is NOT one of the body's three major buffer systems?
    A. protein buffer system
    B. carbonic acid–bicarbonate buffer system
    C. Anheuser-Busch buffer system
    D. phosphate buffer system
    E. none of the above

15. The "kidney stone belt" is primarily found in what part of the United States?
    A. New England
    B. West coast
    C. South and East
    D. Northern plains
    E. none of the above

16. The most common substance found in kidney stones is:
    A. uric acid.
    B. calcium.
    C. creatinine.
    D. magnesium.
    E. none of the above.

17. A risk factor (risk factors) for kidney stones is/are:
    A. male.
    B. familial patterns.
    C. immobilization.
    D. opiate use.
    E. all of the above.

18. The kidneys are located in what body compartment?
    A. pelvic
    B. abdominal
    C. cranial
    D. thoracic
    E. none of the above

19. Which of the following substances rise(s) in the bloodstream with a fall in glomerular filtration rate (GFR)?
    A. blood/urea/nitrogen (BUN)
    B. creatinine
    C. antidiuretic hormone (ADH)
    D. all of the above
    E. A and C

20. You are treating a dialysis patient in ventricular fibrillation that is refractory to first- and second-line antidysrhythmic agents. The patient has not dialyzed in over 10 days. What is the most likely problem?
    A. voronary insufficiency
    B. hyperkalemia
    C. hyponatremia
    D. hypokalemia
    E. none of the above

21. Which of the following is least affected by hydration status?
    A. creatinine
    B. blood/urea/nitrogen (BUN)
    C. sodium
    D. serum osmolality
    E. none of the above

22. The most common extracellular buffer is the:
    A. phosphate system.
    B. protein buffer system.
    C. carbonic acid–bicarbonate system.
    D. A and B.
    E. none of the above.

23. The most common intracellular buffer is the:
    A. phosphate system.
    B. protein buffer system.
    C. carbonic acid–bicarbonate system.
    D. A and B.
    E. none of the above.

24. The overelimination of bicarbonate typically results in:
    A. actual acidosis.
    B. actual alkalosis.
    C. relative acidosis.
    D. relative alkalosis.
    E. none of the above.

25. Treatment for methanol poisoning includes all of the following EXCEPT:
    A. ethanol administration.
    B. airway management.
    C. respiratory support.
    D. intravenous access.
    E. administration of methanol-specific antibody (Mab).

26. A patient has an Na^+ of 157 mEq/L, a K^+ of 4.0 mEq/L, a CL^- of 101 mEq/L, and a HCO_3^- of 22 mEq/L. What is the anion gap?
    A. 22 mEq/L
    B. 27 mEq/L
    C. 34 mEq/L
    D. 56 mEq/L
    E. none of the above

Scenario

Questions 27–28 refer to the following scenario:,
You are called to transfer a 27-year-old female to a University medical center. She has a history of juvenile-onset diabetes mellitus and has developed multiple complications including blindness and chronic renal failure. She is unresponsive with the following vital signs:

Blood pressure = 130/74 mmHg
Respirations = 36 per minute
Pulse = 110 per minute
SpO_2 = 100% (50% Venturi mask)

She has the following labs:
CBC: WBC = 18.1 mm^3
   HgB = 9.6 g/dL
   HCT = 28%
BMP: Na^+ = 156 mEq/L
   K^+ = 5.7 mEq/L
   Cl^- = 110 mEq/L
   HCO_3^- = 8 mEq/L
   BUN = 55 mg/dL
   Creat = 4.1 mg/dL
   Gluc = 806 mg/dL

27. Which of the following arterial blood gas values would be inconsistent with the patient's condition?
    A. high pH
    B. low PCO_2
    C. low bicarbonate
    D. normal PO_2
    E. none of the above

28. An insulin drip is started following an insulin bolus of 20 IU. What should you expect to occur with the patient's K^+ level?
   A. It will rise.
   B. It will remain constant.
   C. It will fall and possibly require supplemental K^+.
   D. All of the above are common.
   E. none of the above

29. Which of the following would you expect to be elevated in a patient in diabetic ketoacidosis (DKA)?
   A. blood/urea/nitrogen (BUN)
   B. bicarbonate ion
   C. pH
   D. $PaCO_2$
   E. none of the above

30. Which of the following is generally NOT indicated in the treatment of DKA?
   A. fluids
   B. supplemental potassium
   C. insulin
   D. beta agonists
   E. sodium bicarbonate

31. Paraldehyde is used to treat:
   A. opiate withdrawal.
   B. delirium tremens.
   C. opiate overdose.
   D. rookie EMTs.
   E. none of the above.

32. Lactic acidosis secondary to a cellular toxin would be classified as which of the following types?
   A. Type A
   B. Type B1
   C. Type B2
   D. Type B3
   E. none of the above

33. In regard to ethylene glycol poisoning, which phase is considered the renal toxicity phase?
   A. Phase I
   B. Phase II
   C. Phase III
   D. Phase IV
   E. none of the above

34. Which of the following statements about fomepizole (Antizol) is FALSE?
   A. It antagonizes alcohol dehydrogenase.
   B. It is administered intravenously.
   C. It is used in methanol poisoning.
   D. It is used in ethylene glycol poisoning.
   E. It is used with pediatric patients.

35. Which of the following is NOT a part of the treatment regimen for salicylate poisoning?
   A. hemodialysis
   B. administration of IV crystalloids for dilution
   C. sodium bicarbonate to alkalinize urine
   D. nasogastric tube placement
   E. none of the above

36. Hyperkalemia generally has what effect on the ECG?
   A. peaked T waves
   B. narrowing of the QRS complex
   C. decreased QT interval
   D. decreased PR interval
   E. none of the above

37. Which of the following is inconsistent with acute renal failure?
   A. elevated creatinine
   B. elevated Blood/Urea/Nitrogen (BUN)
   C. elevated glomerular filtration rate (GFR)
   D. A and B
   E. A and C

38. Which of the following lab values typically increases with renal failure?
   A. serum calcium
   B. urine specific gravity
   C. urine pH
   D. phosphate
   E. none of the above

Scenario

Questions 39–40 refer to the following scenario:
You are transporting a male patient with severe right flank pain that radiates to his right testicle. There is obvious hematuria. The patient is in considerable pain and cannot find a comfortable position. He is afebrile with a blood pressure of 156/90 mmHg, a pulse of 110 per minute, and respirations of 24 per minute. He is retching often.

39. Which of the following would be an **INAPPROPRIATE** prehospital treatment for this patient?
   A. Withhold analgesia as it will blunt the patient's abdominal exam when evaluated by the surgeon.
   B. Administer a fluid bolus.
   C. Strain the urine.
   D. Administer fentanyl or morphine.
   E. Administer an antiemetic.

40. The most likely diagnosis for this patient is:
   A. appendicitis.
   B. ectopic pregnancy.
   C. pelvic inflammatory disease.
   D. pyelonephritis.
   E. none of the above.

CHAPTER 26
Infectious Disease Emergencies

1. A disease or condition caused by the invasion and multiplication of pathogenic microorganisms with the body is a:
   A. toxin.
   B. pathogen.
   C. infection.
   D. antigen.
   E. all of the above.

2. Several body systems help prevent disease transmission. Among these are the skin and the:
   A. mucociliary escalator.
   B. gastrointestinal tract.
   C. genitourinary tract.
   D. nasopharyngeal tract.
   E. all of the above.

3. Signs and symptoms normally associated with infection include:
   A. hypothermia.
   B. hyperthermia.
   C. inflammation.
   D. B and C.
   E. all of the above.

4. Bacteria are unicellular microorganisms classified as _____, _____, and _____.
   A. round, square, oval.
   B. round, spiral, rod-shaped.
   C. spiral, oval, square.
   D. square, round, rod-shaped.
   E. oval, square, spiral.

5. Match the following infectious organisms with their appropriate description.

   a. _____ aerobic bacteria
   b. _____ anaerobic bacteria
   c. _____ viruses
   d. _____ rickettsia
   e. _____ fungi
   f. _____ protozoa
   g. _____ metazoa/helminth
   h. _____ prions

   A. parasitic worm
   B. protein particles lacking nucleic acid
   C. unicellular, pathogenic, parasitic organisms
   D. saprophytic, parasitic, spore producing
   E. live in lice or ticks
   F. grow/multiply only in living cells
   G. survive only in the presence of oxygen
   H. survive in the absence of oxygen

6. *Staphylococcus, Streptococcus, Tuberculosis,* and *Meningococcus* are several of which type of organism?
   A. aerobic bacteria
   B. rickettsia
   C. protozoa
   D. prion
   E. anaerobic bacteria

7. Of the following, which are viruses?
   1. syphilis
   2. measles
   3. yellow fever
   4. tularemia
   5. Q-Fever
   6. Blastomycosis

   A. 1, 3, and 4
   B. 2, 3, and 6
   C. 2, 4, and 5
   D. 2 and 3
   E. 2 and 5

8. You are airlifting a 26-year-old male from a national park in New Mexico. Your patient had been hiking with friends for 10 days and developed a high fever over the past 24 hours. As you assessed him, you found a reddish rash that also involves the patient's palms and soles. The patient is in an altered mental state and dehydrated; however, there are no signs of trauma, and his friends deny that anyone else is ill. Later tests confirm your suspicion that the patient is suffering from Rocky Mountain spotted fever, a disease caused by _____, bacteria that are commonly transmitted to humans by tick bites.
   A. protozoa
   B. rickettsia
   C. prions
   D. scabies
   E. metazoa

9. Actinomycetes is also known as:
   A. thrush.
   B. rickets.
   C. rat bite fever.
   D. trichomoniasis.
   E. none of the above.

10. Microorganisms categorized as "other" (don't fit typical pathogen classification schemes) and that are capable of causing infectious disease may include:
    A. lice.
    B. scabies.
    C. malaria.
    D. Kawasaki (syndrome).
    E. all of the above.

11. The routes of transmission for infection include contact, droplet, vehicle, _____, and _____.
    A. source, airborne
    B. source, vector
    C. vector, dressing
    D. dressing, source
    E. vector, airborne

12. For a disease to be infectious, what three basic elements must be present?
    1. a source organism
    2. a contaminated object
    3. an incubation period
    4. a susceptible host
    5. a means of transmission

    A. 1, 2, and 3
    B. 1, 4, and 5
    C. 3, 4, and 5
    D. 2, 3, and 5
    E. 1, 3, and 5

13. _____ applies to all blood, body fluids, secretions, excretions, nonintact skin, and mucous membranes, with one exception: _____.
    A. Universal Precautions, plasma
    B. BSI precautions, urine
    C. Standard Precautions, sweat
    D. all of the above
    E. none of the above

14. In the OSHA "Standard Precaution" document, which of the following items are among those included for discussion?
    1. handwashing
    2. gloves
    3. respiratory protection
    4. linens
    5. mouth/eye/face protection
    6. patient care equipment

    A. 1, 2, 3, and 5
    B. 1, 2, 4, 5, and 6
    C. 1, 3, 4, 5, and 6
    D. 2, 3, 4, 5, and 6
    E. 1, 2, 3, 4, 5, and 6

15. According to the OSHA Airborne Precautions standard, transport in an ambulance should include a minimum of _____ air exchanges per _____ in the patient compartment and _____ level respirator masks.
    A. 6–12, minute; N-95
    B. 5–10, hour; M-95
    C. 6–12, hour; N-95
    D. 5–10, minute; N-95
    E. 6–12, hour; M-95

16. The OSHA "droplet" precautions specifically include positioning of potentially infectious respiratory patients a minimum of _____ from other persons.
    A. 13 feet
    B. 3 feet
    C. 3 yards
    D. 30 feet
    E. none of the above

17. The Centers for Disease Control (CDC) recommends use of antimicrobial soap after removal of _____ and after contact with a _____ surface.
    A. mask, wet
    B. stitches, hard
    C. gloves, soft
    D. stitches, contaminated
    E. gloves, contaminated

18. Match the following United States Standards with their subject matter:
    a. _____ 29 CFR 1910.1030
    b. _____ 29 CFR 1910.135
    c. _____ 29 CFR 1904; 1910.1020
    d. _____ 29 CFR 1910.1200
    e. _____ P.L. 106-430

    A. Needlestick Injury and Prevention Act
    B. record keeping and reporting of injuries
    C. respiratory protection
    D. hazard communication
    E. bloodborne pathogen exposure

19. According to the CDC, the diseases that require airborne precautions (in addition to standard precautions) include:
    A. chickenpox (varicella).
    B. tuberculosis.
    C. herpes zoster.
    D. measles (rubeola).
    E. all of the above.

20. It is 9:00 PM on Friday and you are assessing a 12-year-old male presenting with uncontrolled diarrhea and vomiting. His mother tells you he came home from school "not feeling well" and shortly thereafter began vomiting. She also tells you that three of his other schoolmates are in the waiting room with the same symptoms.

    After further assessment and interview you find that the patient's entire sixth-grade class went on a field trip today, and several of the class members ate at a seafood restaurant on the wharf. Based on your assessment, the history, and presentation, your differentials should include:
    A. *Neisseria meningitides.*
    B. *E. coli.*
    C. Shigella.
    D. Rotovirus.
    E. B, C, and D.

21. The CDC recommendations for immunization of health care workers includes hepatitis B (HBV) as well as:
    A. typhoid and pneumococcal (23valent).
    B. influenza, tetanus, and diphtheria.
    C. MMR (measles [rubeola], mumps, and rubella/German/red measles).
    D. vaccinia and varicells.
    E. all of the above.

22. The terminal classical manifestation of HIV infection is _____ and the time from infection to death is typically _____.
    A. HBV; 5–10 years
    B. AIDS; 10–12 years
    C. HIV-2; 5–10 years
    D. HIV-1; 10–12 years
    E. AIDS; 1–2 years

23. Of the two classifications, _____ appears more pathogenic than _____, which is rarely found outside of West Africa.
    A. HIV-2; HIV-1
    B. HIV-1; HIV-2
    C. AIDS; HIV-1
    D. HIV-2; Ebola
    E. Ebola; HIV-2

24. Opportunistic infections that may manifest in end-stage AIDS complex include, but are not limited to, the following:
    1. *Pneumocystis carinii* pneumonia.
    2. Kaposi sarcoma.
    3. toxoplasmosis.
    4. non-Hodgkins lymphoma.
    5. candidiasis.

    A. 1, 2, and 3
    B. 1, 3, and 4
    C. 1, 2, 3, and 5
    D. 1, 2, 3, 4, and 5
    E. none of the above

25. According to recent studies, the risk of infection after a single needlestick contaminated by known AIDS is less than 0.5%, as compared to the 25% risk of infection from _____.
    A. cytomegalovirus
    B. toxoplasmosis
    C. hepatitis B
    D. cholera
    E. all of the above

26. Your 32-year-old patient is being treated for a cascade of nonspecific symptoms that include nausea, diarrhea, abdominal pain, jaundice, fatigue, and low-grade fever. As you talk with the patient, he reveals that he recently returned from a Caribbean cruise. Armed with this information, differentials you should consider would include:
    A. epiglottitis.
    B. hepatitis.
    C. RSV.
    D. pancreatitis.
    E. all of the above.

27. Of the five most common hepatic viruses, three are contracted via contact with infected body fluids. The others, contracted through the fecal/oral route, are:
    A. hepatitis A and B.
    B. hepatitis B and C.
    C. hepatitis A and E.
    D. hepatitis C and D.
    E. hepatitis D and E.

28. Preventive measures and immunization against _____ are the only protections health care workers may have against other, more serious versions of the disease.
    A. cholera
    B. smallpox
    C. Ebola
    D. hepatitis B
    E. diphtheria

29. Most adults contract 2–5 upper respiratory infections each year. According to published statistics, these tend to last _____ and result in 40% of all lost work time.
    A. 1–3 days
    B. 3–6 days
    C. 5–7 days
    D. 6–10 days
    E. 10+ days

30. The major complications associated with respiratory infections include development of bacterial superinfections, many of which manifest as:
    A. bacterial sinusitis.
    B. otitis media.
    C. bronchitis and/or pneumonia.
    D. all of the above.
    E. A and C.

31. You are intercepting a ground unit on scene at 0500 hours, for a 10-year-old patient with difficulty breathing and a BCT of 104° F. The patient is anxious, in tripod position, drooling, and unable to speak normally. His mother tells you he woke up complaining of a sore throat about 2 hours ago and she called 911 when it got "worse." The patient is already receiving oxygen therapy, but as you assume patient care, you suspect the patient is suffering from:
    A. asthma.
    B. epiglottitis.
    C. croup.
    D. influenza.
    E. RSV.

32. Signs and symptoms that may distinguish influenza from the common cold include:
    A. headache.
    B. high fever.
    C. chills.
    D. myalgia.
    E. all of the above.

33. Primary respiratory exposure to pneumococcus, *Klebsiella,* or *Legionalla* are among the reasons one may contract:
    A. influenza.
    B. croup.
    C. pneumonia.
    D. epiglottitis.
    E. none of the above.

34. Community acquired pneumonia (CAP) is usually caused by gram-positive agents, such as:
    A. *Streptococcus pneumonia.*
    B. *Streptococcus pyogenes.*
    C. *Staphylococcus aureus.*
    D. *Moraxella catarrhalis.*
    E. all of the above.

35. The treatment of pneumonia is usually supportive in nature, but may also involve the use of pharmacologic agents. These may include, but are not limited to:
    A. oral macrolides.
    B. quinolones.
    C. cephalosporins.
    D. all of the above.
    E. A and C.

36. *Mycobacterium tuberculosis* is a _____ infection primarily spread by pulmonary contact.
    A. bacillus
    B. viral agent
    C. bacterial agent
    D. prion
    E. bloodborne

37. Some of the signs and symptoms a patient may exhibit when infected with pulmonary tuberculosis are:
    A. fever and chills.
    B. cough (especially productive).
    C. chest pain and fatigue.
    D. all of the above
    E. B and C

38. With the exception of laryngeal tuberculosis (TB), "extrapulmonary" lesions are generally considered non-infectious to others, unless there is:
    A. a direct bloodborne vector.
    B. an actively draining lesion.
    C. direct pulmonary contact.
    D. unprotected sexual contact.
    E. direct oral contact.

39. Persons with a competent immune system may be considered positive for tuberculosis if serial PPD tests (within 2 years) incur induations with a measurable difference that equal to or greater than:
    A. 10 mm.
    B. 3 mm.
    C. 15 mm.
    D. 5 mm.
    E. 7 mm.

40. "Active" tuberculosis is currently treated for a period of 6 to 9 months with an initial drug regimen that may include any or all of the following drugs.
    1. rifampin
    2. streptomycin
    3. Indural
    4. isonazide
    5. Ceclor
    6. gentamycin

    A. 1
    B. 2 and 3
    C. 4
    D. 1, 2, and 3
    E. 1, 2, and 4

41. Severe acute respiratory syndrome (SARS) first appeared in what country?
    A. Japan
    B. Russia
    C. China
    D. Thailand
    E. Ecuador

42. SARS is what type of virus?
    A. meningeal
    B. corona
    C. spirochete
    D. all of the above
    E. none of the above

43. The signs and symptoms of SARS may include:
    A. altered mental status.
    B. dyspnea and cough.
    C. cyanosis or hypoxia.
    D. headache and diarrhea.
    E. all of the above.

44. You are assessing a 20-year-old male at your university walk-in clinic, who is complaining of a stiff neck, headache, and sensitivity to light. He has a mid-grade fever and a sore throat, as well. You know he lives in one of the "animal" dorms on campus, and when you ask if anyone else there is ill, he says "Yeah, three or four other guys started feeling bad today, too." You discuss the case with the college physician via telephone, who orders a WBC, throat culture, C-reactive protein, and isolation. Depending on the outcome of these lab tests, you also expect the physician will want to come in and do a lumbar puncture to rule out:
    A. RSV.
    B. epiglottitis.
    C. bacterial meningitis.
    D. HIV.
    E. Guillain-Barré syndrome.

45. In addition to antibiotic therapy for meningococcal infections, the physician may order vasopressors and other drugs designed to mitigate the onset of:
    A. DIC.
    B. RSV.
    C. BSE.
    D. HIV.
    E. AIDS.

46. Differential diagnosis with reference to rubeola and rubella would include the presence or absence of:
    A. cough.
    B. conjunctivitis.

C. maculopapular rash.

D. all of the above.

E. A and C.

47. The mumps virus causes an acute infection that primarily affects the:

    A. tonsils.
    B. larynx.
    C. epiglottis.
    D. parotid glands.
    E. lymph glands.

48. Of the following, which is most dangerous to a developing fetus?

    A. rubella
    B. mumps
    C. varicella
    D. rubeola
    E. chlamydia

49. Hepatitis A, *E-coli,* and *Yersinia* are among the infections commonly responsible for:

    A. chicken pox.
    B. RSV.
    C. gastroenteritis.
    D. diverticulitis.
    E. Crohn's disease.

50. Susceptible persons suffering from gastroenteritis may encounter complications such as:

    A. shock.
    B. DIC.
    C. kidney failure.
    D. all of the above.
    E. A and C.

51. *Clostridium tetani* is a gram-_____, spore forming, anaerobic _____ that can cause tetanus.

    A. negative, bacillus
    B. positive, prion
    C. negative, spirochete
    D. positive, varicella
    E. none of the above

52. When transporting a patient with confirmed _____, the critical care paramedic must pay close attention to the patient's airway, body position, and vital signs because the patient may not be able to indicate problems (even by blinking his eyes), cough, swallow, or move his extremities.

    A. "locked-in" syndrome
    B. tetanus
    C. varicella
    D. shigella
    E. all of the above

53. You have been called to a military barracks to treat a semiconscious 21-year-old female who is very warm to the touch, slightly jaundiced, and reeking of a putrid odor. Her roommate tells you that she has been getting "sicker" over the past 4–5 days. When questioned further, the roommate denies the patient takes recreational drugs of any kind and states flatly that she does not drink. You notice the patient has a stain on the back of her skirt, and lifting it up to investigate you see what appears to be a pus-like discharge from the vaginal area. You ask the roommate if the patient uses tampons or if there is a possibility she may be or has been pregnant. The roommate states she does not know about a pregnancy but is sure the patient does use tampons.

    You continue your assessment and clinical treatment with oxygen, airway protection, and IV access as your partner obtains vital signs. During this process, you are mentally running the list of differentials; however, the one highest on your list is:

    A. spontaneous abortion.
    B. tetanus.
    C. toxic shock syndrome.
    D. chlamydia.
    E. septicemia.

54. _____ is a potentially lethal condition in which bacteria are spread from an infected part of the body through the bloodstream, causing an overwhelming systemic response to the toxin(s).
   A. Toxic shock syndrome
   B. Septicemia
   C. Tetanus
   D. Chlamydia
   E. Meningitis

55. A person diagnosed with chicken pox, herpes zoster, or shingles is considered to be infectious from the _____ through the _____ day after exposure.
   A. 5th, 15th
   B. 10th, 15th
   C. 10th, 21st
   D. 12th, 21st
   E. none of the above

56. The definitive diagnosis for streptococcal toxic shock syndrome (TSS) includes a confirmation of group A streptococci from any number of specific body fluids and two or more of the following:
   1. renal impairment.
   2. liver dysfunction.
   3. ARDS.
   4. leptospirosis.
   5. erythmatous macular rash.
   6. tissue necrosis.
   7. coagulopathy.
   8. hemoglobinemia.

   A. 1, 3, 5, and 7
   B. 1, 2, 3, 4, and 5
   C. 1, 2, 3, 5, 6, and 7
   D. 1, 2, 4, 5, 6, and 8
   E. 1, 2, 3, 4, 5, 6, and 8

57. Necrotizing fasciitis has been linked to several bacteria, including:
   1. group A streptococcus.
   2. polymicrobial colonization.
   3. *Staphylococcus aureus*.
   4. *Haemophilus aprophilus*.
   5. *Haemophilus influenza*.

   A. 1, 3, and 5
   B. 1, 2, 3 and 4
   C. 2, 3, and 4
   D. 2, 3, 4, and 5
   E. 1, 3, 4, and 5

58. You have been asked to transport a patient diagnosed 6 days ago with necrotizing fasciitis. The patient is critical and has been sedated and intubated prior to your arrival. As a critical care paramedic, you know that this infection can evolve into blistering necrosis of the skin, as well as _____ shock, secondary to _____.
   A. compensated, cardiac arrest
   B. irreversible, septicemia
   C. tachycardic, hypovolemic state
   D. bradycardic, increased ICP
   E. none of the above

59. Antibiotic-resistant organisms (ARO's) currently include:
   A. vancomycin-resistant enterococcus.
   B. methicillin-resistant *S. aureus*.
   C. vancomycin-resistant streptococcus.
   D. all of the above.
   E. A and B.

60. Bioterrorism dates back to the 14th century, when deceased victims of *Yersinia pestis*, also known as _____, were dumped in enemy cities during wartime.
   A. *S. aureus*
   B. streptococcus
   C. plague
   D. *Francisella tularemia*
   E. Lassa fever

61. Anthrax is a spore-forming, gram-_____ _____ manifested by signs and symptoms that vary with the type of infectious exposure.
    A. negative, virus
    B. positive, prion
    C. positive, rod-bacillus
    D. negative, rod-bacillus
    E. positive, virus

62. Symptoms of anthrax poisoning usually present within 48 hours and are usually treated with supportive therapy, drugs such as penicillin, and:
    A. tetracylcine.
    B. errythromycin.
    C. ciprofloxacin.
    D. all of the above.
    E. A and B.

63. Smallpox, a variola virus, exhibits signs and symptoms of all of the following, EXCEPT:
    1. fever.
    2. myalgia.
    3. dysarthria.
    4. vomiting.
    5. diarrhea.
    6. chills.
    7. predominant facial papular rash.
    8. headache.
    9. lymph engorgement.
    10. predominant trunk maculopapular rash.
    A. 3 and 10
    B. 5 and 7
    C. 1, 2, 4, and 6
    D. 3, 5, 9, and 10
    E. 2, 3, 7, and 9

64. The bacterial disease *Yersinia pestis,* or "plague," is vectored by infected fleas on _____ and transmitted by _____.
    A. rats, bites
    B. bats, nits
    C. mice, rice
    D. rats, lice
    E. all of the above

65. Botulism is a spore-forming, anaerobic bacillus caused by the bacteria *Clostridium botulinum*. It manifests in three different and specific forms. They are:
    A. wound, inhaled, food-borne.
    B. infant, wound, inhaled.
    C. wound, infant, food-borne.
    D. food-borne, inhaled, infant.
    E. none of the above.

66. There are multiple systems associated with botulism. Of the following, match the vectors with the associated common signs and symptoms. (One or more choices may be appropriate.)
    a. _____ food-borne
    b. _____ wound
    c. _____ infant
    A. difficulty swallowing
    B. descending weakness/paralysis
    C. dry mouth
    D. respiratory failure
    E. droopy eyelids
    F. constipation/diarrhea
    G. respiratory/cardiac arrest
    H. lethargy/anorexia
    I. nausea/vomiting
    J. blurred/double vision

67. "Rabbit fever" and "deer fly fever" are otherwise known as:
    A. filovirus.
    B. tularemia.
    C. malaria.
    D. arenavirus.
    E. none of the above.

68. The *Francisella* (or *Pasturella*) *tularensis* is a gram-negative:
   A. coccobacillus.
   B. rod-shaped spore.
   C. spongiform virus.
   D. all of the above.
   E. none of the above.

69. Even though tularemia is not commonly transmitted from person to person, it is highly contagious. The known vectors include all of the following EXCEPT:
   A. airborne via mucous membranes.
   B. contaminated flea or animal bite.
   C. contaminated water and feces.
   D. bloodborne via infected blood and tissue.
   E. contaminated alcoholic beverages containing sugar cane.

70. Signs and symptoms of tularemia are varied and include GI tract complaints consistent with other toxic infections; however, tularemia is hallmarked by additional specific symptoms that can include:
   A. painful pharyngitis.
   B. swollen, painful lymph nodes.
   C. pleuropneumonitis.
   D. all of the above.
   E. A and C.

71. Match the following viral classes/syndromes with the listed specific transmitter(s) and their main attributed sign(s)/symptom(s):
   a. _____ rilovirus
   b. _____ arenavirus
   c. _____ hantavirus
   d. _____ cholera
   e. _____ Q-Fever
   f. _____ brucellosis

   1. bloodborne
   2. aerosolized/inhaled
   3. direct
   4. food
   5. water

   A. hemorrhagic
   B. renal failure
   C. respiratory
   D. severe dehydration
   E. fever, malaise
   F. secondary infection

72. Treatment for the filo- and arenaviruses, such as Ebola, Marburg, and Lassa, includes supportive therapy, and possible antibiotic treatment with:
   A. cephalosporin.
   B. ribavirin.
   C. amoxicillin.
   D. all of the above.
   E. none of the above.

73. The hantaviruses exhibit GI symptoms similar to most viruses but also include _____, _____, and severe respiratory complications.
   A. hemorrhagic, renal
   B. renal, pancreatic
   C. hemorrhagic, pancreatic
   D. all of the above
   E. none of the above

74. *Vibrio cholerae* produces a(n) _____, resulting in explosive diarrhea and severe dehydration.
   A. cephalotoxin
   B. enterotoxin
   C. spirocele
   D. spore
   E. all of the above

75. Treatment of *Vibrio cholerae* includes rapid fluid and electrolyte replacement as well as drug therapy with any of the following EXCEPT:
   A. tetracycline.
   B. ciprofloxacin.

C. erythromycin.
D. sulfamethoxazole.
E. penicillin.

76. The treatment for Q-Fever includes but is not limited to:
    A. supportive therapy.
    B. antitussives.
    C. antibiotics.
    D. all of the above.
    E. A and B.

77. The treatment for brucellosis is supportive in nature but also includes aggressive and long-term therapy with _____ in order to kill the bacilli involved.
    A. antiviral agents
    B. antibiotic agents
    C. antifungal agents
    D. all of the above
    E. none of the above

78. The cytotoxin _____ is made from the mash left during the processing of castor beans.
    A. saxitoxin
    B. SEB
    C. ricin
    D. trochothecane
    E. none of the above

79. Treatment for cytotoxin exposure includes:
    A. vaccine Cyto S-6.
    B. antidotes derived from the soy bean.
    C. antiviral therapy.
    D. antibiotic therapy.
    E. respiratory and circulatory support.

80. Saxotoxin is a _____ associated with _____.
    A. neurotoxin, marine dinoflagellates
    B. endotoxin, blue-green algae
    C. prion, tropical fish tanks
    D. cytotoxin, crabs and blue-ringed octopus
    E. none of the above

81. Transmitted by ingestion and usually lethal, saxotoxins produce signs and symptoms ranging from numbness and tingling of the neck and extremities to extreme:
    A. respiratory distress.
    B. respiratory paralysis.
    C. aphasia.
    D. all of the above.
    E. none of the above.

82. Treatment for saxotoxin exposure includes induced vomiting, respiratory support, and basic supportive care. The use of _____ is contraindicated, and may increase the likelihood of death.
    A. Pam-E
    B. atropine
    C. MARK-1 kits
    D. all of the above
    E. none of the above

83. Staphylococcus enterotoxin (B), or SEB, is an agent responsible for _____.
    A. blood poisoning
    B. food poisoning
    C. water poisoning
    D. atmospheric poisoning
    E. skin poisoning

84. SEB can be aerosolized, producing more severe GI and neurological symptoms than those caused by food-borne transmission. Treatment is supportive and may include:
    A. cardiovascular therapy.
    B. respiratory therapy, including intubation and ventilation.
    C. antitoxin administration.
    D. all of the above.
    E. A and B.

85. Trichothecene mycotoxins are produced by:
    A. spirochetes.
    B. rod-shaped bacteria.
    C. filamentous fungi.
    D. marine dinoflagellates.
    E. blue-green algae.

86. Mycotoxin exposure can result from inhalation, ingestion, or _____ and can cause extreme GI symptoms, hemorrhage, and _____ symptoms.
    A. absorption, musculoskeletal
    B. radiation, neurological
    C. radiation, musculoskeletal
    D. absorption, cardiorespiratory
    E. none of the above

87. Treatment for exposure to mycotoxins is supportive in nature and may include:
    A. basic life support.
    B. symptomatic therapy as it presents.
    C. intensive care monitoring.
    D. all of the above.
    E. none of the above.

88. When responding to aerosolized incidents involving known toxins, critical care paramedics should use _____ and _____ hazmat suits as their minimal level of protection.
    A. NIOSH-approved SCBA, level A
    B. NIOSH-approved N-95 respirators, level B
    C. NIOSH-approved SCBA, level B
    D. OSHA-approved SCBA, level C
    E. none of the above

89. Which of the following is/are factor(s) in a host's likelihood of becoming infected with a disease?
    A. general health and hygiene
    B. immune status
    C. age
    D. breaks in first lines of defense
    E. all of the above

90. Vaccines are available for which of the following diseases?
    A. hepatitis A
    B. hepatitis B
    C. hepatitis C
    D. A and B
    E. B and C

CHAPTER 27
Pediatric Medical Emergencies

27: PEDIATRIC MEDICAL EMERGENCIES

DIRECTIONS Each of the questions or incomplete statements below is followed by suggested answers or completions. Select the **one answer** that is best in each case.

1. In infants and toddlers, greater body-surface-to-mass ratio, less adipose tissue, and underdeveloped skeletal muscles all combine to predispose the pediatric patient to:
   A. greater incidence of occult injury.
   B. greater incidence of musculoskeletal trauma.
   C. hypothermia.
   D. greater incidence of multiple systems trauma.
   E. none of the above.

2. The most appropriate method for limiting heat loss in the critically ill or injured child is to:
   A. administer warmed IV fluids.
   B. apply external warming blankets.
   C. apply hot packs to the groin, neck and axillae.
   D. increase the ambient temperature.
   E. none of the above.

3. Which of the following is NOT a factor contributing to the pediatric patient's propensity for rapid decompensation?
   A. higher basal metabolic rate
   B. lower pulmonary reserve capacity
   C. less glycogen reserves in the liver
   D. smaller relative size of the heart
   E. none of the above

4. Pediatric patients consume oxygen at roughly _____ the rate of adults.
   A. triple
   B. half
   C. twice
   D. equal
   E. none of the above

5. The increased basal metabolic rate and lower glycogen reserves in pediatric patients make it crucial that the critical care paramedic routinely monitor:
   A. arterial blood gases and evaluation of blood pH.
   B. capillary blood glucose.
   C. serum electrolytes.
   D. cardiac enzymes.
   E. none of the above.

6. Which of the following is NOT an anatomical factor that may contribute to the higher probability of airway occlusion in the pediatric patient?
   A. larger tongue and epiglottis
   B. adenoidal hypertrophy common in many children
   C. larger relative diameter of the nasopharynx
   D. natural subglottic narrowing of the trachea
   E. larger relative tongue size

7. Which of the following anatomical characteristics unique to pediatric patients makes proper positioning of critical importance in maintaining airway patency?
   A. more pliable trachea
   B. obligatory nose breathing
   C. proportionately larger head size
   D. larger tongue
   E. all answers but B

8. The anatomical subglottic narrowing of the pediatric patient's airway:
   A. makes the airway more susceptible to occlusion from edema.
   B. makes the glottis more difficult to visualize.
   C. serves as a physiologic cuff for uncuffed endotracheal tubes.

D. is the primary reason for failed intubation attempts in pediatric patients.

E. A and C.

9. Diaphragmatic "see-saw" breathing in pediatric patients with increased respiratory effort is a direct result of:
   A. naturally increased pliancy of the thoracic cage.
   B. greater development of abdominal musculature.
   C. underdeveloped accessory muscles.
   D. A and C.
   E. lower pulmonary reserve capacity.

10. Poorly developed thoracic musculature, increased flexibility of the rib cage, and increased reliance on diaphragmatic excursion in the pediatric patient make which of the following an intervention of increased importance in children receiving positive pressure ventilation?
    A. endotracheal intubation
    B. gastric decompression via nasogastric or orogastric tube
    C. positive end expiratory pressure (PEEP)
    D. chest tube placement
    E. none of the above

11. Which of the following compensatory mechanisms is limited in the hypovolemic pediatric patient?
    A. increased systemic vascular resistance
    B. increased heart rate
    C. increased cardiac contractile force and stroke volume
    D. increased respiratory rate
    E. none of the above

12. The heightened ability of children to increase systemic vascular resistance as a compensatory mechanism for low volume states often results in:
    A. hypertension.
    B. left ventricular hypertrophy.
    C. normotension even with significantly impaired end-organ perfusion.
    D. pulmonary hypertension.
    E. reflex bradycardia.

13. Which of the following is NOT likely to be a potential cause of respiratory compromise in the pediatric patient?
    A. foreign bodies
    B. edema
    C. bronchospasm
    D. congestive heart failure
    E. none of the above

14. Cardiopulmonary arrest in infants and children is most often:
    A. the end result of respiratory or airway insufficiency.
    B. due to primary ventricular fibrillation.
    C. due to congenital defects.
    D. due to abuse and neglect.
    E. none of the above.

15. Respiratory failure in the infant can be recognized clinically by the presence of increased respiratory effort coupled with:
    A. tachycardia.
    B. audible wheezes.
    C. diaphoresis.
    D. altered mental status such as extreme irritability or stupor.
    E. acrocyanosis.

16. Findings indicative of increased respiratory effort in pediatric patients include all of the following EXCEPT:
    A. nasal flaring.
    B. intercostal retractions.
    C. pallor.
    D. grunting.
    E. tachypnea.

17. Respiratory failure can be defined as:
    A. markedly increased respiratory effort.
    B. decompensation of respiratory compensatory mechanisms.
    C. hypoxemia.
    D. tachypnea.
    E. none of the above.

18. Lethargy and bradycardia in the pediatric patient with respiratory compromise:
    A. indicate late respiratory failure and impending arrest.
    B. indicate cardiovascular insufficiency as the primary cause of instability.
    C. indicate isolated central nervous system dysfunction.
    D. require immediate endotracheal intubation and positive pressure ventilation.
    E. none of the above.

19. Lethargy or stupor in the pediatric patient with adequate respiratory effort and mechanics and good peripheral perfusion may indicate:
    A. hypoglycemia or other metabolic disorder.
    B. CNS depression.
    C. intracranial pathology.
    D. shock.
    E. all answers but D.

20. Croup is most commonly encountered:
    A. during late fall and early winter.
    B. with clinical symptoms of drooling and difficulty swallowing.
    C. in children under 6 years of age.
    D. A and C.
    E. in children over 2 years of age.

21. The hallmark finding of croup is respiratory distress accompanied by:
    A. barking cough.
    B. grunting.
    C. drooling.
    D. runny nose.
    E. none of the above.

22. Clinical findings of epiglottitis include:
    A. rapid onset of fever and difficulty swallowing.
    B. stridor and barking cough.
    C. sore throat.
    D. A and C.
    E. none of the above.

23. Initial treatment of croup includes all of the following EXCEPT:
    A. humidified oxygen.
    B. aerosolized racemic epinephrine.
    C. administration of broad-spectrum antibiotics.
    D. aerosolized or intravenous corticosteroids.
    E. avoiding extensive examination of the airway.

24. The Croup Scale ranks the severity of croup signs on a numeric scale from 0–3 based on _____, retractions, color, breath sounds and level of consciousness.
    A. stridor
    B. pulse oximetry readings
    C. arterial blood gases
    D. fever
    E. none of the above

25. A score of 6–8 on the Croup Scale defines the symptoms as:
    A. mild.
    B. moderate.
    C. severe.
    D. life-threatening.
    E. none of the above.

26. Endotracheal intubation in the patient suspected of epiglottitis should only be performed with extreme caution:
    A. with a bronchoscope.
    B. when the patient adopts a tripod position.

C. when the patient cannot maintain his respiratory effort.

D. when edema causes respiratory occlusion.

E. all of the above.

27. Pathologic changes resulting from asthma include:
    A. inflammation and narrowing of bronchioles.
    B. upper airway edema and stridor.
    C. increased mucous production.
    D. A and C.
    E. increased tidal volume.

28. Inhaled anticholinergics used in the treatment of acute bronchospasm in asthma include:
    A. metaproterenol.
    B. ipratropium bromide.
    C. levalbuterol.
    D. methylprednisolone.
    E. ephedrine.

29. Asthma patients with severely diminished tidal volume may require:
    A. subcutaneous injection of beta agonists.
    B. aerosolized corticosteroids.
    C. aerosolized Ipratropium.
    D. immediate intubation.
    E. none of the above.

30. An adolescent with one-word dyspnea, severe intercostal and subxiphoid retractions, and a peak expiratory flow rate (PEFR) of less than 50% of normal would be classified with:
    A. moderate bronchospasm.
    B. severe bronchospasm.
    C. mild bronchospasm.
    D. silent asthma.
    E. *status asthmaticus.*

31. Aggressive treatment of bronchospasm in the pediatric patient in severe respiratory distress is imperative because intubation and positive pressure ventilation:
    A. may not be effective in providing adequate oxygenation.
    B. may make it impossible to wean the child from the ventilator.
    C. may exacerbate air trapping and hypercapnia.
    D. is likely to induce iatrogenic pneumothorax.
    E. none of the above.

32. Bronchiolitis, a viral infection of the lower respiratory tract that often mimics asthma in children under 24 months of age, is most commonly caused by:
    A. *Haemophilus influenzae.*
    B. *Streptococcal pneumonia.*
    C. inhaled allergens.
    D. respiratory syncytial virus (RSV).
    E. none of the above.

33. Bronchiolitis can sometimes be distinguished from asthma in that:
    A. asthma rarely occurs in children under 2 years of age.
    B. bronchiolitis usually causes coughing in young children, whereas asthma does not.
    C. bronchiolitis usually presents with fever and gradual onset of symptoms.
    D. asthma usually results in wheezing, whereas bronchiolitis does not.
    E. none of the above.

34. Treatment of bronchiolitis is aimed at correcting hypoxia, reversing bronchospasm, _____, and identifying the causative pathogen, if possible.
    A. keeping peak expiratory flow rate (PEFR) within 90% of normal
    B. reducing airway inflammation
    C. administering appropriate antibiotics
    D. controlling fever
    E. all of the above

35. Hypoperfusion due to inadequate vascular tone is termed:
    A. distributive shock.
    B. psychogenic shock.
    C. cardiogenic shock.
    D. hypovolemic shock.
    E. sticker shock.

36. Initial stabilizing treatment in distributive shock often includes the use of:
    A. inotropes.
    B. diuretics.
    C. large volume fluid resuscitation.
    D. vasopressors, particularly alpha agonists.
    E. antibiotics.

37. Potential causes of cardiogenic shock in the pediatric patient may include:
    A. dysrhythmias.
    B. traumatic injury to the myocardium.
    C. exacerbation of previously undiagnosed congenital defects.
    D. all of the above.
    E. none of the above.

38. History findings common in children presenting with cardiogenic shock include:
    A. exertional dyspnea.
    B. postural syncope.
    C. volume loss.
    D. tendency to fatigue easily.
    E. all but C.

39. Clinical findings in infants with cardiogenic shock include hypoperfusion often accompanied by:
    A. signs of CHF.
    B. hives.
    C. facial edema.
    D. poor skin turgor.
    E. sunken anterior fontanelle.

40. Management of the hypotensive pediatric patient in cardiogenic shock often includes:
    A. careful fluid boluses.
    B. vasopressors.
    C. inotropes.
    D. A and C.
    E. beta agonist bronchodilators.

41. ECG findings in the pediatric patient in cardiogenic shock often include:
    A. prolonged QT syndrome.
    B. left ventricular hypertrophy.
    C. extreme right axis deviation.
    D. intraventricular conduction delay.
    E. none of the above.

42. Obstructive shock may typically result from all of the following EXCEPT:
    A. sickle cell crisis.
    B. pulmonary embolus.
    C. tension pneumothorax.
    D. cardiac tamponade.
    E. none of the above.

43. Management of obstructive shock is aimed at:
    A. clot lysis.
    B. volume replacement.
    C. reestablishment of adequate vascular tone.
    D. augmentation of myocardial contractility.
    E. identification and correction of the initial obstructive defect.

44. Hemodynamic instability in septic shock is primarily caused by:
    A. mast cell degranulation and histamine release.
    B. decreased myocardial contractility.
    C. systemic vasodilation in response to release of bacterial endotoxins.

D. interruption of nervous stimuli resulting in loss of vascular tone.
E. intravascular volume depletion.

45. Protective laryngospasm in pediatric drownings often results in:
    A. asphyxiation and dry drowning.
    B. activation of the mammalian dive reflex.
    C. atelectasis and pulmonary shunting.
    D. reactive bronchospasm and wheezing.
    E. none of the above.

46. Management of the pediatric near-drowning patient includes all of the following EXCEPT:
    A. prevention of hypothermia.
    B. administration of diuretics.
    C. airway maintenance and oxygen administration.
    D. cervical spine precautions as appropriate.
    E. positive pressure ventilation as needed.

47. The leading cause of death in children less than one year of age is:
    A. sudden infant death syndrome (SIDS).
    B. congenital anomalies.
    C. seizures.
    D. respiratory syncytial virus (RSV).
    E. abuse or neglect.

48. Congenital cardiac defects are classified according to:
    A. what chamber(s) they affect.
    B. which valve(s) they affect.
    C. how they affect blood flow.
    D. how they affect the great vessels.
    E. none of the above.

49. Which of the following is NOT a congenital cardiac defect that obstructs blood flow?
    A. coarctation of the aorta
    B. aortic valve stenosis
    C. hypoplastic left heart syndrome
    D. patent *ductus arteriosus*
    E. pulmonary atresia

50. Congenital cardiac defects that result in decreased pulmonary blood flow include:
    A. ventricular septal defects.
    B. atrial septal defects.
    C. tetralogy of Fallot.
    D. patent *ductus arteriosus*.
    E. A and D.

51. The infant in respiratory failure with evidence of diaphragmatic herniation on the chest radiograph should initially be treated with:
    A. bronchodilators.
    B. bag-mask ventilation.
    C. endotracheal intubation.
    D. gastric decompression.
    E. surgery.

52. When performing RSI on the pediatric patient, the critical care paramedic should:
    A. premedicate the patient with atropine.
    B. secure the tube.
    C. use a lateral head restraint.
    D. all of the above.
    E. only A and B.

53. Ideally, the critical care paramedic should treat hypoglycemia in infants with dextrose 25% solution, not dextrose 50% solution, because:
    A. hypotonicity of dextrose 50% solutions results in rapid interstitial shift of intravascular volume.
    B. hypertonicity of dextrose 50% solution results in increased serum osmolarity, which can lead to cerebral edema.
    C. dextrose 25% solution is less caustic to veins than dextrose 50%.
    D. infants cannot handle the extra sugar in dextrose 50%.
    E. none of the above.

54. If immediate peripheral vascular access cannot be obtained to administer resuscitation medications in the pediatric arrest patient, the critical care paramedic should:
    A. administer all medications via the endotracheal tube.
    B. cannulate the femoral vein.
    C. cannulate the subclavian vein.
    D. cannulate the intraosseous space.
    E. continue attempts at peripheral vascular access until it is obtained.

55. Which of the following statements about the *ductus arteriosus* is FALSE?
    A. It connects the aorta with the pulmonary artery.
    B. It connects the aorta with the superior vena cava.
    C. It closes at or around birth.
    D. Persistent *ductus arteriosus* (PDA) causes a "machinery murmur."
    E. PDA allows infant survival in a number of congenital heart disorders.

CHAPTER 28

High-Risk Obstetrical/Gynecological Emergencies

DIRECTIONS Each of the questions or incomplete statements below is followed by suggested answers or completions. Select the **one answer** that is best in each case.

1. Fertilization usually takes place in the:
   A. vagina.
   B. uterus.
   C. distal fallopian tube.
   D. proximal fallopian tube.
   E. none of the above.

2. Which hormone stimulates the corpus luteum to release progesterone?
   A. human chorionic gonadotropin (HCG)
   B. antidiuretic hormone (ADH)
   C. estrogen
   D. erythropoietin
   E. none of the above

3. A fetal heart beat is usually present by week _____.
   A. 4
   B. 8
   C. 12
   D. 14
   E. 16

4. Which of the following hormones is NOT produced by the placenta?
   A. relaxin
   B. human placental lactogen (HPL)
   C. estrogen
   D. human chorionic gonadotropin (HCG)
   E. none of the above

5. Human gestation is typically:
   A. 32 weeks.
   B. 266–280 days.
   C. 43 weeks.
   D. 230–240 days.
   E. none of the above.

6. Which of the following statements is TRUE?
   A. There is one umbilical artery.
   B. There are two umbilical arteries.
   C. There is one umbilical vein.
   D. A and C.
   E. B and C.

7. The first extraembryonic membrane to appear is the:
   A. amnion.
   B. allantois.
   C. chorion.
   D. yolk sac.
   E. none of the above.

8. Which extraembryonic membrane contains the fluid that surrounds the developing fetus?
   A. amnion
   B. allantois
   C. chorion
   D. yolk sac
   E. none of the above

9. Most developmental milestones begin during the _____ trimester.
   A. first
   B. second
   C. third
   D. B and C
   E. all of the above

10. Which of the following statements regarding pregnancy is FALSE?
    A. The maternal respiratory rate increases.
    B. The maternal glomerular filtration rate (GFR) increases by roughly 50%.
    C. The maternal blood volume increases by approximately 40–50%.
    D. The maternal hematocrit increases.
    E. none of the above

11. Expulsion of the fetus is called:
    A. conception.
    B. contraception.
    C. gravidity.
    D. parturition.
    E. compulsion.

12. Which of the following factors leads to labor and delivery?
    A. placental production of estrogen
    B. placental production of relaxin
    C. fetal growth
    D. maternal oxytocin release
    E. all of the above

13. Identical twins are called:
    A. dizygotic twins.
    B. monozygotic twins.
    C. fraternal twins.
    D. Kate and Ashley.
    E. none of the above.

14. The sex of the fetus is determined by the:
    A. mother.
    B. father.
    C. brother.
    D. sister.
    E. grandparents.

15. The patient's chart reads "G4/P3 (3-0-0-2)." Which of the following interpretations of this information is NOT correct?
    A. The patient has 3 living children.
    B. The patient is pregnant.
    C. The patient has had no abortions.
    D. The patient has had 3 term infants.
    E. none of the above

16. Which of the following statements concerning fundal height (FH) measurement is true?
    A. Each inch equals one week of fetal growth.
    B. It is measured with the patient in the lateral recumbent position.
    C. The measurement occurs from the fundus to the point where fetal heart tones are best heard.
    D. It is most accurate late in pregnancy.
    E. Each centimeter equals roughly one week of gestational age.

17. Fetal tachycardia is defined as:
    A. heart rate less than 60 for 10 minutes.
    B. heart rate greater than 100 for 2 minutes.
    C. heart rate greater than 160 for 10 minutes.
    D. an increase in heart rate by 20 or more beats per minute.
    E. none of the above.

18. Which of the following primarily affect(s) fetal heart rate variability?
    A. sympathetic tone
    B. parasympathetic tone
    C. placental compression
    D. A and B
    E. A and C

19. Which of the following statements concerning beat-to-beat variability is usually FALSE?
    A. It primarily reflects parasympathetic tone.
    B. Loss may indicate fetal hypoxia.
    C. Normal variability is associated with proper oxygenation.
    D. It is increased with maternal narcotic usage.
    E. none of the above

20. Fetal head compression usually causes a(n):
    A. fall in heart rate early in a contraction.
    B. increase in heart rate early in a contraction.
    C. fall in heart rate late in a contraction.
    D. increase in heart rate late in a contraction.
    E. none of the above.

21. Variable decelerations usually result from:
    A. uteroplacental insufficiency.
    B. head compression.
    C. umbilical cord compression.
    D. pressurized aircraft cabins.
    E. none of the above.

22. Which of the following types of decelerations in fetal heart rate is the most worrisome?
    A. early
    B. late
    C. variable
    D. prominent beat-to-beat variability
    E. none of the above

23. Which of the following is NOT a cause of uteroplacental insufficiency?
    A. abruptio placentae
    B. placenta previa
    C. maternal smoking
    D. prematurity
    E. diabetes

24. Which of the following is the first step in managing fetal distress?
    A. IV fluid boluses
    B. administration of magnesium sulfate
    C. administration of supplemental oxygen
    D. placement of fetal scalp electrode
    E. none of the above

25. Which of the following fetal heart rate patterns is considered ominous?
    A. sinusoidal pattern
    B. variable deceleration
    C. transient tachycardia
    D. early deceleration
    E. none of the above

26. Which of the following is NOT a consistent finding in abruptio placentae?
    A. vaginal hemorrhage
    B. uterine tenderness
    C. abdominal pain
    D. uterine contractions
    E. none of the above

27. Approximately _____ of all cases of second trimester vaginal bleeding are due to placenta previa.
    A. 100%
    B. 80%
    C. 60%
    D. 40%
    E. 20%

28. Which of the following findings is NOT consistent with placenta previa?
    A. vaginal bleeding
    B. second or third trimester
    C. abdominal pain
    D. history of recent sexual intercourse
    E. none of the above

29. Which of the following is a significant risk factor for premature labor?
    A. post-term pregnancy
    B. premature rupture of membranes (PROM)
    C. history of maternal heroin use
    D. diabetes
    E. none of the above

30. The process of slowing or terminating labor is called:
    A. fibrinolysis.
    B. uterolysis.
    C. fetolysis.
    D. tocolysis.
    E. none of the above.

31. Which of the following agents CANNOT be used in an attempt to slow or stop labor?
    A. magnesium sulfate
    B. oxytocin

C. beta adrenergic agonists
D. calcium channel blockers
E. none of the above

32. Which of the following statements about breech deliveries is true?
    A. The fetus is almost always in the face-down position.
    B. They account for 10–15% of all deliveries.
    C. The morbidity is 60% higher than with cephalad presentations.
    D. The fetal airway is rarely a concern.
    E. none of the above

33. The maneuver where the mother's legs are sharply flexed to open the diameter of the pelvis is called:
    A. McLaren's maneuver.
    B. McClinton's maneuver.
    C. McDonald's maneuver.
    D. McRobert's maneuver.
    E. none of the above.

34. Which of the following is NOT a risk factor for shoulder dystocia?
    A. post-datism
    B. maternal obesity
    C. maternal diabetes
    D. large for gestational age (LGA) fetus
    E. cephalic position

35. The definitive treatment for a prolapsed umbilical cord is:
    A. circumcision.
    B. forceps delivery.
    C. predelivery cross-clamp and cutting of cord.
    D. Cesarean section.
    E. none of the above.

36. Which of the following statements about uterine rupture is true?
    A. The shape of the previous cesarean section scar on the skin is a good predictor of uterine rupture.
    B. An "inverted T-shaped" cesarean section uterine scar has the highest association with uterine rupture.
    C. The type of cesarean section scar on the skin always correlates with the uterine scar.
    D. Transverse cesarean scars (Pfannenstiel's incision) are highly associated with uterine rupture.
    E. none of the above

37. The condition where the placenta invades the uterine myometrium is called:
    A. placental abruption.
    B. placenta cementus.
    C. placenta accrete.
    D. placenta proximus.
    E. none of the above.

38. Which of the following is NOT a category of hypertension during pregnancy?
    A. gestational hypertension with preeclampsia
    B. chronic hypertension
    C. gestational hypertension
    D. preeclampsia
    E. chronic gestational hypertension

39. Which of the following is NOT a feature of HELLP syndrome?
    A. elevated platelets
    B. hemolysis
    C. elevated liver function test
    D. low platelets
    E. none of the above

40. Which of the following is NOT a finding of severe preeclampsia?
    A. proteinuria
    B. pulmonary edema
    C. oliguria
    D. systolic blood pressure > 160 mmHg
    E. high platelet count

41. You are treating an eclamptic patient with prolonged seizures. Which of the following treatments would be correct?
    A. high-flow oxygen
    B. 2–4 mg magnesium sulfate IV
    C. delivery of the fetus
    D. A and B
    E. A and C

42. Risk factors for the development of gestational diabetes include:
    A. maternal obesity
    B. history or preeclampsia
    C. > 40-pound weight gain during pregnancy
    D. A, B, and C
    E. none of the above

43. Which of the following is/are among the risk factors for amniotic fluid embolism?
    A. large fetus
    B. maternal age > 32 years
    C. multiparity
    D. abruptio placentae
    E. all of the above

44. The mortality rate for amniotic fluid embolism is:
    A. 10%.
    B. 20–30%.
    C. 50–60%.
    D. 60–70%.
    E. 80–90%.

45. Which of the following lab tests would NOT be useful when assessing a patient who is suffering postpartum hemorrhage?
    A. CBC
    B. type and cross match
    C. C-reactive protein
    D. PT
    E. PTT

Scenario

Questions 46–50 refer to the following scenario:
You are transporting a 24-year-old female G2/P1(0-1-0-1) with an EDC six weeks from today. She is edematous and has the following vital signs:

Blood pressure = 170/110 mmHg
Pulse = 96 per minute
Respirations = 20 per minute
SpO_2 = 99% on 35% venturi mask

46. Which of the following best describes the patient's intravascular volume status?
    A. increased
    B. decreased
    C. normal
    D. A and D
    E. none of the above

47. Which of the following is the biggest factor in the increase in her blood pressure?
    A. increased heart rate
    B. increased stroke volume (SV)
    C. increased cardiac output (CO)
    D. increased systemic vascular resistance (SVR)
    E. none of the above

48. Which of the following medications can be used to treat her elevated blood pressure?
    A. sodium nitroprusside
    B. magnesium sulfate

C. hydralazine
D. A and B
E. B and C

49. Which of the following treatments is appropriate for this patient?
    A. Try and transport without lights and sirens.
    B. Check cervical dilation and effacement prior to transport
    C. Administer crystalloid IV fluids.
    D. Place the patient in the left lateral recumbent position.
    E. Dim the lights.

50. What are the hallmarks of the mild form of this patient's condition?
    A. hypertension
    B. edema
    C. protein in the urine
    D. all of the above
    E. only A and B

CHAPTER 29

Neonatal Emergencies

DIRECTIONS Each of the questions or incomplete statements below is followed by suggested answers or completions. Select the **one answer** that is best in each case.

1. If the ambient room temperature is comfortable for the critical care paramedic, it is usually:
   A. too cold for the neonate.
   B. just right for the neonate.
   C. too warm for the neonate.
   D. irrelevant if the neonate is dried and wrapped well in receiving blankets.
   E. none of the above.

2. The neonate's inability to maintain thermoregulation can be attributed to:
   A. higher body surface to mass ratio.
   B. less adipose tissue.
   C. immature hypothalamus.
   D. poor muscle tone limiting ability to shiver effectively.
   E. all answers but C.

3. Hypoglycemia is a common problem among neonates. How often should the critical care paramedic assess the newborn's blood sugar level?
   A. every 2 hours
   B. within 1–2 hours after birth, then every 30 minutes to 1 hour until normal glucose levels are attained
   C. every 3 hours
   D. within half an hour after birth, then every 15 minutes until normal glucose levels are attained
   E. every 15 minutes as a part of routine vital signs monitoring

4. Signs of hypoglycemia in the neonate include all of the following EXCEPT:
   A. twitching and seizures.
   B. muscular hypotonia.
   C. eye rolling.
   D. increased agitation.
   E. apnea and/or irregular respirations.

5. Normal blood glucose levels in the neonate are:
   A. 70–80 mg/dL.
   B. minimum 60 mg/dL.
   C. 80–100 mg/dL.
   D. 50–60 mg/dL.
   E. 100–120 mg/dL.

6. Proper positioning is of vital importance in managing the neonate's airway because:
   A. the neonate has poor muscle tone and cannot breathe effectively unless supine.
   B. a prominent occiput predisposes the neonate to a position of neck flexion.
   C. poorly developed cartilaginous tracheal rings make the trachea much more pliable and susceptible to kinking.
   D. B and C.
   E. the tongue is proportionately larger.

7. The larger, more pliable epiglottis of the neonate makes it necessary to:
   A. use a straight (Miller) laryngoscope blade to directly elevate the epiglottis for visualization of the vocal cords.
   B. use a curved (MacIntosh) laryngoscope blade to avoid direct contact and possible injury to the delicate, poorly supported epiglottis.
   C. hyperextend the neck in order to visualize the glottic opening.
   D. hyperextend the neck in order to deliver effective BVM ventilations.
   E. none of the above.

8. The more anterior and cephalad position of the neonate's larynx may make it necessary to:
   A. hyperflex the neck in order to displace the larynx posteriorly.
   B. place approximately 2 inches of padding underneath the neonate's occiput to maintain a sniffing position.
   C. posteriorly displace the larynx with cricoid pressure in order to visualize the glottic opening.
   D. use a curved (MacIntosh) laryngoscope blade.
   E. none of the above.

9. A unique anatomical feature that makes the neonate more susceptible to aspiration into both lungs is the:
   A. larger, more pliable trachea that allows foreign objects to pass more easily.
   B. poor smooth-muscle tone, inhibiting protective laryngospasm.
   C. decreased angle of the left mainstem bronchus.
   D. increased angle of the right mainstem bronchus.
   E. none of the above.

10. Due to immature thoracic musculature and increased pliancy of the ribs and sternum, infants must compensate for respiratory compromise primarily by:
    A. increasing respiratory rate.
    B. increasing tidal volume (VT).
    C. gasping.
    D. diaphragmatic breathing.
    E. none of the above.

11. Signs of increased work of breathing such as accessory muscle use, retractions, and excessive diaphragmatic breathing are significant because:
    A. they herald significantly increased metabolic work with relatively little gain in tidal volume.
    B. they indicate the neonate is successfully increasing tidal volume.
    C. limited energy reserves make the neonate with increased work of breathing prone to tire more quickly.
    D. they always signify significant hypoxia.
    E. A and C.

12. The neonate is predominantly dependent on _____ to maintain cardiac output.
    A. contractile force
    B. preload and stroke volume
    C. heart rate
    D. respiratory rate
    E. all of the above

13. The _____ is the fetal structure directly connected to the inferior vena cava that allows oxygenated blood and nutrients to be pumped from the body without first passing through the kidneys.
    A. *ductus venosus*
    B. *ductus arteriosus*
    C. foramen ovale
    D. umbilical artery
    E. foramen magnum

14. The _____ is the fetal structure that allows blood to pass directly from the right atrium to the left atrium.
    A. *ductus venosus*
    B. *ductus arteriosus*
    C. foramen ovale
    D. umbilical artery
    E. foramen magnum.

15. The _____ is the fetal structure that allows blood to flow directly from the pulmonary artery to the aorta, bypassing the lungs.
    A. *ductus venosus*
    B. *ductus arteriosus*
    C. foramen ovale
    D. umbilical artery
    E. foramen magnum

16. Respiratory failure in the neonate is best described as:
    A. an ominous finding that heralds impending respiratory arrest.
    B. increased work of breathing that is still able to sustain adequate minute ventilation.
    C. deterioration of respiratory compensatory mechanisms and inability to sustain adequate minute ventilation.
    D. both A and C.
    E. agonal breathing.

17. At 5 minutes after birth, a newborn exhibits central cyanosis, poor muscle tone, no crying, and intercostal retractions with excessive diaphragmatic breathing, even after stimulation and warming. Her condition is best described as:
    A. respiratory failure.
    B. respiratory arrest.
    C. respiratory distress.
    D. normal.
    E. none of the above.

18. At 5 minutes after birth, a newborn exhibits acrocyanosis, active flexion of extremities, and vigorous crying with intercostal retractions and excessive diaphragmatic breathing, even after stimulation and warming. Her condition is best described as:
    A. respiratory failure.
    B. respiratory arrest.
    C. respiratory distress.
    D. normal.
    E. none of the above.

19. Persistent pulmonary hypertension of the newborn (PPHN) results in increased pulmonary vascular resistance and sustained fetal circulation in which:
    A. the *ductus venosus* remains open and patent.
    B. the *ductus arteriosus* and foramen ovale remain open.
    C. a passage in the ventricular septum remains, allowing intermixing of blood between right and left ventricles.
    D. type II respiratory distress syndrome results.
    E. none of the above.

20. Treatment of PPHN is aimed at:
    A. decreasing pulmonary vascular resistance with pulmonary vasodilators such as inhaled nitric oxide.
    B. sustaining oxygenation and serum alkalosis through hyperventilation.
    C. sustaining oxygenation and maintaining serum alkalosis with administration of sodium bicarbonate.
    D. A and C.
    E. decreasing pulmonary vascular resistance with systemic vasodilators such as sodium nitroprusside.

21. Administration of inhaled nitric oxide in newborns diagnosed with PPHN may help promote the shift from intrauterine to extrauterine circulation, which in turn results in:
    A. decreased pulmonary vascular resistance.
    B. pressure imbalance between right and left side of the heart.
    C. increased systemic vascular resistance.
    D. closure of the foramen ovale and *ductus arteriosus*.
    E. all of the above.

22. Meconium aspiration into the lower airways occurs in approximately _____ of live births.
    A. 1 in 100
    B. 1 in 10
    C. 15 in 100
    D. 30%
    E. none of the above

Scenario

Questions 23–25 refer to the following scenario:
Your NICU transport team has been called to the labor and delivery unit of a community hospital to assist in the delivery and subsequent transport of a full-term infant of a mother suffering from eclampsia. The obstetrician, who was awaiting your arrival, immediately performs an emergency Caesarean section and, after clamping and cutting the umbilical cord, hands off the infant to your team. You quickly move the male infant to the radiant warmer and begin your assessment. You note that the infant is cyanotic and limp, and the obstetrician informs you of the presence of thin, nonparticulate meconium staining of the amniotic fluid. After drying, positioning, and suctioning of the mouth and nose, you note that he exhibits active flexion of his extremities and cries vigorously. His heart rate is 96 and respiratory rate is 60, with mild intercostal retractions. His trunk pinks up, but his hands and feet remain dusky and cyanotic.

23. Which of the following actions is **NOT** appropriate for this infant?
    A. deep tracheal suctioning using a meconium aspirator
    B. blow-by oxygen and continued assessment
    C. measurement of blood glucose
    D. continued warming and temperature maintenance
    E. none of the above

24. After 5 minutes, the neonate's APGAR score is 10, yet the infant continues to be tachypneic, with a respiratory rate of 68. Lung auscultation reveals coarse crackles. In the context of the neonate's APGAR score, this neonate's tachypnea is:
    A. evidence of significant meconium aspiration.
    B. transient tachypnea of the newborn (TTN), caused by delayed clearing of excess fluid from the lungs.
    C. indicative of cardiogenic shock.
    D. indicative of a patent *ductus arteriosus*.
    E. none of the above.

25. At 10 minutes post delivery, the infant begins to exhibit brief periods of apnea and lies limply in the radiant warmer. His heart rate is 124 and his core temperature is 98 degrees. You should suspect:
    A. respiratory failure and impending respiratory arrest.
    B. hypovolemia.
    C. hypoglycemia.
    D. sepsis.
    E. asphyxiation due to meconium aspiration.

26. Premature infants are at increased risk for neonatal respiratory distress syndrome due to inadequate:
    A. development of accessory muscles.
    B. stimuli from underdeveloped CO_2 chemoreceptors.
    C. amounts of surfactant.
    D. glycogen reserves.
    E. none of the above.

27. Inadequate amount of surfactant in premature neonates contributes to all of the following **EXCEPT**:
    A. poor lung compliance.
    B. atelectasis.

C. hypoxia.
D. respiratory alkalosis.
E. all answers but D.

28. As supportive care for the neonate with hyaline membrane disease, the critical care paramedic typically provides which of the following?
    A. surfactant replacement therapy
    B. large doses of corticosteroids to accelerate lung development
    C. ventilatory support and supplemental oxygen
    D. inhaled nitric oxide
    E. none of the above

29. Grunting respirations, a reflexive response produced by exhalation against a partially closed glottis, provide PEEP for the neonate in respiratory distress. This is beneficial for which of the following conditions?
    A. atelectasis
    B. poorly developed accessory musculature
    C. increased pliancy of the thoracic cage
    D. hyperventilation
    E. none of the above

30. The mortality rate for neonates with congenital diaphragmatic herniation is:
    A. 85%.
    B. 40–60%.
    C. 25–30%.
    D. 10%.
    E. none of the above.

31. The neonate with congenital diaphragmatic herniation may present clinically with all of the following EXCEPT:
    A. respiratory distress.
    B. unequal lung sounds.
    C. scaphoid abdomen in the first few hours after birth.
    D. wheezing.
    E. none of the above.

32. For the neonate with congenital diaphragmatic herniation, which of the following interventions may NOT be appropriate?
    A. sedation and neuromuscular blockade
    B. endotracheal intubation
    C. bag-valve-mask ventilation
    D. gastric decompression using an orogastric tube
    E. none of the above

33. The most common type of congenital heart defect, occurring in roughly 25% of live births, is:
    A. ventricular septal defect.
    B. atrial septal defect.
    C. patent *ductus arteriosus.*
    D. tetralogy of Fallot.
    E. coarctation of the aorta.

34. Which of the following is NOT a typical clinical feature of congenital defects in the neonate that produce left-to-right shunting?
    A. chamber enlargement
    B. signs of congestive heart failure
    C. fatigue and diaphoresis at feeding
    D. cyanosis
    E. all of the above

35. Incomplete closure of the foramen ovale in neonates results in a congenital:
    A. ventricular septal defect.
    B. atrial septal defect.
    C. patent *ductus arteriosus.*
    D. pulmonary stenosis.
    E. none of the above.

36. A large ventricular septal defect, if evident in the first few hours after birth, most likely will result in which clinical finding?
    A. cyanosis
    B. right ventricular enlargement
    C. global chamber enlargement
    D. right atrial enlargement
    E. left ventricular hypertrophy evident on the ECG

37. Supportive care of the neonate with a large ventricular septal defect and congestive heart failure generally consists of:
    A. inotropes.
    B. vasodilators.
    C. surgical repair of the hole.
    D. fluid restriction and diuretics.
    E. none of the above.

38. Patent *ductus arteriosus*, as a disease process in and of itself, is generally described as:
    A. failure of the *ductus arteriosus* to close after adequate pulmonary circulation has been established.
    B. a direct result of inadequate initial ventilatory pressure due to meconium aspiration.
    C. a direct result of inadequate initial ventilatory pressure due to lack of alveolar surfactant.
    D. a direct result of inadequate systemic vascular resistance.
    E. none of the above.

39. Clinical signs of patent *ductus arteriosus* include all of the following EXCEPT:
    A. respiratory distress.
    B. cyanosis.
    C. fatigue during feeding.
    D. widened pulse pressure.
    E. tachycardia.

40. The neonate with pulmonic stenosis may present with all of the following EXCEPT:
    A. enlargement of the right ventricle.
    B. enlargement of the left ventricle.
    C. dilation of the pulmonary artery.
    D. hypotension.
    E. fatigue during feeding.

41. A neonate with bounding upper extremity pulses and thready or absent lower extremity pulses should be suspected of having:
    A. patent *ductus arteriosus*.
    B. pulmonic stenosis.
    C. aortic stenosis.
    D. coarctation of the aorta.
    E. ventricular septal defect.

42. The congenital heart defects that result in right-to-left shunting, poor pulmonary perfusion, and/or structural deformity of the heart are known collectively as:
    A. obstructive heart defects.
    B. inappropriate flow defects.
    C. cyanotic heart defects.
    D. tetralogy of Fallot.
    E. none of the above.

43. The presence of atrial septal defects, ventricular septal defects, and patent *ductus arteriosus* in neonates with transposition of the great vessels, while fairly common, are usually:
    A. significant comorbid factors.
    B. beneficial, in that they allow intermixing of blood between the right and left sides of the heart.
    C. a grim prognostic finding.
    D. benign.
    E. none of the above.

44. Tetralogy of Fallot is the complex of defects consisting of subaortic ventricular septal defect, right ventricular infundibular stenosis, aortic valve positioned to override the right ventricle, and:
    A. aortic stenosis.
    B. coarctation of the aorta.
    C. patent *ductus arteriosus*.
    D. right ventricular hypertrophy.
    E. atrial septal defect.

45. The most common cyanotic heart defect seen in children beyond infancy is:
    A. tetralogy of Fallot.
    B. transposition of great vessels.
    C. patent *ductus arteriosus.*
    D. coarctation of the aorta.
    E. aortic stenosis.

46. To make a diagnosis of tetralogy of Fallot, which of the following must be present?
    A. significant left-to-right shunting
    B. ventricular septal defect large enough to allow equalization of right and left ventricular pressures
    C. significantly compromised aortic blood flow
    D. pulmonary stenosis causing significant reduction in outflow from the right ventricle
    E. B and D

47. In the neonate with a cyanotic heart defect, which of the following best indicate(s) a chronic condition in which aggressive oxygenation is unnecessary?
    A. normal respiratory effort
    B. bradycardia
    C. normal respiratory rate
    D. normal heart rate
    E. all answers but B

48. Necrotizing enterocolitis (NEC) in the neonate most commonly results from:
    A. ischemic damage to the intestinal lining and bacterial growth.
    B. ingestion of contaminated formula.
    C. ingestion of breast milk in the mother with a bacterial infection.
    D. congenital diaphragmatic herniation.
    E. none of the above.

49. NEC may present with which of the following clinical findings?
    A. decreased or absent bowel sounds
    B. bloody diarrhea
    C. fever
    D. vomiting
    E. all answers but C

50. Treatment of the neonate with NEC includes all of the following EXCEPT:
    A. gastric decompression with an orogastric tube.
    B. fever control.
    C. antibiotics.
    D. fluid maintenance.
    E. correction of electrolyte imbalance.

51. The most common cause of neonatal sepsis is:
    A. lack of sterile technique during delivery.
    B. depressed and/or immature immune system.
    C. maternal gastrointestinal or urinary tract infections.
    D. administration of corticosteroids in the mother in the days preceding birth.
    E. none of the above.

52. Acrocyanosis in the crying newborn is:
    A. normal.
    B. a sign of significant hypoxia.
    C. a sign of cyanotic heart disease.
    D. a sign of hypoperfusion.
    E. none of the above.

53. A relatively benign condition resulting from the neonate's immature liver being unable to efficiently process bilirubin is known as:
    A. cyanosis.
    B. jaundice.
    C. beta-carotene imbalance.
    D. polycythemia.
    E. none of the above.

54. The most common treatment for neonates with extremely high bilirubin levels is:
    A. blood transfusions.
    B. liver transplant.
    C. fluorescent phototherapy.
    D. tincture of time.
    E. none of the above.

55. Rapid sequence induction is rarely used in neonates because:
    A. pharmacologic agents should be avoided in this patient population.
    B. preinduction sedation is usually effective in calming the neonate and reducing the work of breathing, thereby making intubation unnecessary.
    C. depolarizing neuromuscular blockers cause significant serum hyperkalemia in newborns.
    D. neonates are not strong enough to fight the tube.
    E. none of the above.

56. A commonly used alternative vascular access route (other than intraosseous) that may be considered in the newborn is cannulation of the:
    A. internal jugular vein.
    B. subclavian vein.
    C. femoral vein.
    D. umbilical vein.
    E. none of the above.

57. The most common complication (other than infection) of umbilical vein cannulation is:
    A. liver necrosis resulting from insertion of the catheter into the hepatic portal circulation.
    B. volume overload.
    C. perforation of the vein.
    D. loss of patency due to premature closure of the ductus venosus.
    E. none of the above.

58. To maintain temperature control when transporting the neonate, the critical care paramedic should:
    A. increase the ambient cabin temperature.
    B. use warmed blankets and hot water bottles.
    C. use chemical heat packs placed directly against the neonate's skin.
    D. use a neonatal transport isolette.
    E. all of the above.

59. Hypoglycemia in the newborn should initially be treated with:
    A. 20 mL/kg boluses of D5½ NS solution.
    B. 0.5–1.0 g/kg (5–10 mL/kg) of $D_{10}W$ solution.
    C. 0.5–1.0 g/kg (5–10 mL/kg) of $D_{25}W$ solution.
    D. 0.5–1.0 g/kg (5–10 mL/kg) of $D_{50}W$ solution.
    E. maintenance infusion of $D_{10}W$ at 80 mL/kg/day.

60. Administration of high concentration ($D_{25}W$ or $D_{50}W$) dextrose solutions in the neonate:
    A. is often required due to their higher basal metabolic rate and poor glycogen reserves.
    B. is usually only necessary if the mother was taking insulin at the time of birth.
    C. may cause serum hyperosmolarity and cerebral edema.
    D. is acceptable if limited to one dose.
    E. none of the above.

CHAPTER 30

Environmental Emergencies

30: ENVIRONMENTAL EMERGENCIES

DIRECTIONS Each of the questions or incomplete statements below is followed by suggested answers or completions. Select the **one answer** that is best in each case.

1. The critical thermal maximum is generally considered to be:
   A. > 45° C (113° F).
   B. > 43° C (109.4° F).
   C. < 41° C (105.8° F).
   D. > 50° C (122° F).
   E. none of the above.

Make the conversions for questions 2–6:

2. 98.3° F = _____ ° C
3. 35° C = _____ ° F
4. 105° F = _____ ° C
5. 37° C = _____ ° F
6. 91° F = _____ ° C

   A. 98.6
   B. 32.8
   C. 95.0
   D. 40.6
   E. 36.8

7. The part of the diencephalon responsible for body temperature is the:
   A. thalamus.
   B. pons.
   C. hypothalamus.
   D. hyperthalamus.
   E. none of the above.

8. The thermostat for the body is in the _____ region.
   A. anterior
   B. posterior
   C. tuberal
   D. preoptic
   E. suprachiasmatic nucleus

9. Thermoreceptors are located in which body area?
   A. skin
   B. interior vessel walls
   C. core of the body
   D. hypothalamus
   E. all of the above

10. Factors that predispose a person to temperature-related disorders include all of the following EXCEPT:
    A. age of the patient.
    B. health of the patient.
    C. medications.
    D. ethnicity of the patient.
    E. exposure time.

11. Absolute zero is _____.
    A. –460° F
    B. –273° C
    C. 100° C
    D. 0° F
    E. A and B

12. The most common mechanism of heat loss is:
    A. radiation.
    B. conduction.
    C. evaporation.
    D. convection.
    E. none of the above

13. Biochemical processes that use energy specifically to generate heat are termed:
    A. electron transport.
    B. oxidative phosphorylation.
    C. futile cycles.
    D. gluconeogenesis.
    E. protein synthesis.

14. Which of the following statements is FALSE?
    A. All objects not at absolute zero radiate heat.
    B. An object can never actually reach absolute zero due to the first law of thermodynamics.

C. Heat loss occurs from electromagnetic radiation (infrared waves).
D. Heat always moves from a warmer object to a cooler object.
E. Approximately 15% of heat loss is by conduction.

15. Heat loss from air currents passing over the body is called:
    A. radiation.
    B. conduction.
    C. evaporation.
    D. convection.
    E. none of the above.

16. Activation of the sweat glands (sudoriferous and merocrine) usually begins at temperatures greater than _____ degrees F.
    A. 105
    B. 100
    C. 98
    D. 91
    E. none of the above

17. Which of the following increase(s) the basal metabolic rate (BMR)?
    A. thyroxine (T4)
    B. triiodothyronine (T3)
    C. thyroid-stimulating hormone (TSH)
    D. all of the above
    E. A and B

18. Mechanisms that cool the body include all of the following EXCEPT:
    A. vasodilation.
    B. sweating.
    C. slowing of BMR.
    D. piloerection.
    E. none of the above.

19. Stimulation of the *arrector pili* muscles causes:
    A. goose bumps.
    B. activation of the merocrine sweat glands.
    C. activation of the apocrine sweat glands.
    D. all of the above.
    E. B and C.

20. The process of adapting to a new climate is termed:
    A. acclimatization.
    B. sojourning.
    C. cohabitation.
    D. sweating.
    E. none of the above.

21. Which of the following statements is FALSE?
    A. Hyperthermia is a normal physiological response.
    B. The two most common manifestations of hyperthermia encountered in prehospital care are heat exhaustion and heat stroke.
    C. Fever is a normal physiological response.
    D. Heat tetany is due to hyperventilation.
    E. none of the above.

22. Complications of heat exhaustion include:
    A. tachycardia.
    B. headache.
    C. orthostasis.
    D. fatigue and weakness.
    E. all of the above.

23. Heat syncope results from:
    A. sodium loss.
    B. postural hypotension.
    C. systemic hypertension.
    D. hyperventilation.
    E. none of the above.

24. Which of the following is NOT a sign of heat stroke?
    A. core temperature > 40.5° C (104.9° F)
    B. profuse sweating
    C. altered mental status
    D. all of the above
    E. A and C

25. When cooling a victim of heat stroke, the temperature at which active cooling should stop is:
    A. 35° C.
    B. 37° C.
    C. 40° C.
    D. 33° C.
    E. none of the above.

26. Altered mental status is apparent in ____ % of heat stroke patients.
    A. 0
    B. 20
    C. 40
    D. 50
    E. 80

27. Risk factors for hypothermia include all of the following EXCEPT:
    A. alcoholism.
    B. myxedema.
    C. sepsis.
    D. shock.
    E. none of the above.

28. Which of the following is a sign of severe hypothermia?
    A. lack of shivering
    B. lethargy
    C. lack of coordination
    D. A and C
    E. none of the above

29. Which of the following medications do NOT increase the risk of heat stroke?
    A. diuretics
    B. beta blockers
    C. phenothiazines
    D. tricyclic antidepressants
    E. none of the above

30. Most hypothermia patients who die during active rewarming die from:
    A. subarachnoid hemorrhage.
    B. pulseless electrical activity.
    C. ventricular fibrillation.
    D. asystole.
    E. none of the above.

31. Which of the following would be a mechanism of evaporative heat loss?
    A. immersion
    B. snowfall
    C. damp ground
    D. damp clothing
    E. none of the above

32. Hypothermia is typically defined as a core temperature below:
    A. 30° C.
    B. 35° C.
    C. 37° C.
    D. 85° F.
    E. none of the above.

33. Approximately what percentage of hypothermia patients have some ECG abnormality?
    A. 10%
    B. 20%
    C. 40%
    D. 60%
    E. 90%

34. Which of the following statements about frostbite is FALSE?
    A. Wetness may facilitate development of frostbite.
    B. Wind may facilitate development of frostbite.
    C. A freezing environment is not a prerequisite for development of frostbite.
    D. A high altitude may facilitate development of frostbite.
    E. none of the above

35. You are treating a frostbite victim who has waxy skin with multiple vesicles (blisters) filled with blood. This would be classified as _____ frostbite.
    A. first-degree
    B. second-degree
    C. third-degree
    D. fourth-degree
    E. none of the above

36. Which of the following ECG changes is NOT usually associated with hypothermia?
    A. bradycardia (vagally mediated)
    B. T-wave inversion
    C. atrioventricular blocks
    D. prolonged QT intervals
    E. widened QRS complexes

37. Osborne waves are best seen in which of the following ECG leads?
    A. II, III, and AVF
    B. I and III
    C. AVR and AVF
    D. V1–V6
    E. none of the above

38. The breakdown of skeletal muscle in heat stroke is termed:
    A. myoglobinemia.
    B. cardiomyopathy.
    C. hydrophonia.
    D. glomerulonephritis.
    E. rhabdomyolysis.

39. When treating a hypothermic patient in cardiac arrest, which of the following should the critical care paramedic do?
    A. Begin passive rewarming after intubation.
    B. Withhold medications if the core temperature is < 30° C.
    C. Repeat defibrillation every 5 minutes while core temperature is < 30° C.
    D. Slow CPR to 30 compressions a minute.
    E. none of the above

40. A wet drowning is differentiated from a dry drowning by:
    A. gasping, which will cause either laryngospasm or inhalation of fluid.
    B. temperature of the water.
    C. nature of the water (salt or fresh).
    D. age of the victim.
    E. gender of the victim.

41. Approximately what percentage of drownings are dry drownings?
    A. 85%
    B. 10%
    C. 15%
    D. 50%
    E. 60%

42. Which of the following statements is FALSE?
    A. In freshwater drowning, the water moves from the alveolar space to the vascular space.
    B. In salt water drowning, the water moves from the alveolar space to the vascular space.
    C. Fresh water causes destruction of surfactant.
    D. Fresh water results in atelectasis.
    E. In saltwater, immediate washout of surfactant occurs.

43. Treatment of drowning includes all of the following EXCEPT:
    A. CPAP.
    B. PEEP.
    C. intubation.
    D. decompression of the stomach.
    E. permissive hypotension.

44. The difference between the temperatures of two objects is called:
    A. thermal difference.
    B. kinetic imbalance.
    C. thermal equilibrium.
    D. thermal gradient.
    E. kinetic gradient.

45. Which of the following is NOT necessarily a risk factor for nonexertional heat stroke?
    A. extremes in age
    B. underlying chronic illness
    C. exercising in a warm environment
    D. use of certain medications
    E. none of the above

CHAPTER 31
Diving Emergencies

DIRECTIONS

Each of the questions or incomplete statements below is followed by suggested answers or completions. Select the **one answer** that is best in each case.

1. Placing divers underwater at deep depths for an extended period of time is called:
   A. commercial diving.
   B. saturation diving.
   C. equilibrium diving.
   D. artificial diving.
   E. none of the above.

2. 1 atm = _____ mmHg
   A. 360
   B. 720
   C. 760
   D. 1,033
   E. 101.3

3. Pressure is measured in what units?
   A. Pascals
   B. Newtons
   C. pounds per square inch
   D. Daltons
   E. A and C

4. Which of the following statements is true?
   A. As the force increases, the pressure increases.
   B. As the force decreases, the pressure increases.
   C. As the area decreases, the pressure increases.
   D. As the area increases, the pressure increases.
   E. A and C.

5. A diver at 33 feet would be exposed to _____ atmosphere(s).
   A. 1
   B. 2
   C. 3
   D. all of the above
   E. none of the above

6. Which of the following statements about nitrogen is FALSE?
   A. On the surface, nitrogen is considered an inert gas.
   B. Under pressure, nitrogen can have a narcotic effect.
   C. The absorption of nitrogen at depth can cause decompression sickness on ascent.
   D. Nitrogen has an egg-like odor.
   E. none of the above

7. Which of the following factors affect buoyancy?
   A. weight of the object
   B. specific gravity of the liquid
   C. density of the object
   D. A and B
   E. B and C

8. What is the specific gravity of fresh water?
   A. 0.1
   B. 1.0
   C. 10.0
   D. 1:1
   E. none of the above

9. When an object is placed into water, it will displace an amount of water equal to the weight of the water displaced by the object. This phenomenon was discovered by:
   A. Archimedes.
   B. Blaise Pascal.
   C. Sir Isaac Newton.
   D. Johann Carl Friedrich Gauss.
   E. Jean Poiseuille.

10. Most recreational divers breathe:
    A. heliox.
    B. pure oxygen.

C. compressed air.
D. perfluorocarbon.
E. none of the above.

11. Navy SEALS use specialized canisters to remove carbon dioxide from rebreathed air and decrease expelled bubbles. These canisters are referred to as:
    A. washers.
    B. scrubbers.
    C. extractors.
    D. limiters.
    E. capnometers.

12. A long-term effect of excessive pressure while diving is:
    A. dysbaric osteonecrosis (DON).
    B. nitrogen narcosis.
    C. raptures of the deep.
    D. dysbarism.
    E. none of the above.

13. Most cases of nitrogen narcosis occur at depths greater than _____ feet.
    A. 10
    B. 33
    C. 50
    D. 100
    E. 233

14. Which of the following is NOT a sign or symptom of nitrogen narcosis?
    A. deficits in reasoning
    B. problems with judgment
    C. priapism
    D. feeling of well-being
    E. unconsciousness

15. Which of the following will NOT worsen the effects of nitrogen narcosis?
    A. alcohol
    B. depressants (including sea-sickness medications)
    C. hallucinogens
    D. hypothermia
    E. none of the above

16. Which of the following is the best treatment for nitrogen narcosis?
    A. acetazolamide (Diamox)
    B. recompression
    C. phenytoin
    D. mannitol
    E. none of the above

17. Decompression sickness is also known as:
    A. the bends.
    B. dysbarism.
    C. caisson disease.
    D. diver's paralysis.
    E. all of the above.

18. The gas that causes decompression sickness is:
    A. water vapor.
    B. oxygen.
    C. nitrogen.
    D. carbon dioxide.
    E. none of the above.

19. Which of the following is NOT a common sign or symptom of decompression sickness?
    A. joint pain
    B. muscle pain
    C. headache
    D. vertigo
    E. dysrhythmia

20. The "chokes" is a condition that results from:
    A. gas expansion in the cranial vault.
    B. pulmonary capillary occlusions.
    C. laryngeal edema from gas expansion in the respiratory tree.
    D. hypothermia in the esophagus.
    E. none of the above.

21. The definitive treatment for decompression sickness is:
    A. intra-arterial hydrogen peroxide.
    B. hyperbaric recompression.
    C. CPAP/BiPAP.
    D. loop diuretics.
    E. vasodilators.

22. Seizures or severe cramping in decompression sickness should be treated with:
    A. diazepam.
    B. midazolam.
    C. phenytoin.
    D. A and B.
    E. B and C.

23. Which of the following is NOT true of high-pressure neurologic syndrome (HPNS)?
    A. It begins as paraparesis.
    B. It is associated with the breathing of helium.
    C. It is almost exclusively seen in commercial diving.
    D. It is also known as "helium tremors."
    E. It occurs at depths exceeding 400 feet.

24. Prevention of HPNS includes:
    A. introduction of mild nitrogen narcosis.
    B. decreasing the concentration of hydrogen.
    C. increasing the concentration of oxygen.
    D. administration of a mild sedative prior to the dive.
    E. A and D.

25. The Divers Alert Network (DAN) is associated with:
    A. Margaritaville in Key West, Florida.
    B. Harvard University in Cambridge, Massachusetts.
    C. Scripps Institute in San Diego, California.
    D. Duke University in Durham, North Carolina.
    E. Cairns University in Cairns, Queensland, Australia.

26. Poorly maintained, poorly vented, or older gasoline-powered air compressors:
    A. have a tendency to suck in their own exhaust.
    B. allow the entrance of carbon monoxide into the dive gas mix.
    C. decrease the amount of oxygen in the dive gas mix.
    D. A and B.
    E. A and C.

27. Injuries associated with ascent include:
    A. mediastinal emphysema.
    B. arterial gas embolism.
    C. pulmonary expansion injury.
    D. pulmonary barotrauma.
    E. all of the above.

28. The definitive treatment for pulmonary overexpansion injuries is:
    A. decompression in a chamber.
    B. CPAP/BiPAP.
    C. potassium-sparing diuretics.
    D. vasodilators.
    E. none of the above.

29. Signs and symptoms of saltwater aspiration syndrome include all of the following EXCEPT:
    A. dyspnea.
    B. cough.
    C. diplopia.
    D. hemoptysis.
    E. radiographic changes.

30. Which of the following marine animals can bite?
    A. dolphins
    B. seals

C. moray eels

D. whales

E. all of the above

31. Treatment for a sea-snake bite should include all of the following EXCEPT:
    A. submersion in hot water (105–115° F) for 30–90 minutes to deactivate the poison.
    B. immediate administration of analgesics.
    C. administration of antivenom.
    D. ventilations and chest compressions as needed.
    E. the pressure-immobilization technique.

32. _____ is the taxonomic phylum that includes jellyfish.
    A. Cnidaria
    B. Porifera
    C. Annelida
    D. Mollusca
    E. none of the above

33. _____ are organelles that line the tentacles of stinging creatures like the Portuguese man-of-war and shoot out venomous threadlike fibers.
    A. Cytokines
    B. Nematocysts
    C. Células Tacañas
    D. Cellules Cuisantes
    E. none of the above

34. Paramedics in coastal regions of Queensland, Australia, carry an antivenom for a jellyfish known as _____ or _____ that has been considered to be the most deadly animal in the world with the ability to invade blood vessels and cause death in seconds.
    A. Portuguese man-of-war, fire coral
    B. fire coral, lion's mane
    C. lion's mane, sea wasp
    D. sea wasp, box jellyfish
    E. box jellyfish, sea anemone

35. Treatment for a jellyfish sting should include all of the following EXCEPT which of the following?
    A. Remove as many tentacles as possible by rinsing with seawater.
    B. Rinse with fresh water to prevent venom discharge.
    C. Deactivate stinging cells with vinegar.
    D. Apply urine if other chemicals are unavailable.
    E. Apply shaving cream and shave the tentacles away.

36. Which of the following statements about ciguatera is FALSE?
    A. It is found in small plankton that inhabit ocean reefs.
    B. It accumulates as larger reef fish eat smaller reef fish.
    C. Signs and symptoms develop with 15 minutes to 3 hours of ingestion.
    D. Prehospital treatment includes the antidote CAG.
    E. It causes an unexplained reversal of hot and cold perception.

37. Which of the following statements about scombroid poisoning is FALSE?
    A. It does not occur in sushi and sashimi.
    B. It is found in tuna and related open-water species.
    C. It results from decomposition of the muscle of the fish and subsequent bacterial activity.
    D. It involves development of large amounts of histamines.
    E. Occasionally there is a metallic or peppery taste to tainted fish.

38. The most common cause of death in divers is:
    A. nitrogen narcosis.
    B. marine animal injury.
    C. drowning.
    D. coronary artery disease.
    E. none of the above.

39. Which of the following is NOT a major factor in diving deaths?
    A. human error
    B. environmental causes
    C. equipment failure
    D. demonic possession
    E. none of the above

40. During decompression treatment in a hyperbaric chamber, most patients are taken to a pressure of:
    A. 1 atmosphere.
    B. 2–3 atmospheres.
    C. 10–12 atmospheres.
    D. 14–16 atmospheres.
    E. 4 atmospheres and pressure is then increased every 10 minutes by 1 atmosphere until improvement is seen.

CHAPTER 32
Toxicological Emergencies

32: TOXICOLOGICAL EMERGENCIES

DIRECTIONS Each of the questions or incomplete statements below is followed by suggested answers or completions. Select the **one answer** that is best in each case.

1. What is the contact number for United States poison control centers?
   A. 1-800-223-1212
   B. 1-800-222-1222
   C. 1-800-222-1223
   D. 1-800-233-1233
   E. 1-800-222-1333

2. The many roles of poison control centers (PCCs) include:
   A. assistance to citizens and medical professionals.
   B. telephone triage.
   C. information dissemination.
   D. management direction for toxicological emergencies.
   E. all of the above.

3. Drug abuse may be defined as:
   A. intentional abuse of medications.
   B. intentional abuse of illicit drugs.
   C. drug use that results in addiction, physical dependence, and/or tolerance.
   D. all of the above.
   E. A and B only.

4. The syndrome characterized by one or more behaviors that may include impaired control over drug use, compulsive use, and continued use despite obvious harm, and cravings is called:
   A. tolerance.
   B. physical dependence.
   C. addiction.
   D. toxidrome.
   E. withdrawal.

5. The syndrome in which withdrawal symptoms can be caused by abrupt cessation, rapid dose reduction, decreased blood level of drug, or administration of an antagonist is called:
   A. tolerance.
   B. physical dependence.
   C. addiction.
   D. toxidrome.
   E. abuse.

6. A state of adaptation in which exposure to a drug induces changes that result in a diminution of one or more of the drug's effects over time is called:
   A. tolerance.
   B. physical dependence.
   C. addiction.
   D. abuse.
   E. withdrawal.

7. A syndrome that requires both a preexisting physical adaptation to a specific drug and decreasing concentrations or availability of that drug is called:
   A. tolerance.
   B. abuse.
   C. addiction.
   D. toxidrome.
   E. withdrawal.

8. A constellation of clinical signs and symptoms that together reliably suggest an exposure to a specific drug class is called:
   A. abuse.
   B. physical dependence.
   C. addiction.
   D. toxidrome.
   E. withdrawal.

9. The major illicit drug groups include:
   1. hallucinogens.
   2. sympathomimetics.

3. narcotics.
4. sedative-hypnotics.
5. marijuana.

A. 1, 2, and 3
B. 2, 3, and 4
C. 1, 3, 4, and 5
D. 1, 2, 4, and 5
E. 1, 2, 3, 4, and 5

10. _____ are compounds that involve serotonergic effects and lead to distorted sensorium, hallucinations, and "to touch within" effects.
    A. Hallucinogens
    B. Opioids
    C. Hypnotics
    D. Benzodiazepines
    E. Amphetamines

11. Commonly abused hallucinogens may include LSD as well as:
    A. psilocybin.
    B. Ecstasy.
    C. mescaline.
    D. all of the above.
    E. B and C.

12. Clinical effects of hallucinogens include all of the following EXCEPT:
    A. confusion.
    B. ataxia.
    C. hypotension.
    D. labile emotions.
    E. teeth clenching.

13. A class of drugs that mimic the effects of endogenous epinephrine and norepinephrine is:
    A. hallucinogens.
    B. narcotics.
    C. hypnotics.
    D. sympathomimetics.
    E. benzodiazepines.

14. Toxic effects of drugs such as cocaine, amphetamine, and methamphetamine can include:
    A. intracranial hemorrhage.
    B. seizure.
    C. myocardial infarction.
    D. hyperthermia.
    E. all of the above.

15. The components of a toxidrome profile include:
    A. classification of drug.
    B. specific toxins.
    C. signs/symptoms.
    D. treatment.
    E. all of the above.

16. Treatment for the cholinergic toxidrome may include:
    A. pralidoxime (2-pam).
    B. glycopyrrolate.
    C. atropine.
    D. all of the above.
    E. A and B.

17. The drug class that includes codeine is:
    A. anticholinergic.
    B. opioid (narcotic).
    C. cholinergic.
    D. sympathomimetic.
    E. none of the above.

18. Opiates are naturally occurring compounds derived from:
    A. foxglove.
    B. impatiens.
    C. poppies.
    D. goldenrod.
    E. roses.

19. Fentanyl and morphine are members of what class of drugs?
    A. anticholinergics
    B. cholinergics
    C. GABA-agonists
    D. sympathomimetics
    E. opioids

20. You have just landed at the scene of a single-vehicle rollover in the desert. Your 18-year-old patient was the restrained driver. He has no visible injuries, but has presented to the BLS crews on scene as unconscious and in respiratory arrest. The patient has been packaged with spinal precautions prior to your arrival and is being ventilated via BVM with 100% O_2.

    You begin your initial assessment and prepare to secure the airway prior to lift-off. You find no obvious trauma, but the patient is pale, cool, and diaphoretic. Vital signs are HR = 124 per minute; RR = 0 per minute; BP = 88/46 mmHg; SpO_2 = 96%; pupils = pinpoint.

    Based on your assessment, your continuing care plan might include:
    A. O_2/BVM, ETT, IV access, ECG, PASG, vasopressor (prn).
    B. O_2/BVM, IV access, 0.4mg naloxone IVP, ECG, ETT/other (prn).
    C. ETT, O_2/BVM, ECG, CPR, IV access, cardiac drugs (prn).
    D. ETT, O_2/BVM, ECG, SpO_2, IV access, drugs (prn).
    E. none of the above.

21. Benzodiazepines, barbiturates, chloral hydrate, propofol, and diphenhydramine are all included in what drug toxidrome?
    A. cholinergic
    B. opioid
    C. sedative-hypnotic
    D. hypoxic
    E. none of the above

22. Administration of naloxone to a patient compromised by the use of speedballs may have undesired effects, including:
    A. agitation.
    B. tachycardia.
    C. hypertension.
    D. all of the above.
    E. A and B.

23. Dihydropyridines, benzothiapines, and phenylalkylamines are what type of medications?
    A. salicylates (ASAs)
    B. calcium channel blockers (CCBs)
    C. monoamine oxidase inhibitors (MAOIs)
    D. selective serotonin reuptake inhibitors (SSRIs)
    E. nonsteroidal anti-inflammatory drugs (NSAIDs)

24. Your 15-year-old patient is exhibiting signs of severe hypotension and tachycardia. She denies any previous medical history, allergies, or regular medications. Her grandmother states that the patient has been acting strangely since breakfast, is known to have abused prescription medications in the past, and a bottle of the grandmother's cardiac medication is missing. Investigating, you find an empty pill bottle in the patient's bedroom. Based on presentation and discovery of the pill bottle, you have a high index of suspicion that the patient has ingested a toxic dose of:
    A. hydrocodone.
    B. verapamil.
    C. diphenhydramine.
    D. digoxin.
    E. none of the above.

25. Digitalis toxicity is a result of interference with the:
    A. sodium-potassium pump.
    B. normal calcium levels in blood.

C. efficient breakdown of CO_2.

D. blood glucose levels.

E. none of the above.

26. Your patient is suffering from nausea, vomiting, and generalized malaise. Her vital signs are consistent with mild cardiogenic shock, and the ECG is showing an apparent Mobitz Type I heart block. Her medications include 81 mg ASA/day, a potassium supplement, digitalis, furosemide, and nitro (prn). As you begin oxygen therapy and check vital signs, you begin to form your list of differentials. Included is/are:

    A. congestive heart failure.
    B. electrolyte imbalance.
    C. digitalis toxicity.
    D. all of the above.
    E. B and C.

27. Your 68-year-old patient is diagnosed with digitalis toxicity. The physician has ordered 6.0 mg glucagon, IVP. Observing the patient post administration, you note increasing hypotension. The physician further orders a bolus of 250 mL 0.9% NaCl, but the patient's BP is not improving. Based on your knowledge of this situation, you suspect the physician's next order will be for administration of:

    A. sodium bicarbonate.
    B. placement of an intra-arterial balloon pump.
    C. norepinephrine.
    D. desipramine.
    E. none of the above.

28. The mnemonic associated with the tricyclic toxidrome is known as "three Cs and an A," which stands for:

    A. coma, cardiogenic shock, calcium overload, and alkalosis.
    B. coma, convulsions, cardiac dysrhythmias, and acidosis.
    C. cardiac dysrhythmias, calcium deficiency, catatonia, and acidosis.
    D. calcium deficiency, catatonia, convulsions, and alkalosis.
    E. catatonia, convulsions, calcium overload, and acidosis.

29. The most important toxic effect of tricyclic antidepressants (TCAs) is _____, causing QRS prolongation, cardiac dysrhythmias, and seizures.

    A. beta inhibition
    B. adrenergic blockage
    C. calcium channel innervation
    D. sodium channel blockade
    E. potassium channel inhibition

30. _____ relieve depression by blocking metabolization of the neurotransmitters dopamine, norepinephrine, and serotonin.

    A. TCAs
    B. MAOIs
    C. SSRIs
    D. CCBs
    E. ASAs

31. MAOIs can have serious adverse effects in conjunction with use or ingestion of other substances. Among these substances are:

    A. foods containing tyramine.
    B. SSRIs.
    C. amphetamines.
    D. all of the above.
    E. B and C.

32. In the emergent setting, the critical care paramedic's treatment for a victim of MAOI toxicity could include:

    A. oxygen.
    B. benzodiazepines.
    C. sodium channel blockers.
    D. all of the above.
    E. A and B only.

33. Commonly used _____ include buproprion, trazadone, fluoxetine, and mirtazipine.
    A. MAOIs
    B. TCAs
    C. SSRIs
    D. CCBs
    E. ASAs

34. You are working in a psychiatric center and are called to assess a 28-year-old male patient with a history of suicidal ideation and clinical depression. He is presenting with an altered mental state, severe hypertension, and mild hyperthermia and is myoclonic. After conferring with the doctor, you decide to treat him with oxygen by nasal cannula, IV hydration, IM benzodiazepine, and rapid sequence induction (RSI) with an endotrachial tube to protect his airway. You chose this pathway, because you believe the patient is suffering from:
    A. TCA toxicity.
    B. serotonin syndrome.
    C. lithium toxicity.
    D. MAOI toxicity.
    E. none of the above.

35. The drug lithium has a very narrow therapeutic window. If your patient is suffering from toxic exposure, you may need to treat the patient for side effects that include:
    A. tremor, ataxia and rigidity.
    B. delirium and myoclonus.
    C. coma, hypotension, and seizures.
    D. nausea, vomiting and dizziness.
    E. all of the above.

36. Benzodiazepines, phenytoin, carbamazepine, valproic acid, and gabapentin all fall into what class of drugs?
    A. MAOIs
    B. SSRIs
    C. anticonvulsants
    D. antidepressants
    E. antihypertensives

37. The most common toxic effects of benzodiazepines are:
    A. CNS depression.
    B. respiratory compromise.
    C. hyperthermia.
    D. A and B.
    E. A and C.

38. Your 8-year-old male patient is presenting in the ED for a severe headache that started earlier at school. The patient is known to have "absence seizures," but the school nurse called his mother because this time he became extremely lethargic and was also complaining of pain in his legs and arms. Today is the first manifestation like this, so his mother brought him directly from school to the ED for evaluation.

    As you begin your interview, the patient starts to exhibit signs of an uncontrollable tremor on the right side of his body. You place the patient in a left lateral position and ask the mother about his medications. She tells you he started taking phenytoin 4 months ago. When you ask if she has the bottle, she tells you her son has control of his medications, and she thinks it is probably at home.

    The patient is now semiconscious and very cold to the touch. As you begin to manage the airway, you realize you may be looking at signs and symptoms that are consistent with:
    A. CVA.
    B. subdural bleed.
    C. accidental overdose.
    D. psychotic break.
    E. none of the above.

39. When trying to determine the stage of acetaminophen (APAP) overdose, it is important to establish a:
    A. reason.
    B. type.
    C. time line.

D. route.

E. none of the above.

40. Match the following signs and symptoms with the appropriate stage of APAP overdose.

   a. _____ recovery or hepatic failure, death
   b. _____ hepatic/renal failure, coagulopathy, hypoglycemia, and/or shock
   c. _____ upper right quadrant pain
   d. _____ nausea, vomiting, abdominal pain

   A. stage I (0.5–24 hrs)
   B. stage II (24–48 hrs)
   C. stage III (2–3 days)
   D. stage IV (2 days to 8 weeks)

41. Definitive treatment for acetaminophen overdose is administration of:

   A. sodium bicarbonate.
   B. calcium carbonate.
   C. *n*-acetylcysteine.
   D. apapcysteine.
   E. A and B.

42. An over-the-counter (OTC) drug class that specifically interferes with energy production and causes metabolic acidsois is:

   A. ASA.
   B. APAP.
   C. NSAID.
   D. AVPU.
   E. none of the above.

43. Acute salicylate poisoning can progress from upset stomach to death in rapid progression when large doses are ingested; however, it can have the same results with chronic low-level use. Among other things, salicylates can cause vomiting, tachycardia, and diaphoresis, and all of the following EXCEPT:

   A. hypothermia.
   B. cardiac dysrhythmias.
   C. pulmonary edema.
   D. delirium.
   E. seizures.

44. As a critical care paramedic, you know that treatment for salicylate overdose is time dependent and important for preservation of vital function. Treatment in the field includes oxygen therapy, IV hydration, and possible administration of sodium bicarbonate. Definitive treatment may also include:

   A. serum acidization.
   B. urine desalinization.
   C. possible hemodialysis.
   D. all of the above.
   E. A and C.

45. Your 16-year-old female patient has ingested an entire bottle of cold medication containing dextromethorphan. She is exhibiting dizziness, nystagmus, and ataxia and is having hallucinations. Your treatment is mostly supportive, but her condition may progress to the point that you need to begin more aggressive therapy. Among the debilitating issues that may be present are:

   A. rhabdomyolysis.
   B. serotonin syndrome.
   C. hyperthermia.
   D. all of the above.
   E. A and C.

46. OTC "natural" or "herbal" products carry several risks. Among them are the lack of verification of individual ingredients, their ratios, and lack of testing for biological effects, as well as little-to-no knowledge of:

   A. long term side effects.
   B. drug interaction(s).
   C. potential manufacturing deficits.
   D. all of the above.
   E. A and B.

47. Abnormal sequelae that may be a result of herbal ingestion are varied and range from relatively benign (GI symptoms) to lethal (cardiac dysrhythmias). It is important to know what potential problems there may be with concomitant drug use, whether OTC or prescription. Among these potential problems are:
    A. symptoms of digitalis toxicity.
    B. bradycardia.
    C. heart blocks not responsive to atropine.
    D. hypokalemia.
    E. A, B, and C.

48. According to experts, the extent of dermal and mucosal injury from caustic agents normally depends on several factors, including:
    1. alkalinity.
    2. concentration.
    3. temperature.
    4. acidity.
    5. volume.
    6. duration of exposure.

    A. 1, 2, 3, and 4
    B. 2, 3, 4, and 5
    C. 1, 2, 5, and 6
    D. 1, 2, 3, and 5
    E. 2, 4, 5, and 6

49. The leading cause of death in the United States from nonpharmaceutical exposures is from ingestion of:
    A. corrosives.
    B. alkalis.
    C. acids.
    D. desiccants.
    E. none of the above.

50. Sodium hypochlorite, ammonia, hair dyes, and lime are examples of alkalines that can cause:
    A. coagulation necrosis.
    B. hyperthermic necrosis.
    C. liquefaction necrosis.
    D. all of the above.
    E. none of the above.

51. The formation of eschar after an acidic exposure may:
    A. extend the damage.
    B. limit the damage.
    C. cause less scarring.
    D. smell bad.
    E. have no effect.

52. Signs and symptoms of corrosive inhalation or ingestion can include:
    A. cough and stridor.
    B. esophageal or gastric rupture.
    C. chest pain.
    D. all of the above.
    E. A and C.

53. The primary concern of the critical care paramedic when managing patients with caustic exposure is:
    A. the safety of all involved.
    B. airway management.
    C. IV access.
    D. respiratory support.
    E. cleansing the exposure site.

54. It is 2300 hours. You are working in a pediatric intensive care unit and intake a 4-year-old male patient who is being admitted for pain, drooling, anorexia, and dysphagia. The parents state these symptoms have come on over the past 2 weeks and seem more intense during the night. You ask the parents about the potential for the patient having swallowed something unobserved, such as a toy or a cleaning agent. The parents deny this possibility, and since the child is sedated they leave for the night. Based on previous calls in the field, you recognize that the patient's signs and

symptoms may be due to a corrosive exposure. The next day when you return for your shift you are not surprised to be told that testing revealed the patient swallowed a:
   A. paper clip.
   B. penny.
   C. watch battery.
   D. marble.
   E. tiddly wink.

55. The toxic alcohols _____, _____, and _____ are all associated with significant morbidity and mortality.
   A. ethanol, methanol, isopropranolol
   B. ethylene glycol, ethanol, methanol
   C. isopropanol, methanol, ethylene glycol
   D. ethanol, isopropanol, methanol
   E. none of the above

56. Match the following substances with their most commonly available sources.
   a. _____ ethanol
   b. _____ methanol
   c. _____ ethylene glycol
   d. _____ isopropanol
   A. automotive antifreeze
   B. rubbing alcohol, disinfectant solutions
   C. beer, wine, liquors, colognes
   D. windshield fluid/antifreeze, paint removers, moonshine

57. Apparently intoxicated patients should be evaluated for a constellation of other syndromes including potential for trauma, other substance abuse and:
   A. chronic medical conditions.
   B. hazardous/toxic exposures.
   C. psychiatric disorders.
   D. environmental exposures.
   E. all of the above.

58. The agency that requires that the material safety data sheet (MSDS) for every potentially hazardous substance accompany it, be printed on the label, or be made accessible to all employees is:
   A. MSHA.
   B. OSHA.
   C. NIOSH.
   D. EPS.
   E. DOT.

59. The MSDS for a hazardous material should include (at minimum) the chemical name, brand name, health effects, and:
   A. ISBN number.
   B. CAS number.
   C. NTSA number.
   D. DOT number.
   E. NFPA number.

60. The clinical effects of _____ build over time, are varied, and can mimic many medical conditions, including viral illnesses. The most prevalent and common symptoms are headache, dizziness, nausea and vomiting, confusion, and hypoxia.
   A. hydrogen sulfide
   B. toluene
   C. carbon monoxide
   D. benzene
   E. all of the above

61. Gases that have a nearly immediate effect on the respiratory and cardiac system may include:
   A. benzene.
   B. toluene.
   C. hydrogen sulfide.
   D. cyanide.
   E. all of the above.

62. Patients exposed to a high level of carbon monoxide can expect to experience delirium and syncope once the CO level reaches _____% in the bloodstream.
    A. 10–20
    B. 20–30
    C. 30–40
    D. 40–50
    E. 60–70

63. Your patient has been exposed to cyanide and is experiencing severe hypoxia. En route to the hospital you can expect the patient to exhibit continued deterioration, including symptoms of metabolic acidosis, cardiovascular collapse, coma, and death.
    Your immediate concern(s) and treatment should be:
    A. accessing an antidote kit.
    B. gaining a secure airway.
    C. starting an IV.
    D. diesel bolus.
    E. A and B.

64. You are transporting a 52-year-old female patient who has had prolonged vapor and dermal exposure to hydrofluoric acid while cleaning rust out of the porcelain toilets in the ladies' gym. She is coughing uncontrollably and complaining of excruciating pain in her hands and eyes. In addition to supportive treatment, oxygen therapy, and IV access, your treatment modality could include:
    A. milk.
    B. cheese.
    C. magnesium.
    D. calcium carbonate.
    E. all of the above.

65. Modern warfare agents fall into two groups. They are:
    A. airborne and chemical.
    B. chemical and biological.
    C. biological and bloodborne.
    D. bloodborne and airborne.
    E. airborne and biological.

66. Tabun, Sarin, and Soman are nerve agents that are _____ compounds.
    A. vesicant
    B. lacrimator
    C. organophosphate
    D. A and B
    E. B and C

67. For any warfare agents, prehospital and clinical concerns should be to prevent secondary contamination to health care workers and to initiate immediate:
    A. drug therapy.
    B. decontamination.
    C. IV access.
    D. A and C.
    E. all of the above.

68. You respond to the local police department to treat a person exposed to capsaicin spray. On your arrival the patient appears to be having severe respiratory distress far beyond the expected response. He is also complaining of itching. The patient has no known prior medical history, and you suspect he is experiencing an:
    A. overreaction.
    B. anaphylactic reaction.
    C. undocumented reaction.
    D. all of the above.
    E. none of the above.

69. Warfarin and other similar agents are intended to:
    A. inhibit platelet aggregation.
    B. inhibit the sodium-potassium pump.
    C. inhibit serotonin reuptake.
    D. increase platelet aggregation.
    E. none of the above.

70. Patients experiencing symptomatic tachycardia or who are in asystole after known

exposure to hydrocarbons should receive basic life support measures and **SHOULD** be treated with _____, but **NOT** with _____.

A. beta drugs, norepinephrine
B. beta blockers, epinephrine
C. alpha drugs, norepinephrine
D. alpha blockers, epinephrine
E. calcium channel blockers, epinephrine

71. Metals capable of causing acute-onset toxicity include, but are not limited to:
    1. lead
    2. cadmium
    3. arsenic
    4. iron
    5. mercury
    6. nickel

    A. 1, 3, 4, and 5
    B. 2, 4, and 6
    C. 1, 2, 4, and 6
    D. 2, 3, and 5
    E. 1, 2, 3, 4, 5, and 6

72. Treatment of scombroid poisoning includes oxygen therapy, antiemetics, and:
    A. beta blockers.
    B. calcium channel blockers.
    C. diphenhydramine.
    D. A and C.
    E. none of the above.

73. Of the following, which are potentially lethal to humans in any quantity?
    1. Christmas cactus
    2. poison ivy
    3. oleander
    4. water hemlock
    5. psilocybin spp
    6. *gyromitra esculenta*

    A. 1, 3, and 5
    B. 2, 4, and 6
    C. 3, 4, and 6
    D. 1, 5, and 6
    E. 2, 3, 4, and 5

74. Venomous snakes in the United States fall into two categories: pit vipers and coral snakes. Pit vipers include:
    A. water moccasins.
    B. rattlesnakes.
    C. copperheads.
    D. all of the above.
    E. B and C.

75. The use of a tourniquet, ice, or suction is _____ in case of snake bite.
    A. indicated
    B. mandatory
    C. contraindicated
    D. optional
    E. advised

76. Most patients being treated for snake envenomation will benefit from IV fluids, analgesics, and antiemetics; however, patients receiving antivenin are at high risk for _____ and should be monitored closely by the critical care paramedic during transport.
    A. gastroenteritis
    B. hyperthermia
    C. anaphylaxis
    D. phlebitis
    E. rhinitis

77. *Hymenoptera* is a large order of animals that includes:
    A. bees.
    B. wasps.
    C. ants.
    D. all of the above.
    E. A and B.

78. Lactrodectism is another term for _____ envenomation.
    A. rattlesnake
    B. African bee
    C. black widow spider
    D. brown recluse spider
    E. all of the above

79. Emergency treatment for black widow spider envenomation may include:
    A. supportive therapy.
    B. analgesics.
    C. benzodiazepines.
    D. antivenin.
    E. all of the above.

80. The most significant effects of brown recluse spider envenomation, aside from tissue necrosis at the injection site, include:
    A. systemic hemolysis.
    B. renal shutdown.
    C. cardiac arrest.
    D. all of the above.
    E. A and C.

81. You are treating an envenomation site with 5% acetic acid, or vinegar. What kind of event are you involved in?
    A. spider bite
    B. sea snake bite
    C. nematocyst attack
    D. African bee attack
    E. none of the above

CHAPTER 33
Weapons of Mass Destruction

DIRECTIONS: Each of the questions or incomplete statements below is followed by suggested answers or completions. Select the **one answer** that is best in each case.

1. _____ is a term that describes both common and unusual industrial agents, along with other potentially toxic chemicals, readily available in society.
   A. Chemical, biological, radiological, nuclear, explosive (CBRNE)
   B. Agents of opportunity (AO)
   C. Toxic Industrial Materials/Toxic Industrial Chemicals (TIM/TIC)
   D. Weapons of mass destruction (WMD)
   E. all of the above

2. The mnemonic _____ is used to represent nuclear, biological, radiological, explosive, and/or chemical agents.
   A. RAID
   B. WMD
   C. CBRNE
   D. all of the above
   E. none of the above

3. Experts generally agree that the most likely threats of chemical terrorism involve:
   A. TIC/TIM incidents.
   B. weapons of mass destruction.
   C. search and rescue services.
   D. agents of opportunity.
   E. none of the above.

4. _____ are agents or substances that can cause illness or injury to one, several, or many exposed victims.
   A. Specialized environmental radiation substances (SERS)
   B. Weapons of mass destruction (WMD)
   C. Airborne infectious medical surfactants (AIMS)
   D. Cardiogenic respiratory anaphylactic prions (CRAP)
   E. Radiological airborne infectious diseases (RAID)

5. To ensure that the crew is not exposed to any hazardous substance, any casualty of a CBRNE incident must be thoroughly decontaminated and must not be a risk for:
   A. out-gassing.
   B. pre-gassing.
   C. in-gassing.
   D. slo-gassing.
   E. off-gassing.

6. TIC and TIM stand for:
   A. toxic industrial carbons; temperature-involved materials.
   B. toxic industrial chemicals; toxic industrial materials.
   C. thermal-involved chemicals; toxic industrial materials.
   D. temperature-immolated chemicals; toxic infiltrating materials.
   E. toxic infiltrating chemicals; temperature-immolated materials.

7. Patients who have ingested or aspirated hazardous substances may give off toxic vapors from the:
   A. cardiovascular or digestive system.
   B. respiratory or immune system.
   C. gastrointestinal or pulmonary tract.
   D. muscle or nerve cells.
   E. urinary or digestive tract.

8. Treatment modalities during transport of plague, smallpox, or inhalational anthrax victims are likely to be no different than for a _____ patient.
   A. SARS
   B. avian flu
   C. chickenpox
   D. all of the above
   E. A and B

9. Nerve agents are chemical weapons (CWs) or industrial chemicals that inhibit the uptake of _____ and affect central nervous system (CNS) function.

   A. cholinesterase
   B. adrenaline
   C. serotonin
   D. acetylcholinesterase
   E. none of the above

10. Chemical weapons, like all other hazardous materials, may exist as solids, liquids, or gases, depending on:

    A. storage modality.
    B. temperature.
    C. pressure.
    D. all of the above.
    E. B and C.

11. Classic military nerve agents include:
    1. Soman.
    2. Tabun.
    3. Sarin.
    4. mustard.
    5. phosgene.
    6. VX.

    A. 1, 2, 3, and 5
    B. 2, 3, 4, and 5
    C. 2, 3, 4, and 6
    D. 1, 2, 3, and 6
    E. 1, 2, 3, 4, 5, and 6

12. ACh is a neurotransmitter that affects the _____ receptor site(s).

    A. muscarinic
    B. nicotinic
    C. enbolic
    D. all of the above
    E. A and B

13. If there is no timely intervention when a nerve gas binds permanently to acetylcholinesterase, a process known as _____ occurs, resulting in permanent binding that cannot be reversed.

    A. crowning
    B. aging
    C. synthesizing
    D. refraction
    E. none of the above

14. A key difference between pesticide types is that aging with **ORGANOPHOSPHATE PESTICIDES** _____, while aging with **CARBAMATE PESTICIDES** _____.

    A. occurs at various rates; occurs incompletely
    B. is similar to military nerve agents; is almost always reversible
    C. occurs very slowly; is never reversible
    D. is slower than with military nerve agents; occurs quickly and completely
    E. A and B

15. Patients exposed to organophosphate compounds will suffer clinical effects associated with uncontrolled stimulation of the:
    1. smooth muscles.
    2. skeletal muscles.
    3. central nervous system.
    4. peripheral nervous system.
    5. exocrine glands.
    6. endocrine glands.

    A. 1, 2, 3, and 5
    B. 2, 3, 4, and 5
    C. 3, 4, 5, and 6
    D. 1, 3, 5, and 6
    E. 1, 2, 3, 4, 5, and 6

16. The mnemonic "SLUDGE" is intended to represent signs and symptoms of organophosphate poisoning. The letters stand for:
    A. salivation, levitation, uremia, dysrhythmia, glomerulitis, expectoration.
    B. salination, lividity, uteralgia, defecation, gangrene, elimination.
    C. salivation, lacrimation, urinary incontinence, diarrhea, gastric upset, excessive secretions.
    D. salubrity, levity, upper respiratory secretions, diuresis, glossitis, electrolysis.
    E. none of the above.

17. Treatment for patients with significant exposure to organophosphate compounds should include:
    1. airway management.
    2. bronchodilators.
    3. atropine.
    4. benzodiazepine therapy.
    5. 2-PamCL.
    6. corticosteroid therapy.

    A. 1, 2 and 3
    B. 1, 2, and 4
    C. 2, 3, and 4
    D. 1, 3, 4, and 5
    E. 2, 3, 5, and 6

18. Pulmonary agents, such as chlorine and phosgene, are commonly distributed in _____ form.
    A. liquid
    B. vapor
    C. solid
    D. all of the above
    E. none of the above

19. Chlorine, when it reacts with water, rapidly forms _____ and _____ acids.
    A. hypochloride, hypochlorous
    B. hypochlorous, hydrochloric
    C. hydrochloride, hypochlorate
    D. hydrochloric, hypochlorite
    E. hydrochlorus, hypochlorate

20. Inhaled _____ immediately reacts with moisture in the airway tissues to form acid with resulting chemical burns. Inhaled _____ also converts to acid but at a much slower rate so that tissue damage and symptoms may not be recognized for some time after exposure.
    A. phosgene, chlorine
    B. chloride, carbon monoxide
    C. phosgene, chlorine
    D. chlorine, phosgene
    E. carbon monoxide, phosgene

21. Treatment of bronchospasm resulting from toxic pulmonary exposure may include administration of _____. However, initial empiric use of _____ is **NOT** recommended.
    A. beta-2 bronchodilators, antibiotics
    B. PEEP, diuretics
    C. albuterol, erythromycin
    D. needle decompression, epinephrine
    E. rapid sequence induction, glucose

22. Cyanide exposure can result from:
    A. smoke inhalation.
    B. electroplating processes.
    C. X-ray film recovery.
    D. battlefield CW.
    E. all of the above.

23. Cyanide affects the body by causing:
    A. inactivation of cellular enzymes.
    B. lactic acidosis.
    C. cellular asphyxiation.
    D. all of the above.
    E. none of the above.

24. Which of the following is **NOT** true regarding cyanide inhalation victims?
    A. Exposure to cyanide, even at low levels, is immediately deadly.
    B. The body can naturally combat and survive low-level cyanide exposure.
    C. A victim who does not exhibit immediate signs of toxicity will most likely recover without intervention.
    D. Higher dose exposures require immediate emergency medical care.
    E. Body systems are able to metabolize and eliminate low cyanide concentrations.

25. Treatment for cyanide poisoning includes standard basic life support procedures. In the USA, the critical care paramedic may also initiate drug therapy to include:
    A. dicobalt EDTA.
    B. 3% sodium nitrite.
    C. sodium thiosulfate.
    D. B and C
    E. A and C

26. Vesicants are defined as chemical agents that _____ human tissue.
    A. immobilize
    B. blister
    C. energize
    D. liquefy
    E. dessicate

27. Mustard gas destroys human tissue by binding with:
    A. proteins, DNA, and BUN.
    B. DNA, RNA, and electrolytes.
    C. proteins, DNA, and RNA.
    D. DNA, RAD, and electrolytes.
    E. none of the above.

28. Antibiotics are often administered _____ after mustard exposures.
    A. prophylactlcally
    B. topically
    C. intravenously
    D. all of the above
    E. A and B

29. Toxic exposure to Lewisite may result in:
    A. hypovolemic shock.
    B. immunosuppression.
    C. hepatic and renal necrosis.
    D. A and B.
    E. A and C.

30. Incapacitating and irritant agents may include:
    1. tear gas.
    2. oleoresin capsicum.
    3. chlorobenzylidenemalononitrile.
    4. Lewisite.
    5. mustard gas.

    A. 1, 2, and 3
    B. 2, 3, and 4
    C. 3, 4, and 5
    D. 1, 4, and 5
    E. 2, 4, and 5

31. Radiological dispersal devices (RDDs) are designed for the purposeful dissemination of radioactive materials across an area without the means of:
    A. nuclear detonation.
    B. blasting agents.
    C. explosives.
    D. all of the above.
    E. none of the above.

32. Types of ionizing radiation are:
    1. alpha.
    2. beta.
    3. delta.
    4. gamma.
    5. theta.
    6. epsilon.

    A. 1, 2, and 3
    B. 2, 3, and 4
    C. 1, 2, and 4
    D. 3, 4, and 5
    E. 1, 2, 3, and 6

33. _____ is defined as the moment radiation interacts with atoms and energy is deposited.
    A. Contamination
    B. Injury
    C. Ionization
    D. Exposure
    E. All of the above

34. If radiation injuries have occurred in conjunction with an explosion, radiation injuries may not be your patient's only or most serious problem. The critical care paramedic must remain vigilant in the investigation and management of secondary injuries such as:
    A. tympanic membrane damage.
    B. thermal burns.
    C. blunt trauma.
    D. penetrating trauma.
    E. all of the above.

35. Match the following phases of acute radiation syndrome (ARS) with their known sequelae.

    a. _____ prodromal
    b. _____ latent
    c. _____ manifest illness

    A. anemia
    B. nausea/vomiting/diarrhea
    C. bone marrow dysfunction
    D. fatigue/weakness
    E. fever/headache
    F. symptoms subside

36. Your patient has received whole-body exposure to 2,500 RADs of ionizing radiation. You know the patient is likely to develop _____ within 10 minutes and _____ within 1 hour.
    A. nausea, ataxia
    B. diarrhea, confusion
    C. ataxia, vomiting
    D. burning sensation, death
    E. all of the above

37. Standard pharmacological therapy for radiation illness includes:
    A. antiemetics.
    B. antibiotics.
    C. analgesics.
    D. all of the above.
    E. A and C.

38. Ferric ferrocyanide, stable iodine, and calcium edentate may be used to promote _____ or _____ of internal radiological contaminants.
    A. dilution, blocking
    B. neutralizing, dispersal
    C. derangement, dissolution
    D. absorption, deterrence
    E. none of the above

39. Explosive devices produce three categories of injuries: primary, secondary, and tertiary. Match each category to the mechanisms of injury typically associated with it.

    a. _____ primary
    b. _____ secondary
    c. _____ tertiary

    A. blunt force projectiles
    B. penetrating force projectiles
    C. impact from body being thrown
    D. pressure wave
    E. crushing/pinning from structural collapse
    F. heat

40. Incendiary devices, which burn at extremely high temperatures, might contain:
    A. gasoline.
    B. magnesium.

C. napalm.
D. all of the above.
E. B and C.

41. _____ agents include any living organism or toxin that can be used as a weapon.
   A. Radiological
   B. Biological
   C. Chemical
   D. Nuclear
   E. Environmental

42. According to the Centers for Disease Control, *variola major* and hantavirus are, respectively, examples of category _____ and _____ biological agents.
   A. C and D
   B. A and B
   C. A and C
   D. B and C
   E. none of the above

43. Cutaneous, gastrointestinal, and inhalational are the three generally accepted _____ syndromes.
   A. plague
   B. anthrax
   C. hantavirus
   D. *variola*
   E. *rickettsia*

44. The many antibiotics that have been used in the treatment of anthrax exposure include:
   A. penicillin derivatives.
   B. vancomycin.
   C. thiopental.
   D. all of the above.
   E. A and B.

45. Patients infected with *Yersenia pestis* can progress in stages from _____ to _____ to _____.
   A. septicemia, buboes, bacteremia
   B. buboes, bacteremia, septicemia
   C. bacteremia, septicemia, buboes
   D. septicemia, bacteremia, buboes
   E. bacteremia, buboes, septicemia

46. _____ plague is not considered transmittable, but may develop into _____ plague.
   A. Bubonic, septicemic
   B. Septicemic, bacteremic
   C. Septicemic, pneumonic
   D. Pneumonic, bubonic
   E. Bacteremic, bubonic

47. Tularemia is caused by *Francisella tularensis*, which can be carried, most notably, by:
   A. cats and dogs.
   B. rabbits and squirrels.
   C. mice and ticks.
   D. A and B.
   E. B and C.

48. _____ is the antibiotic of choice in the treatment of tularemia.
   A. Amoxicillin
   B. Ampicillin
   C. Streptomycin
   D. Sulfamethosazole/trimethoprim
   E. Penicillin

49. _____ is one of the most infective agents known, requiring as few as 10 organisms to cause the disease.
   A. Hantavirus
   B. Tularemia
   C. Anthrax
   D. Botulism
   E. Encephalitis

50. Your patient works on a ranch in Montana. He is experiencing fever, chills, malaise, and diarrhea. On physical examination you find ascites and unexplained oral lesions. You suspect that the patient is suffering from:

   A. gastrointestinal anthrax.
   B. pneumonic plague
   C. ulceroglandular tularemia
   D. bacterial pneumonia
   E. dengue fever

CHAPTER 34

Organ Donation and Retrieval

34: ORGAN DONATION AND RETRIEVAL

DIRECTIONS Each of the questions or incomplete statements below is followed by suggested answers or completions. Select the **one answer** that is best in each case.

1. The entities designated by the federal government to recover organs for transplantation are called:
   A. tissue banks.
   B. organ procurement organizations.
   C. cell savers.
   D. coroner's organ and tissue center.
   E. Organs 'R Us.

2. The complete, irreversible cessation of all brain and brainstem activity is called:
   A. neurologic death.
   B. clinical death.
   C. brain death.
   D. politics.
   E. A and C.

3. Which of the following is NOT a clinical finding for brain death?
   A. apnea
   B. no brainstem reflexes
   C. no motor response to painful stimuli
   D. explained loss of consciousness
   E. none of the above

4. Which of the following is NOT a part of a brain death examination?
   A. coma
   B. absence of pupillary reflex
   C. absent rectal sphincter tone
   D. absence of ocular movements
   E. absence of response to corneal stimulation

5. Which of the following statements about the apnea test is FALSE?
   A. The patient is preoxygenated with 100% oxygen.
   B. Normal baseline PCO_2 (> 40 mmHg) levels are obtained.
   C. The ventilator is disconnected and the patient given 6 liters per minute of oxygen via endotracheal cannula.
   D. If ventilations are observed, the test is continued.
   E. none of the above

6. Following death pronouncement, which of the following statements is TRUE?
   A. Physicians who pronounced the patient brain dead should begin harvesting organs per accepted protocols.
   B. The hospital ethics committee should meet to determine who should receive the donated organs.
   C. Brain transplants are reserved for only the most severe cases.
   D. Organs cannot be sold.
   E. none of the above

7. Who should obtain consent from the legal next-of-kin for organ donation?
   A. hospital chaplain
   B. organ procurement coordinator
   C. attending physician
   D. hospital operating room supervisor
   E. none of the above

8. Which is NOT a purpose of the medical/social/behavioral history obtained during the family interview?
   A. to identify patients at high risk for HIV/AIDS
   B. to identify patients at high risk for hepatitis
   C. to identify whether the deceased took risks such as sky diving
   D. to identify underlying medical conditions that may affect the safety and quality of the organs or tissues.
   E. none of the above

9. In the United States, the organization that oversees organ donation and transplantation is the:
   A. United Network for Organ Sharing (UNOS).
   B. American College of Surgeons (ACS).
   C. State Anatomical Board (SAB).
   D. Centers for Disease Control and Prevention (CDC).
   E. none of the above.

10. An organ donor has Type B blood. Which of the following recipient blood types would be compatible in the ABO system?
    A. A
    B. B
    C. AB
    D. O
    E. B and C

11. What is the most common complication in the brain-dead organ donor?
    A. hypertension
    B. conductive system disturbances
    C. hypotension
    D. hypernatremia
    E. hyponatremia

12. Diabetes insipidus is caused by the lack of which hormone following cerebral death?
    A. antidiuretic hormone (ADH)
    B. aldosterone
    C. oxytocin
    D. calcitonin
    E. none of the above

13. Diabetes insipidus in the organ donor is best treated with:
    A. pitocin.
    B. corticosteroids.
    C. thyroid hormone.
    D. vasopressin.
    E. phenylephrine.

14. Which of the following would make a donor heart nontransplantable?
    A. ejection fraction < 40%
    B. hypertrophic heart
    C. dominant right coronary artery
    D. A and B
    E. A and C

15. When organs are being harvested, which of the following is NOT a function of the anesthesiologist or anesthetist attending the donor?
    A. maintain IV fluids
    B. administer analgesics
    C. monitor hemodynamic parameters
    D. titrate medications
    E. none of the above

16. The typical organ preservation time for a human heart is:
    A. 2 hours.
    B. 4 hours.
    C. 24 hours.
    D. 18 hours.
    E. none of the above.

17. Which of the following tissues has the longest preservation time?
    A. liver
    B. corneas
    C. fresh skin
    D. dura
    E. none of the above

18. Which of the following organs is NOT usually suitable for donation?
    A. liver
    B. pancreas
    C. brain
    D. kidney
    E. none of the above

19. It is possible for a single bone donor to help up to _____ people, depending on the usage and planning of the grafts.
    A. 1
    B. 5
    C. 10
    D. 35
    E. 75

20. The most common veins harvested for transplantation are the:
    A. greater saphenous.
    B. inferior vena cava.
    C. femoral vein.
    D. all of the above.
    E. A and C.

21. Which of the following conditions would NEGATE a possible EMS referral for organ donation?
    A. obvious trauma incompatible with life
    B. extended downtime with evidence of rigor mortis or dependent lividity
    C. use of a field termination protocol
    D. all of the above
    E. A and C

22. Which of the following heart valves is least often used for valve repairs?
    A. tricuspid valve
    B. aortic valve
    C. pulmonic valve
    D. mitral valve
    E. none of the above

23. Dura mater can be recovered up to _____ following death.
    A. 4 hours
    B. 24 hours
    C. 30 hours
    D. 40 hours
    E. 5 years

24. The typical organ preservation time for a kidney is:
    A. 4 hours.
    B. 8–12 hours.
    C. 24 hours.
    D. 24–72 hours.
    E. none of the above.

25. Which of the following statements about organ transplantation is FALSE?
    A. There are more possible recipients than donors.
    B. The demand for organs is increasing.
    C. Organ transplantation is the primary therapy for end-stage failure of the heart, lungs, liver, kidney, pancreas, or small intestine.
    D. Only 48% of suitable organ donors become organ donors.
    E. Donated organs must be transported in a red ice chest manufactured by Igloo, available from any Wal-Mart.

CHAPTER 35
Quality Improvement in Critical Care Transport

35: QUALITY IMPROVEMENT IN CRITICAL CARE TRANSPORT

DIRECTIONS Each of the questions or incomplete statements below is followed by suggested answers or completions. Select the **one answer** that is best in each case.

1. A fundamental tenet of quality in EMS is:
   A. survival to discharge.
   B. customer satisfaction.
   C. cost/benefit ratio.
   D. system costs.
   E. none of the above.

2. Which of the following is a part of the Deming cycle?
   A. consumer research (plan)
   B. product production (do)
   C. assurance that product was produced according to plan (check)
   D. market the product (act)
   E. all of the above

3. Who should be excluded from quality management endeavors in EMS?
   A. CEO
   B. dispatchers
   C. civil service personnel
   D. supply staff
   E. none of the above

4. Who described the 80/20 rule in quality management?
   A. Juran
   B. Bledsoe
   C. Deming
   D. Taigman
   E. Benner

5. Six-sigma programs strive for:
   A. quality.
   B. customer satisfaction.
   C. less than 0.02 defective products per million.
   D. a cross-functional team.
   E. all of the above.

6. The activity of actively looking for changes in clinical literature that might affect patient care is:
   A. the Peter principle.
   B. quality assault.
   C. environmental scanning.
   D. employee punishment.
   E. none of the above.

7. Which of the following would NOT be a key results area (KRA) of a quality program?
   A. customer satisfaction
   B. employee satisfaction
   C. safety
   D. employee ethnicity
   E. financial performance

8. Which of the following is NOT a component of the QCDSM model?
   A. safety
   B. merchandising
   C. quality
   D. delivery
   E. cost

9. The American Heart Association Emergency Cardiac Care algorithms are:
   A. flowcharts.
   B. cause-and-effect charts.
   C. trend charts.
   D. histograms.
   E. Pareto charts.

10. You are a supervisor for a critical care transport (CCT) team. You have had complaints that it is taking a crew too long to "get out of the chute" and start on the call. You have checked the times for the crew in question and found that they are indeed taking longer

than other crews. What tool might help you evaluate variables affecting their times?

A. histogram
B. flowchart
C. Fishbone diagram
D. trend chart
E. Pareto chart

11. Which of the following statements about quality improvement (QI) programs is FALSE?

A. They should be punitive for those doing poorly.
B. All personnel should be involved.
C. There should be no fear of retribution for bringing a quality issue up.
D. There must be a commitment from management down.
E. Goals should be set.

12. When employees are pressured into meeting unobtainable goals, which of the following are possible employee responses?

A. work to improve the system
B. distort the data
C. distort the system
D. all of the above
E. A and C

13. Which of the following statements about quality is CORRECT?

A. Ninety-four percent of the problems in any organization are due to the system and thus are management's responsibility.
B. Leadership is not necessarily supervision.
C. A good leader does not look for someone to blame when there is a problem.
D. When there is a problem, a good leader focuses on the system as a whole.
E. all of the above

14. Your EMS system recently changed to a different type of ECG monitor. During the first month, quality indicators revealed that several paramedics were not obtaining required 12-Lead ECGs properly. This may be described as:

A. common cause variation.
B. special cause variation.
C. alternative minimum tax.
D. Physio/Phillips/Zoll syndrome.
E. none of the above.

15. In EMS, the patients are considered:

A. customers.
B. clients.
C. prospects.
D. necessary evils.
E. none of the above.

CHAPTER 36

Communications and Documentation

DIRECTIONS

Each of the questions or incomplete statements below is followed by suggested answers or completions. Select the **one answer** that is best in each case.

1. Which of the following statements regarding communications is **NOT** correct?
   A. Effective communications optimize patient care and transport.
   B. "Communications" refers to the open transference of patient information by verbal, written, or electronic means.
   C. HIPAA guidelines do not apply to prehospital and interhospital documentation.
   D. Accurate communications and documentation can help protect a critical care paramedic in the event of a lawsuit.
   E. none of the above

2. Which of the following statements about an EMS communications system is **FALSE**?
   A. The communications center should be protected from atmospheric, industrial, and seismic disturbances.
   B. The communications center is the nerve center for critical care transport.
   C. The communications center is often the first contact potential patients have with the critical care agency.
   D. Communications personnel have influence in "go/no-go" flight decisions.
   E. none of the above

3. Most commercial air traffic communications fall within which of the following radio bands?
   A. VHF AM
   B. VHF FM
   C. VHF low-band
   D. UHF AM
   E. none of the above

4. A radio system that can transmit data and voice simultaneously, allowing an ongoing conversation between individuals, is called a _____ system.
   A. simplex
   B. full duplex
   C. multiplex
   D. A and C
   E. none of the above

5. VHF low-band communications fall into what spectrum?
   A. 1–2 MHZ
   B. 30–50 MHZ
   C. 118–136 MHZ
   D. 148–174 MHZ
   E. 403–941 MHZ

6. Which is **NOT** part of the phonetic code used in aircraft communications?
   A. Foxtrot
   B. Quebec
   C. Hospital
   D. Niner
   E. Mike

7. Which of the following statements is **NOT** correct regarding whom the critical care paramedic (CCP) must communicate with?
   A. The CCP must communicate with other health care providers.
   B. The CCP must communicate with receiving facilities.
   C. The CCP must communicate with the transferring facility.
   D. The CCP must communicate with air traffic controllers.
   E. none of the above

8. All of the following describe points in a flight that typically require contact with the communications center EXCEPT:
   A. at shutdown of engines.
   B. every 10 minutes during flight.
   C. on landing at final destination.
   D. when the aircraft lifts off.
   E. at patient contact.

9. Which of the following is NOT a routine part of the patient report to a receiving facility?
   A. age
   B. gender
   C. ethnicity
   D. current mental status
   E. medical insurance status

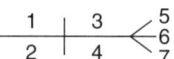

Figure 36–1

Questions 10–14 refer to Figure 36–1.
A charting scheme for a Basic Metabolic Profile (SMA-7) is shown in Figure 36–1. Choose the lab value (from the list lettered A to I) that matches each numbered position in Figure 36–1.

10. Position 1 = _____
11. Position 2 = _____
12. Position 3 = _____
13. Position 4 = _____
14. Position 5 = _____
15. Position 6 = _____
16. Position 7 = _____

   A. BUN
   B. potassium
   C. carbon dioxide
   D. sodium
   E. bicarbonate
   F. chloride
   G. bilirubin
   H. creatinine
   I. glucose

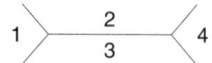

Figure 36–2

Questions 17–20 refer to Figure 36–2.
A charting scheme for a various blood values is shown in Figure 36–2. Choose the value (from the list lettered A to E) that belongs in each numbered position in Figure 36–2.

17. Position 1 = _____
18. Position 2 = _____
19. Position 3 = _____
20. Position 4 = _____

   A. hemoglobin level
   B. segmented neutrophils
   C. platelets
   D. white blood cell count
   E. hematocrit

21. Proper documentation should be:
   A. completed in its entirety.
   B. highly accurate.
   C. legible.
   D. submitted in a timely manner.
   E. all of the above.

22. Purposes for a patient care report (PCR) include all of the following EXCEPT:
   A. supports the billing program.
   B. is used for research.
   C. provides supplemental company income through sales to personal injury lawyers.
   D. provides documentation for legal concerns such as being called to court to testify about care provided.
   E. is used for quality of care evaluation programs.

23. Which of the following is **NOT** a high priority inclusion in a bedside report?
    A. names of all consulting physicians
    B. current vital signs
    C. any uncommon medical technology in use
    D. significant medical history
    E. allergies

24. The declaration of _____ status to an air-traffic controller (ATC) indicates that patient care is underway and the aircraft is given priority over other flights.
    A. life-flight
    B. care-flight
    C. lifeguard
    D. code red
    E. code life

25. In aviation, the abbreviation "IFR" means:
    A. I fly radar.
    B. individual flight rating.
    C. instrument flight regulations.
    D. inadequate fuel reserves.
    E. none of the above.

# CHAPTER 37
The Critical Care Paramedic in the Hospital Environment

DIRECTIONS Each of the questions or incomplete statements below is followed by suggested answers or completions. Select the **one answer** that is best in each case.

1. Paramedics and their critical care peers often work in in-hospital settings that include:
   A. emergency department (ED).
   B. intensive care unit (ICU).
   C. cardiac catheterization lab.
   D. stress lab.
   E. all of the above.

2. In most states, paramedic scope of practice is defined in what area of the statutes?
   A. Nursing Practice Act
   B. Allied Health Practice Act
   C. State Fire Commission
   D. Medical Practice Act
   E. none of the above

3. Unlike nursing, paramedic practice is under the auspices of whom?
   A. State Board of Occupations
   B. State Department of Health
   C. Medical Direction Physician
   D. State Fire Marshal
   E. State Nursing Board

4. All of the following are arguments advanced by the nursing profession as reasons why paramedics should not be allowed to practice in the hospital setting EXCEPT:
   A. Paramedics are unlicensed providers in most states.
   B. Paramedics lack the breadth of education that nursing students typically receive.
   C. Paramedics are more often attuned to skills performance than to holistic care.
   D. Paramedics demand a higher salary than a comparable nurse.
   E. none of the above.

5. Which of the following skills is less frequently or infrequently performed by in-hospital paramedics?
   A. conscious sedation monitoring
   B. ECG monitoring
   C. venous blood sampling
   D. immobilization
   E. patient movement and handling

6. Which of the following interventional radiology responsibilities would be INAPPROPRIATELY delegated to a critical care paramedic?
   A. starting an IV
   B. administering IV contrast under a physician's supervision
   C. assisting with ACLS measures if the patient deteriorates
   D. catheterizing an artery for angiography
   E. none of the above

7. A hospital facility where cardiac stress tests are routinely performed is referred to as a(n):
   A. cardiac catheterization lab.
   B. electrophysiology studies lab.
   C. diagnostic noninvasive cardiology lab.
   D. pulmonary function lab.
   E. morgue.

8. The most common type of task in-hospital paramedics may be asked to perform is:
   A. wound care.
   B. medical emergencies.
   C. rape intervention.
   D. administering medications.
   E. none of the above.

9. Of the following, which is commonly OUTSIDE the scope of practice for in-hospital paramedics?
   A. patient movement
   B. triage
   C. administration of nebulized medications
   D. obtaining venous blood sample
   E. wound care

10. Which of the following statements is TRUE?
    A. The rules and regulations that pertain to a critical care paramedic assessing a patient prior to critical transport are the same as those for the critical care paramedic working the ED.
    B. EMTALA and COBRA have specific rules that allow paramedics to perform triage.
    C. In a hospital setting, medical oversight can be provided to a critical care paramedic only by the EMS medical director.
    D. Any in-hospital critical care paramedic, by law, can provide on-line medical direction to EMT-Paramedics in the field setting.
    E. none of the above

Answer Key

Following each answer you will find page numbers indicating where the question topic is discussed in other Brady texts. The texts cited include *Critical Care Paramedic*, ISBN 0-13-119271-X (CCP), the second edition of *Anatomy & Physiology for Emergency Care*, ISBN 0-13-234298-7 (AP), the third edition of *Paramedic Care: Principles & Practice, Volume 1: Introduction to Advanced Prehospital Care*, ISBN 0-13-513704-7 (PCPP V1), the third edition of *Paramedic Care: Principles & Practice, Volume 3: Medical Emergencies*, ISBN 0-13-513702-0 (PCPP V3), and the seventh edition of *Prehospital Emergency Pharmacology*, ISBN 0-13-513822-1 (PEP).

CHAPTER 1: INTRODUCTION TO CRITICAL CARE TRANSPORT

1. E (CCP, p. 3)
2. B (CCP, p. 4)
3. A (CCP, p. 4)
4. C (CCP, p. 4)
5. E (CCP, p. 4)
6. C (CCP, p. 4)
7. E (CCP, p. 5)
8. A (CCP, p. 7)
9. C (CCP, p. 7)
10. E (CCP, pp. 8–9)
11. C (CCP, p. 9)
12. A (CCP, p. 9)
13. E (CCP, p. 12)
14. C (CCP, p. 13)
15. D (CCP, p. 13)
16. B (CCP, p. 9)
17. D (CCP, p. 7)
18. E (CCP, p. 4)
19. E (CCP, p. 4)
20. A (CCP, p. 10)

CHAPTER 2: CRITICAL CARE GROUND TRANSPORT

1. E (CCP, p. 19)
2. A (CCP, pp. 18–19)
3. C (CCP, p. 19)
4. A (CCP, p. 20)
5. E (CCP, p. 20)
6. C (CCP, p. 20)
7. E (CCP, p. 20)
8. D (CCP, p. 21)
9. B (CCP, p. 20)
10. B (CCP, p. 21)

CHAPTER 3: CRITICAL CARE AIR TRANSPORT

1. D (CCP, p. 27)
2. B (CCP, p. 28)
3. C (CCP, p. 27)
4. C (CCP, p. 27)
5. E (CCP, p. 28)
6. E (CCP, p. 28)

7. B (CCP, p. 29)
8. B (CCP, p. 28)
9. A (CCP, p. 29)
10. B (CCP, p. 29)
11. E (CCP, p. 29)
12. C (CCP, p. 30)
13. D (CCP, p. 31)
14. B (CCP, p. 32)
15. C (CCP, pp. 31–37)
16. E (CCP, p. 36)
17. A (CCP, p. 41)
18. B (CCP, pp. 41, 44)
19. C (CCP, pp. 41–44)
20. C (CCP, p. 46)

CHAPTER 4:
ALTITUDE PHYSIOLOGY

1. E (CCP, p. 50)
2. A (CCP, p. 50)
3. E (CCP, p. 51)
4. B (CCP, p. 51)
5. C (CCP, p. 51)
6. B (CCP, p. 51)
7. E (CCP, p. 53)
8. D (CCP, p. 53)
9. C (CCP, p. 53)
10. E (CCP, p. 53)
11. D (CCP, p. 54)
12. A (CCP, p. 54)
13. C (CCP, p. 56)
14. D (CCP, p. 55)
15. B (CCP, p. 57)
16. C (CCP, p. 58)
17. B (CCP, p. 59)
18. C (CCP, p. 60)
19. A (CCP, p. 61)
20. B (CCP, p. 60)
21. A (CCP, p. 60)
22. E (CCP, pp. 61–62)
23. D (CCP, p. 62)
24. B (CCP, pp. 54, 61)
25. A (CCP, p. 63)
26. C (CCP, p. 63)
27. C (CCP, p. 64)
28. D (CCP, p. 64)
29. C (CCP, p. 64)
30. D (CCP, p. 65)
31. A (CCP, p. 65)
32. E (CCP, pp. 65–66)
33. A (CCP, p. 66)
34. D (CCP, p. 67)
35. B (CCP, p. 67)
36. C (CCP, p. 67)
37. E (CCP, p. 67)
38. A (CCP, p. 68)
39. B (CCP, p. 68)
40. E (CCP, p. 69)
41. E (CCP, p. 69)
42. B (CCP, p. 69)
43. A (CCP, p. 69)
44. E (CCP, pp. 69–70)
45. A (CCP, p. 70)
46. E (CCP, p. 71)
47. D (CCP, p. 71)
48. D (CCP, p. 73)
49. D (CCP, p. 73)
50. A (CCP, p. 59)

CHAPTER 5:
FLIGHT SAFETY AND SURVIVAL

1. E (CCP, p. 79)
2. B (CCP, p. 79)
3. E (CCP, p. 79)
4. C (CCP, pp. 79–80)
5. D (CCP, p. 80)
6. A (CCP, p. 80)
7. E (CCP, p. 80)
8. A (CCP, p. 80)
9. C (CCP, p. 80)
10. D (CCP, p. 81)
11. D (CCP, pp. 81–82)
12. B (CCP, pp. 81–82)
13. C (CCP, p. 83)
14. D (CCP, p. 83)
15. C (CCP, p. 83)
16. A (CCP, p. 83)
17. B (CCP, p. 84)
18. C (CCP, p. 96)
19. C (CCP, p. 85)
20. E (CCP, p. 86)

21. A (CCP, p. 86)
22. C (CCP, p. 86)
23. A (CCP, p. 87)
24. C (CCP, p. 87)
25. B (CCP, p. 87)
26. B (CCP, p. 88)
27. D (CCP, p. 88)
28. E (CCP, pp. 88–89)
29. A (CCP, p. 89)
30. D (CCP, p. 89)
31. B (CCP, p. 89)
32. D (CCP, p. 90)
33. B (CCP, p. 90)
34. E (CCP, p. 91)
35. D (CCP, p. 92)
36. A (CCP, p. 93)
37. C (CCP, p. 93)
38. B (CCP, p. 94)
39. D (CCP, p. 94)
40. E (CCP, p. 94)
41. A (CCP, p. 94)
42. D (CCP, p. 95)
43. B (CCP, p. 95)
44. C (CCP, p. 95)
45. E (CCP, p. 96)
46. A (CCP, p. 96)
47. D (CCP, p. 97)
48. C (CCP, p. 98)
49. B (CCP, p. 98)
50. A (CCP, p. 98)
51. E (CCP, p. 98)
52. B (CCP, p. 99)
53. E (CCP, p. 99)
54. D (CCP, p. 99)
55. E (CCP, p. 100)
56. E (CCP, p. 101)

CHAPTER 6:
PATIENT ASSESSMENT AND PREPARATION FOR TRANSPORT

1. D (CCP, p. 106)
2. B (CCP, p. 107)
3. A (CCP, p. 108)
4. D (CCP, pp. 108, 110)
5. C (CCP, p. 109)
6. C (CCP, p. 110)
7. D (CCP, p. 110)
8. B (CCP, p. 111)
9. A (CCP, p. 111)
10. D (CCP, p. 112)
11. D (CCP, p. 113)
12. C (CCP, p. 113)
13. A (CCP, p. 113)
14. B (CCP, p. 114)
15. C (CCP, p. 114)
16. E (CCP, p. 115)
17. A (CCP, p. 115)
18. B (CCP, p. 115)
19. A (CCP, p. 115)
20. C (CCP, p. 116)
21. E (CCP, pp. 116, 119)
22. C (CCP, p. 117)
23. E (CCP, p. 117)
24. E (CCP, p. 118)
25. B (CCP, p. 118)
26. E (CCP, p. 118)
27. C (CCP, p.120)
28. E (CCP, p. 121)
29. B (CCP, pp. 121–122)
30. B (CCP, p. 122)

CHAPTER 7:
AIRWAY MANAGEMENT AND VENTILATION

1. A (CCP, p. 127)
2. A (AP, p. 441)
3. A (AP, p. 443)
4. E (AP, p. 443)
5. B (AP, p. 556)
6. A (AP, pp. 448–449)
7. C (PCPP V1, p. 548)
8. C (AP, p. 453)
9. A (AP, p. 451)
10. D (AP, p. 454)
11. C (AP, p. 454)
12. E (AP, p. 456)
13. B (CCP, p. 129)
14. C (CCP, p. 129)
15. D (CCP, p. 131)
16. D (CCP, p. 132)

17. E (CCP, p. 133)
18. A (CCP, p. 134)
19. B (CCP, p. 140)
20. B (CCP, p. 142)
21. C (CCP, pp. 143–145)
22. A (CCP, p. 143)
23. A (CCP, p. 143)
24. E (CCP, p. 144)
25. B (CCP, p. 145)
26. A (CCP, p. 145)
27. A (CCP, p. 146)
28. C (CCP, p. 146)
29. E (AP, p. 172)
30. E (PEP, p. 127)
31. B (CCP, p. 146)
32. E (CCP, p. 146)
33. B (CCP, p. 149)
34. C (CCP, p. 150)
35. D (CCP, p. 151)
36. C (CCP, p. 152)
37. D (CCP, p. 153)
38. E (CCP, pp. 151–160)
39. C (CCP, pp. 156–158)
40. D (CCP, p. 160)
41. E (CCP, p. 161)
42. A (CCP, p. 161)
43. A (CCP, p. 162)
44. C (CCP, p. 164)
45. B (CCP, pp. 169–170)
46. C (CCP, p. 168)
47. B (CCP, p. 168)
48. E (CCP, p. 169)
49. E (CCP, pp. 142–151)
50. D (CCP, p. 172)
51. B (CCP, p. 172)
52. B (CCP, p. 174)
53. B (CCP, p. 176)
54. C (CCP, p. 179)
55. A (CCP, p. 179)

CHAPTER 8:
THE SHOCK PATIENT: ASSESSMENT AND MANAGEMENT

1. E (CCP, p. 188)
2. D (CCP, p. 189)
3. A (CCP, p. 189)
4. C (CCP, p. 189)
5. A (CCP, p. 189)
6. A (CCP, p. 189)
7. C (CCP, p. 188)
8. D (CCP, p. 188)
9. E (CCP, p. 188)
10. A (CCP, p. 188)
11. B (CCP, p. 188)
12. E (CCP, p. 189)
13. B (CCP, p. 191)
14. E (CCP, p. 191)
15. D (CCP, p. 191)
16. D (CCP, p. 190)
17. A (CCP, p. 193)
18. E (CCP, p. 193)
19. A (CCP, p. 193)
20. C (CCP, p. 194)
21. A (CCP, p. 194)
22. C (CCP, p. 198)
23. A (CCP, p. 198)
24. D (CCP, p. 198)
25. A (CCP, p. 198)
26. B (CCP, p. 199)
27. D (CCP, p. 199)
28. D (CCP, p. 199)
29. B (CCP, p. 201)
30. C (AP, pp. 262–263)

CHAPTER 9:
CARDIAC AND HEMODYNAMIC MONITORING

1. A (CCP, p. 207)
2. D (CCP, p. 207)
3. C (CCP, p. 209)
4. C (CCP, p. 209)
5. C (CCP, p. 211)
6. B (CCP, p. 210)
7. E (CCP, p. 212)
8. C (CCP, p. 213)
9. A (CCP, p. 216)
10. E (CCP, p. 213)
11. A (CCP, p. 215)
12. D (CCP, p. 216)
13. D (CCP, p. 220)

ANSWER KEY ■ 293

14. B (CCP, p. 221)
15. D (CCP, p. 220)
16. D (CCP, pp. 222, 330)
17. A (CCP, p. 220)
18. B (CCP, p. 222)
19. C (CCP, p. 222)
20. B (CCP, p. 225)
21. B (CCP, p. 225)
22. C (CCP, p. 227)
23. D (CCP, p. 226)
24. C (CCP, p. 228)
25. A (CCP, p. 210)
26. B (CCP, p. 229)
27. C (CCP, p. 214)
28. E (CCP, pp. 228–229)
29. A (CCP, p. 231)
30. C (CCP, p. 231)
31. D (CCP, p. 232)
32. B (CCP, p. 233)
33. A (CCP, p. 232)
34. D (CCP, p. 231)
35. B (CCP, p. 231)
36. D (CCP, p. 234)
37. C (CCP, p. 238)
38. E (CCP, p. 224)
39. D (CCP, p. 241)
40. E (CCP, p. 241)

CHAPTER 10: ECG MONITORING AND CRITICAL CARE

1. B (CCP, p. 248)
2. D (CCP, p. 248)
3. B (CCP, p. 248)
4. A (CCP, pp. 247–248)
5. C (CCP, p. 248)
6. E (CCP, p. 250)
7. C (CCP, p. 250)
8. B (CCP, p. 250)
9. C (CCP, p. 250)
10. B (CCP, p. 250)
11. B (CCP, p. 251)
12. E (CCP, pp. 251–252)
13. C (CCP, p. 253)
14. D (CCP, p. 255)
15. C (CCP, p. 256)
16. D (CCP, p. 257)
17. B (CCP, p. 258)
18. C (CCP, p. 260)
19. D (CCP, p. 260)
20. A (CCP, p. 259)
21. B (CCP, p. 261)
22. D (CCP, p. 262)
23. C (CCP, pp. 262–263)
24. D (CCP, pp. 262–263)
25. A (CCP, p. 263)
26. B (CCP, p. 264)
27. A (CCP, p. 264)
28. C (CCP, p. 264)
29. B (CCP, p. 264)
30. C (CCP, p. 265)
31. C (CCP, p. 266)
32. B (CCP, p. 266)
33. C (CCP, p. 266)
34. E (CCP, p. 266)
35. B (CCP, p. 266)
36. C (CCP, pp. 266–267)
37. A (AP, p. 363)
38. A (AP, p. 368)
39. C (AP, p. 366)
40. E (AP, p. 361)
41–50. Per following chart (CCP, pp. 248–270)

	PARAMETER	INTERPRETATION
41.	Rate	67
	Rhythm	Regular
	P Wave	Present, upright (II)
	PR Interval	0.12 sec
	QRS Complex	0.04 sec
	ST Elevation	I, aVL, aVF, V_1-V_4 (tombstones
	ST Depression	II, III, aVF
	Pathologic Q Waves	None
	Interpretation	Normal sinus rhythm, anteroseptal MI
42.	Rate	66
	Rhythm	Irregular
	P Wave	Present, upright (II)
	PR Interval	0.16 sec
	QRS Complex	0.08 sec
	ST Elevation	V_1-V_6
	ST Depression	III, aVF
	Pathologic Q Waves	None
	Interpretation	Normal sinus rhythm, anteroseptal MI
43.	Rate	66
	Rhythm	Regular
	P Wave	Present, upright (II)
	PR Interval	0.18 sec
	QRS Complex	0.08 sec
	ST Elevation	V_1-V_4 with T wave inversion
	ST Depression	None
	Pathologic Q Waves	None
	Interpretation	Normal sinus rhythm with anterolateral MI
44.	Rate	88
	Rhythm	Regular
	P Wave	Present, notched (II)
	PR Interval	0.20 sec
	QRS Complex	0.12 sec
	ST Elevation	None
	ST Depression	None
	Pathologic Q Waves	None
	Interpretation	Normal sinus rhythm, left axis deviation, LBBB

	PARAMETER	INTERPRETATION
45.	Rate	55
	Rhythm	Irregular
	P Wave	None present
	PR Interval	0
	QRS Complex	0.16 sec
	ST Elevation	None
	ST Depression	None
	Pathologic Q Waves	None
	Interpretation	Atrial fibrillation, RBBB
46.	Rate	73
	Rhythm	Regular
	P Wave	Present, notched (II)
	PR Interval	0.14 sec
	QRS Complex	0.08 sec
	ST Elevation	None
	ST Depression	None
	Pathologic Q Waves	None
	Interpretation	Normal sinus rhythm, left axis deviation
47.	Rate	200
	Rhythm	Regular
	P Wave	Not present
	PR Interval	0
	QRS Complex	0.07 sec
	ST Elevation	None
	ST Depression	None
	Pathologic Q Waves	None
	Interpretation	Supraventricular tachycardia
48.	Rate	> 200
	Rhythm	Irregular
	P Wave	None present
	PR Interval	0
	QRS Complex	0.16 sec
	ST Elevation	None
	ST Depression	None
	Pathologic Q Waves	None
	Interpretation	Ventricular tachycardia

	PARAMETER	INTERPRETATION
49.	Rate	98
	Rhythm	Irregular
	P Wave	None
	PR Interval	0
	QRS Complex	0.12 sec
	ST Elevation	I, II, III, aVF, V_1-V_6
	ST Depression	aVR
	Pathologic Q Waves	None
	Interpretation	Junctional rhythm with bigeminy PVCs, anteroseptal infarct, inferolateral infarct
50.	Rate	70
	Rhythm	Regular
	P Wave	None
	PR Interval	0
	QRS Complex	0.18 sec
	ST Elevation	None
	ST Depression	None
	Pathologic Q Waves	None
	Interpretation	Pacemaker rhythm

CHAPTER 11: CRITICAL CARE PHARMACOLOGY

1. E (CCP, p. 274)
2. A (CCP, p. 274)
3. D (CCP, p. 274)
4. B (CCP, p. 274)
5. D (CCP, p. 275)
6. C (CCP, p. 275)
7. B (CCP, p. 275)
8. C (CCP, p. 275)
9. C (CCP, p. 275)
10. E (CCP, p. 275)
11. A (CCP, p. 275)
12. E (CCP, p. 275)
13. D (CCP, p. 275)
14. B (CCP, p. 276)
15. C (CCP, p. 276)
16. D (CCP, p. 276)
17. E (CCP, p. 276)
18. E (CCP, p. 276)
19. E (CCP, pp. 274–322)
20. C (CCP, pp. 274–322)
21. D (CCP, pp. 274–322)
22. E (CCP, p. 276)
23. E (CCP, p. 277)
24. A (CCP, p. 277)
25. D (CCP, p. 277)
26. A (CCP, p. 277)
27. E (CCP, p. 278)
28. C (CCP, p. 279)
29. B (CCP, p. 280)
30. D (CCP, p. 280)
31. A (CCP, p. 280)
32. D (CCP, p. 280)
33. E (CCP, p. 281)
34. E (CCP, p. 281)
35. C (CCP, p. 282)
36. E (CCP, p. 282)
37. E (CCP, p. 282)
38. B (CCP, p. 282)
39. C (CCP, pp. 282–283)
40. B (CCP, pp. 283–284)
41. E (CCP, p. 285)
42. E (CCP, p. 285)

43. C (CCP, p. 286)
44. A (CCP, p. 286)
45. C (CCP, p. 287)
46. E (CCP, p. 288)
47. B (CCP, p. 288)
48. E (CCP, p. 288)
49. C (CCP, p. 289)
50. D (CCP, p. 289)
51. C (CCP, p. 289)
52. B (CCP, p. 290)
53. C (CCP, p. 290)
54. B (CCP, p. 290)
55. E (CCP, p. 290)
56. C (CCP, p. 288)
57. D (CCP, p. 291)
58. E (CCP, p. 291)
59. E (CCP, p. 292)
60. B (CCP, p. 291)
61. A (CCP, p. 292)
62. D (CCP, p. 292)
63. E (CCP, p. 292)
64. C (CCP, p. 292)
65. B (CCP, p. 292)
66. B (CCP, p. 293)
67. E (CCP, p. 293)
68. E (CCP, pp. 294–297)
69. C (CCP, pp. 294–297)
70. D (CCP, p. 294)
71. D (CCP, p. 295)
72. D (CCP, pp. 294–297)
73. C (CCP, p. 296)
74. D (CCP, p. 297)
75. C (CCP, p. 297)
76. E (CCP, pp. 198–301)
77. C (CCP, p. 298)
78. C (CCP, pp. 298–301)
79. D (CCP, p. 300)
80. C (CCP, pp. 300–301)
81. A (CCP, p. 302)
82. B (CCP, p. 302)
83. D (CCP, p. 303)
84. B (CCP, pp. 300–303)
85. C (CCP, pp. 303–305)
86. D (CCP, pp. 303–305)
87. B (CCP, pp. 305–306)
88. A (CCP, p. 306)
89. D (CCP, p. 306)
90. B (CCP, p. 306)
91. E (CCP, p. 307)
92. C (CCP, p. 308)
93. A (CCP, pp. 309–310)
94. E (CCP, pp. 309–310)
95. A (CCP, pp. 310–311)
96. E (CCP, pp. 311–312)
97. D (CCP, pp. 311–312)
98. B (CCP, pp. 312–314)
99. C (CCP, pp. 312–314)
100. E (CCP, pp. 312–315)
101. A (CCP, p. 314)
102. E (CCP, p. 314)
103. A (CCP, p. 315)
104. B (CCP, p. 316)
105. E (CCP, p. 316)
106. C (CCP, p. 316)
107. D (CCP, pp. 317–318)
108. D (CCP, p. 318)
109. B (CCP, p. 318)
110. D (CCP, pp. 320–321)
111. D (CCP, pp. 321–322)
112. B (CCP, p. 324)
113. C (PEP, pp. 64–85)

Equation:

$$\frac{250 \text{ mL}}{80{,}000 \text{ mcg}} \times \frac{8 \text{ mcg}}{1 \text{ kg/min}}$$

$$\times \frac{60 \text{ min}}{1 \text{ hr}} \times \frac{60 \text{ kg}}{1}$$

$$= \frac{7{,}200{,}000 \text{ mL}}{80{,}000 \text{ hr}} = 9 \text{ mL/hr}$$

114. B (PEP, pp. 64–85)

Equation:

$$\frac{250 \text{ mL}}{800{,}000 \text{ mcg}} \times \frac{8 \text{ mcg}}{1 \text{ kg/min}}$$

$$\times \frac{60 \text{ min}}{1 \text{ hr}} \times \frac{60 \text{ kg}}{1}$$

$$= \frac{7{,}200{,}000 \text{ mL}}{80{,}000 \text{ hr}} = 9 \text{ mL/hr}$$

115. D (PEP, pp. 64–85)

Equation:

$$\frac{50{,}000 \text{ mcg}}{250 \text{ mL}} \times \frac{15 \text{ mL}}{1 \text{ hr}}$$

$$\times \frac{1 \text{ hr}}{60 \text{ min}} = \frac{750{,}000 \text{ mcg}}{15{,}000}$$

$$= 50 \text{ mcg/min}$$

CHAPTER 12: INTERPRETATION OF LAB AND BASIC DIAGNOSTIC TESTS

1. D (CCP, p. 329)
2. D (CCP, p. 329)
3. A (CCP, p. 329)
4. C (CCP, p. 330)
5. B (CCP, p. 330)
6. E (CCP, p. 332)
7. E (CCP, p. 332)
8. D (CCP, p. 332)
9. A (CCP, p. 333)
10. B (CCP, p. 332)
11. D (CCP, p. 334)
12. A (CCP, p. 334)
13. A (CCP, p. 336)
14. D (CCP, p. 336)
15. D (CCP, p. 339)
16. B (CCP, p. 340)
17. A (CCP, p. 339)
18. B (CCP, p. 336)
19. E (CCP, p. 336)
20. C (CCP, p. 338)
21. E (CCP, p. 338)
22. D (CCP, p. 340)
23. A (CCP, pp. 341–342)
24. C (CCP, p. 342)
25. B (CCP, p. 342)
26. D (CCP, p. 342)
27. A (CCP, p. 342)
28. E (CCP, p. 342)
29. C (CCP, p. 342)
30. A (CCP, p. 342)
31. B (CCP, p. 342)
32. C (CCP, p. 344)
33. B (CCP, p. 345)
34. D (CCP, p. 345)
35. E (CCP, p. 346)
36. D (PCPP V1, p. 410)
37. C (CCP, p. 346)
38. D (CCP, p. 347)
39. A (CCP, p. 347)
40. A (CCP, p. 349)
41. C (CCP, p. 352)
42. D (CCP, p. 352)
43. D (CCP, p. 353)
44. D (CCP, p. 353)
45. A (CCP, pp. 350–351)

CHAPTER 13: INTRODUCTION TO TRAUMA

1. E (CCP, p. 359)
2. E (CCP, p. 359)
3. A (CCP, p. 359)
4. B (CCP, p. 361)
5. E (CCP, p. 361)
6. B (CCP, p. 362)
7. D (CCP, p. 363)
8. C (CCP, p. 363)
9. C (CCP, p. 363)
10. A (CCP, p. 363)
11. B (CCP, p. 363)
12. C (CCP, p. 365)
13. C (CCP, p. 365)
14. E (CCP, p. 366)
15. E (CCP, p. 365)
16. E (CCP, p. 366)
17. A (CCP, p. 367)
18. E (CCP, p. 368)
19. D (CCP, p. 367)
20. B (CCP, p. 369)
21. B (CCP, p. 369)
22. E (CCP, p. 369)
23. B (CCP, p. 369)
24. C (CCP, p. 368)
25. D (CCP, p. 367)

CHAPTER 14: NEUROLOGIC TRAUMA

1. E (CCP, p. 374)
2. C (CCP, p. 374)
3. D (CCP, p. 375)

4. C (CCP, p. 375)
 5. E (CCP, p. 375)
 6. C (CCP, p. 375)
 7. E (CCP, p. 377)
 8. B (CCP, p. 377)
 9. C (CCP, p. 377)
10. D (CCP, p. 378)
11. A (CCP, p. 378)
12. E (CCP, pp. 378–379)
13. C (CCP, p. 378)
14. D (CCP, p. 381)
15. C (CCP, p. 381)
16. B (CCP, p. 382)
17. C (CCP, p. 382)
18. B (CCP, p. 382)
19. C (CCP, p. 382)
20. E (CCP, p. 382)
21. C (CCP, p. 383)
22. C (CCP, p. 383)
23. E (CCP, p. 384; AP, p. 233)
24. D (CCP, p. 384)
25. D (CCP, pp. 385–387)
26. B (CCP, p. 388)
27. B (CCP, p. 389)
28. D (CCP, pp. 389–390)
29. C (CCP, p. 390)
30. A (CCP, p. 390)
31. C (CCP, p. 390)
32. E (CCP, p. 391)
33. B (CCP, p. 391)
34. C (CCP, p. 392)
35. E (CCP, p. 392)
36. B (CCP, p. 392)
37. A (See http://www.uic.edu/classes/pmpr/pmpr652/Final/Winkler/ICP.html)
38. B (See http://www.uic.edu/classes/pmpr/pmpr652/Final/Winkler/ICP.html)
39. B (CCP, p. 393)
40. A (CCP, p. 393)
41. D (CCP, p. 393)
42. E (CCP, p. 393)
43. D (CCP, p. 394)
44. B (CCP, p. 394)
45. A (CCP, pp. 394–395)
46. B (CCP, p. 395)
47. E (CCP, p. 395)
48. D (CCP, p. 395)
49. D (CCP, p. 395)
50. B (CCP, p. 396)
51. E (CCP, p. 396)
52. C (CCP, p. 397)
53. C (CCP, p. 379)
54. C (CCP, p. 378)
55. E (AP, p. 261)

CHAPTER 15: THORACIC TRAUMA: ASSESSMENT AND MANAGEMENT

 1. B (CCP, p. 402)
 2. C (CCP, p. 403)
 3. B (CCP, p. 404)
 4. D (CCP, p. 404)
 5. A (CCP, p. 404)
 6. C (CCP, p. 405)
 7. C (CCP, p. 405)
 8. A (CCP, p. 406)
 9. D (CCP, p. 406)
10. B (CCP, p. 406)
11. C (CCP, p. 407)
12. D (CCP, p. 407)
13. D (CCP, p. 407)
14. B (CCP, p. 408)
15. E (CCP, p. 408)
16. C (CCP, p. 410)
17. A (CCP, p. 410)
18. B (CCP, p. 410)
19. E (CCP, p. 410)
20. D (CCP, p. 410)
21. A (CCP, p. 410)
22. C (CCP, p. 410)
23. B (CCP, p. 411)
24. C (CCP, p. 411)
25. E (CCP, p. 412)
26. C (CCP, p. 413)
27. C (CCP, p. 413)
28. E (CCP, p. 413)
29. B (CCP, p. 414)
30. C (CCP, p. 406)
31. B (CCP, p. 414)
32. C (CCP, p. 414)
33. C (CCP, pp. 414–415)
34. B (CCP, p. 414)
35. E (CCP, p. 415)

36. C (CCP, p. 415)
37. D (CCP, p. 415)
38. C (CCP, p. 415)
39. A (CCP, p. 416)
40. D (CCP, p. 417)
41. C (CCP, p. 417)
42. D (CCP, p. 417)
43. E (CCP, p. 417)
44. E (CCP, p. 418)
45. A (CCP, p. 418)
46. B (AP, pp. A13–6)
47. A (AP, pp. A16–8)
48. B (AP, pp. A14–6)
49. B (AP, pp. A13–6)
50. C (AP, pp. A16–8)

CHAPTER 16: ABDOMINAL AND GENITOURINARY TRAUMA

1. B (CCP, p. 423)
2. D (CCP, p. 423)
3. C (CCP, p. 423)
4. D (CCP, p. 423)
5. D (CCP, p. 425)
6. C (CCP, p. 426)
7. B (CCP, p. 426)
8. C (CCP, p. 428)
9. C (CCP, p. 429)
10. A (CCP, p. 429)
11. C (CCP, p. 429)
12. A (CCP, p. 430)
13. D (CCP, p. 430)
14. C (CCP, p. 432)
15. B (CCP, p. 432)
16. A (CCP, p. 432)
17. D (CCP, p. 433)
18. D (CCP, p. 433)
19. C (CCP, p. 434)
20. E (CCP, p. 434)
21. D (CCP, p. 434)
22. C (CCP, p. 434)
23. C (CCP, p. 435)
24. E (CCP, p. 436)
25. B (CCP, p. 438)
26. A (CCP, p. 439)
27. B (CCP, p. 439)
28. E (CCP, p. 439)
29. C (CCP, p. 440)
30. C (CCP, p. 440)
31. D (CCP, p. 440)
32. C (CCP, p. 440)
33. B (CCP, p. 441)
34. E (CCP, p. 438–439)
35. C (CCP, p. 445)
36. D (CCP, p. 445)
37. B (CCP, p. 445)
38. C (CCP, p. 445)
39. C (CCP, pp. 445–446)
40. D (CCP, p. 446)
41. B (CCP, p. 446)
42. E (CCP, p. 445)
43. B (CCP, p. 447)
44. E (CCP, p. 445)
45. B (AP, p. 660)
46. D (AP, p. 614)
47. B (AP, p. 607)
48. A (AP, p. 661)
49. C (AP, p. 661)
50. E (AP, p. 672)

CHAPTER 17: FACE/EAR/OCULAR/ NECK TRAUMA

1. E (CCP, p. 453)
2. A (CCP, p. 453)
3. B (CCP, p. 453)
4. D (CCP, p. 453)
5. B (CCP, p. 453)
6. A (CCP, p. 453)
7. C (CCP, p. 453)
8. C (CCP, p. 453)
9. E (CCP, p. 454)
10. D (CCP, p. 454)
11. E (CCP, p. 455)
12. E (CCP, p. 455)
13. A (CCP, p. 455)
14. B (CCP, p. 455)
15. D (CCP, p. 457)
16. D (CCP, p. 457)
17. C (CCP, p. 457)
18. D (CCP, p. 458)
19. A (CCP, p. 458)

20. D (CCP, p. 458)
21. C (CCP, p. 458)
22. A (CCP, p. 459)
23. D (CCP, p. 459)
24. E (CCP, p. 459)
25. A (CCP, p. 461)
26. C (CCP, p. 463)
27. C (CCP, p. 463)
28. D (CCP, p. 463)
29. A (CCP, p. 463)
30. D (CCP, p. 463)
31. A (CCP, p. 464)
32. C (CCP, p. 464)
33. E (CCP, p. 464)
34. E (CCP, p. 464)
35. C (CCP, p. 465)
36. D (CCP, p. 465)
37. C (CCP, p. 465)
38. B (CCP, p. 467)
39. B (CCP, p. 470)
40. E (CCP, p. 470)
41. D (CCP, p. 471)
42. A (CCP, p. 472)
43. D (CCP, p. 472; AP, p. 254)
44. D (CCP, p. 472)
45. D (CCP, p. 473)
46. E (CCP, p. 473)
47. C (CCP, p. 473)
48. B (CCP, p. 475)
49. C (CCP, p. 478)
50. E (CCP, p. 482)
51. B (CCP, p. 476)
52. D (CCP, p. 476)
53. E (CCP, p. 483)
54. D (CCP, p. 482)
55. A (CCP, p. 481)

CHAPTER 18: BURNS AND ELECTRICAL INJURIES

1. D (CCP, p. 489)
2. A (CCP, p. 489)
3. C (CCP, p. 489)
4. E (CCP, p. 489)
5. D (CCP, p. 489)
6. D (CCP, p. 490)
7. A (CCP, p. 490)
8. B (CCP, p. 490)
9. C (CCP, p. 490)
10. A (CCP, p. 490)
11. B (CCP, p. 491)
12. C (CCP, p. 491)
13. B (CCP, p. 491)
14. A (CCP, p. 491)
15. D (CCP, p. 491)
16. D (CCP, p. 491)
17. D (CCP, p. 491)
18. E (CCP, p. 492)
19. E (CCP, p. 492)
20. E (CCP, p. 492)
21. B (CCP, p. 493)
22. C (CCP, pp. 494, 502)
23. E (CCP, p. 494)
24. C (CCP, pp. 494, 502)
25. A (CCP, p. 497)
26. E (CCP, p. 494)
27. C (CCP, p. 494)
28. E (CCP, p. 495)
29. D (CCP, p. 496)
30. B (CCP, p. 496)
31. E (CCP, p. 466)
32. A (CCP, p. 497)
33. B (CCP, p. 497)
34. E (CCP, p. 500)
35. E (CCP, p. 500)
36. B (CCP, p. 501)
37. D (CCP, p. 502)
38. C (CCP, p. 503)
39. D (CCP, p. 503)
40. A (CCP, p. 497)
41. B (CCP, p. 504)
42. B (CCP, p. 504)
43. D (CCP, p. 504)
44. E (CCP, p. 504)
45. B (CCP, p. 505)
46. C (CCP, p. 505)
47. D (CCP, p. 506)
48. C (CCP, p. 506)
49. B (CCP, p. 508)
50. B (CCP, p. 507)
51. D (CCP, p. 510)
52. D (CCP, p. 510)
53. E (CCP, p. 511)

54. B (CCP, p. 511)
55. E (CCP, p. 511)
56. D (CCP, p. 511)
57. E (CCP, p. 511)
58. B (CCP, p. 512)
59. E (CCP, p. 512)
60. B (CCP, p. 513)
61. C (CCP, p. 513)
62. A (CCP, p. 513)
63. B (CCP, p. 514)
64. D (CCP, p. 514)
65. D (CCP, p. 515)
66. C (CCP, p. 517)
67. E (CCP, p. 518)
68. D (AP, p. 109)
69. A (AP, p. 111)
70. E (AP, p. 111)
71. E (AP, p. 113)
72. E (AP, p. 114)
73. A (AP, pp. 115–116)
74. B (AP, p. 110)
75. C (AP, p. 109)

CHAPTER 19: PRINCIPLES OF ORTHOPEDIC CARE

1. E (AP, p. 152)
2. A (AP, p. 153)
3. B (AP, p. 153)
4. D (AP, p. 153)
5. C (AP, p. 156)
6. C (AP, p. 157)
7. D (AP, p. 158)
8. B (AP, p. 158)
9. A (AP, p. 158)
10. D (AP, p. 159)
11. A (AP, p. 160)
12. E (AP, p. 160)
13. E (CCP, p. 523)
14. D (CCP, p. 523)
15. B (CCP, p. 523)
16. A (CCP, p. 523)
17. C (CCP, p. 523)
18. C (CCP, p. 523)
19. A (CCP, p. 523)
20. B (CCP, p. 523)
21. D (CCP, p. 524)
22. A (CCP, p. 524)
23. C (CCP, p. 525)
24. A (CCP, p. 526)
25. C (CCP, p. 528)
26. D (CCP, p. 529)
27. D (CCP, p. 529)
28. B (CCP, p. 529)
29. A (CCP, p. 529)
30. E (CCP, p. 530)
31. B (CCP, p. 532)
32. E (CCP, p. 532)
33. E (CCP, p. 533)
34. E (CCP, p. 533)
35. B (CCP, p. 534)
36. C (CCP, p. 534)
37. E (CCP, p. 534)
38. D (CCP, p. 534)
39. D (CCP, p. 534)
40. D (AP, p. 255)
41. A (CCP, p. 534)
42. E (CCP, p. 534)
43. A (CCP, p. 535)
44. C (CCP, p. 536)
45. D (CCP, p. 537)
46. B (CCP, p. 538)
47. C (PEP, p. 387)
48. E (CCP, p. 539)
49. D (CCP, p. 540)
50. D (CCP, p. 541)

CHAPTER 20: SPECIAL PATIENTS: PEDIATRIC, GERIATRIC, AND OBSTETRICAL TRAUMA

1. C (CCP, p. 546)
2. D (CCP, p. 546)
3. B (CCP, p. 547)
4. A (CCP, p. 547)
5. D (CCP, p. 548)
6. B (CCP, p. 548)
7. A (CCP, p. 548)
8. C (CCP, p. 549)
9. C (CCP, p. 550)
10. E (CCP, p. 550)
11. B (CCP, p. 550)

12. C (CCP, p. 552)
13. B (CCP, p. 554)
14. C (CCP, p. 552)
15. D (CCP, p. 552)
16. B (CCP, p. 555)
17. B (CCP, p. 555)
18. B (CCP, p. 556)
19. C (CCP, p. 556)
20. A (CCP, pp. 556–557)
21. D (CCP, p. 558)
22. A (CCP, p. 558)
23. D (CCP, p. 558)
24. A (CCP, p. 558)
25. C (CCP, p. 559)
26. C (CCP, p. 559)
27. B (CCP, p. 559)
28. D (CCP, p. 562)
29. D (CCP, p. 562)
30. B (CCP, p. 563)
31. B (CCP, p. 563)
32. C (CCP, p. 564)
33. E (PCPP V1, p. 550)
34. B (CCP, p. 566)
35. D (CCP, p. 567)
36. C (CCP, pp. 567–568)
37. D (CCP, pp. 567–568)
38. B (CCP, pp. 568–569)
39. C (CCP, p. 573)
40. E (CCP, pp. 573–574)
41. B (CCP, p. 575)
42. C (CCP, p. 575)
43. C (CCP, p. 574)
44. E (CCP, p. 554)
45. A (CCP, p. 574)

CHAPTER 21: PULMONARY EMERGENCIES

1. B (CCP, p. 581)
2. B (CCP, p. 584)
3. D (CCP, p. 584)
4. D (CCP, p. 585)
5. B (CCP, p. 585)
6. D (CCP, p. 586)
7. A (CCP, p. 586)
8. C (CCP, p. 586)
9. D (CCP, p. 586)
10. B (CCP, p. 586)
11. A (CCP, p. 586)
12. B (CCP, p. 588)
13. C (CCP, p. 588)
14. E (CCP, p. 588)
15. D (CCP, p. 588)
16. C (CCP, p. 589)
17. D (CCP, p. 589)
18. D (CCP, p. 589)
19. A (CCP, p. 589)
20. C (CCP, p. 589)
21. A (CCP, p. 590)
22. E (CCP, p. 590)
23. E (CCP, p. 590)
24. D (CCP, p. 590)
25. E (CCP, p. 591)
26. A (CCP, p. 591)
27. A (CCP, p. 591)
28. D (CCP, p. 591)
29. D (CCP, p. 592)
30. D (CCP, p. 592)
31. E (CCP, p. 592)
32. B (CCP, p. 592)
33. A (CCP, p. 592)
34. C (CCP, p. 592)
35. A (CCP, pp. 592-593)
36. C (CCP, p. 593)
37. D (CCP, p. 593)
38. A (CCP, p. 593)
39. E (CCP, p. 594)
40. C (CCP, p. 594)
41. C (CCP, p. 594)
42. C (CCP, p. 594)
43. C (CCP, p. 595)
44. B (CCP, p. 595)
45. B (CCP, p. 595)
46. D (CCP, pp. 595–596)
47. D (CCP, p. 596)
48. D (CCP, p. 596)
49. D (CCP, p. 596)
50. D (CCP, p. 598)
51. D (CCP, p. 597)
52. C (CCP, pp. 597–598)
53. D (CCP, p. 598)
54. B (CCP, p. 598)
55. C (CCP, pp. 598–601)
56. C (CCP, p. 602)

57. D (CCP, p. 603)
58. E (CCP, p. 603)
59. B (CCP, p. 603)
60. A (CCP, p. 603)
61. B (CCP, p. 605)
62. A (CCP, pp. 606–607)
63. D (CCP, p. 607)
64. D (CCP, p. 608)
65. A (CCP, p. 609)
66. D (CCP, p. 609)
67. C (CCP, p. 610)
68. D (CCP, p. 610)
69. A (CCP, p. 611)
70. E (CCP, p. 613)
71. D (CCP, p. 613)
72. D (CCP, p. 614)
73. B (CCP, p. 614)
74. C (CCP, p. 614)
75. E (CCP, p. 614)

CHAPTER 22: CARDIOVASCULAR EMERGENCIES

1. A (CCP, p. 623)
2. B (AP, p. 312)
3. C (AP, p. 459)
4. D (AP, p. 394, 482)
5. A (AP, p. 394, 482)
6. B (CCP, p. 623)
7. B (CCP, p. 624)
8. D (CCP, p. 624)
9. E (CCP, p. 624)
10. A (CCP, p. 626)
11. A (CCP, p. 627)
12. A (CCP, p. 627)
13. E (CCP, p. 627)
14. E (CCP, p. 628)
15. A (CCP, p. 628)
16. B (CCP, p. 628)
17. E (CCP, p. 629)
18. A (CCP, p. 630)
19. B (CCP, p. 633)
20. E (CCP, p. 633)
21. C (CCP, p. 633)
22. B (CCP, p. 633)
23. D (CCP, p. 624)
24. D (CCP, pp. 636–637)
25. B (CCP, p. 635)
26. D (CCP, p. 635)
27. C (CCP, p. 635)
28. C (CCP, p. 635)
29. C (CCP, p. 635)
30. A (CCP, p. 635)
31. A (CCP, pp. 636–637)
32. B (CCP, p. 637)
33. D (CCP, p. 638)
34. C (CCP, p. 638)
35. E (CCP, p. 638)
36. D (CCP, p. 639)
37. E (CCP, p. 640)
38. C (CCP, p. 641)
39. E (CCP, pp. 639, 641)
40. E (CCP, p. 642)
41. C (CCP, p. 642)
42. B (CCP, p. 643)
43. C (CCP, p. 643)
44. C (CCP, p. 643)
45. B (CCP, p. 644)
46. D (CCP, p. 644)
47. D (CCP, p. 645)
48. E (CCP, p. 645)
49. D (CCP, p. 636)
50. A (CCP, p. 645)
51. B (CCP, p. 645)
52. E (CCP, p. 645)
53. C (CCP, p. 645)
54. E (CCP, p. 647)
55. E (CCP, p. 647)
56. C (CCP, p. 648)
57. D (CCP, p. 652)
58. D (CCP, p. 652)
59. C (CCP, p. 652)
60. B (CCP, p. 652)
61. A (CCP, p. 653)
62. B (CCP, p. 654)
63. C (CCP, p. 654)
64. D (CCP, pp. 655–656)
65. C (CCP, p. 656)
66. A (CCP, p. 658)
67. E (CCP, p. 659)
68. D (CCP, p. 659)
69. B (CCP, p. 660)

ANSWER KEY ■ 305

70. E (CCP, p. 661)
71. C (CCP, p. 661)
72. C (CCP, p. 662)
73. D (CCP, p. 662)
74. A (CCP, p. 664)
75. A (CCP, p. 664)
76. E (CCP, p. 665)
77. C (CCP, p. 665)
78. A (CCP, pp. 665–668)
79. B (CCP, pp. 665–668)
80. A (CCP, pp. 665–668)
81. E (CCP, pp. 669–670)
82. E (CCP, pp. 671–672)
83. B (CCP, p. 672)
84. B (CCP, p. 672)
85. D (CCP, p. 673)

CHAPTER 23: NEUROLOGIC EMERGENCIES

1. E (CCP, p. 679)
2. C (CCP, p. 679)
3. D (CCP, p. 679)
4. B (CCP, p. 680)
5. C (CCP, p. 680)
6. A (CCP, p. 680)
7. B (CCP, p. 680)
8. C (CCP, p. 680)
9. B (CCP, p. 680)
10. B (CCP, p. 680)
11. A (CCP, p. 681)
12. A (CCP, p. 681)
13. D (CCP, p. 681)
14. D (CCP, p. 681)
15. C (CCP, p. 681)
16. B (CCP, p. 681)
17. A (CCP, p. 681)
18. B (CCP, p. 681)
19. D (CCP, p. 681)
20. C (CCP, p. 682)
21. B (CCP, p. 682)
22. C (CCP, p. 682)
23. C (CCP, p. 682)
24. B (CCP, p. 684)
25. D (CCP, p. 684)
26a. C (CCP, p. 684)
 b. D (CCP, p. 684)
 c. J (CCP, p. 684)
 d. I (CCP, p. 684)
 e. H (CCP, p. 684)
 f. G (CCP, p. 684)
 g. K (CCP, p. 684)
 h. E (CCP, p. 684)
 i. B (CCP, p. 684)
 j. A (CCP, p. 684)
 k. F (CCP, p. 684)
 l. L (CCP, p. 684)
27. A (CCP, p. 684)
28. C (CCP, p. 685)
29. B (CCP, p. 685)
30. C (CCP, p. 685)
31. B (CCP, p. 685)
32. C (CCP, p. 686)
33. E (CCP, p. 686)
34. D (CCP, p. 686)
35. D (CCP, p. 686)
36. B (CCP, p. 686)
37. B (CCP, p. 687)
38. E (CCP, p. 687)
39. C (CCP, p. 687)
40. D (CCP, p. 687)
41. E (CCP, p. 687)
42. D (CCP, p. 687)
43. C (CCP, p. 687)
44. B (CCP, p. 687)
45. C (CCP, p. 688)
46. E (CCP, p. 688)
47. C (CCP, p. 689)
48. B (CCP, p. 689)
49. D (CCP, p. 689)
50. C (CCP, p. 690)
51. C (CCP, p. 690)
52. A (CCP, p. 691)
53. A (CCP, p. 691)
54(1). D (CCP, p. 692)
54(2). F (CCP, p. 692)
54(3). C (CCP, p. 692)
54(4). A (CCP, p. 692)
54(5). B (CCP, p. 692)
54(6). I (CCP, p. 692)
54(7). G (CCP, p. 692)
54(8). H (CCP, p. 692)

54(9). E (CCP, p. 692)
55. D (CCP, p. 694)
56. E (CCP, p. 694)
57. E (CCP, p. 694)
58. B (CCP, p. 694)
59. D (CCP, p. 695)
60. B (CCP, p. 695)
61. D (CCP, p. 696)
62. E (CCP, p. 696)
63. B (CCP, p. 697)
64. D (CCP, p. 697)
65. A (CCP, p. 698)
66. B (CCP, p. 698)
67. B (CCP, p. 699)
68. B (CCP, p. 700)
69. C (CCP, p. 700)
70. E (CCP, p. 701)
71. A (CCP, p. 701)
72. C (CCP, p. 701)
73. E (CCP, p. 701)
74. A (CCP, p. 702)
75. D (CCP, p. 702)
76. B (CCP, p. 702)
77. B (CCP, p. 703)
78. B (CCP, p. 703)
79. C (CCP, p. 704)
80. E (CCP, p. 704)
81. C (CCP, p. 705)
82. E (CCP, p. 705)
83. C (CCP, p. 706)
84. A (CCP, p. 706)
85. D (CCP, p. 706)
86. C (CCP, p. 707)
87. B (CCP, p. 708)
88. A (CCP, p. 708)
89. B (CCP, p. 708)
90. E (CCP, p. 709)
91. C (CCP, p. 709)
92(1). I (CCP, pp. 709–712)
92(2). G (CCP, pp. 709–712)
92(3). J (CCP, pp. 709–712)
92(4). F (CCP, pp. 709–712)
92(5). E (CCP, pp. 709–712)
92(6). D (CCP, pp. 709–712)
92(7). B (CCP, pp. 709–712)
92(8). H (CCP, pp. 709–712)
92(9). A (CCP, pp. 709–712)
92(10). C (CCP, pp. 709–712)
93. C (CCP, p. 710)
94. B (CCP, p. 712)
95. E (CCP, p. 714)
96. D (CCP, p. 714)
97. E (CCP, pp. 714–715)
98. B (CCP, p. 715)
99a. D (CCP, p. 715)
  b. C (CCP, p. 715)
  c. B (CCP, p. 715)
  d. A (CCP, p. 715)
100. C (CCP, p. 715)

CHAPTER 24: GASTROINTESTINAL EMERGENCIES

1. C (AP, p. 596)
2. B (CCP, pp. 321–322)
3. A (CCP, pp. 735–736)
4. D (CCP, p. 732)
5. C (AP, p. 612)
6. C (CCP, p. 720)
7. A (CCP, p. 720)
8. D (CCP, p. 721)
9. B (CCP, p. 724)
10. A (CCP, p. 729)
11. D (CCP, p. 730)
12. E (CCP, p. 730)
13. A (CCP, p. 731)
14. D (CCP, p. 731)
15. B (CCP, p. 731)
16. B (CCP, p. 731)
17. C (CCP, p. 731)
18. D (CCP, p. 731)
19. C (CCP, p. 731)
20. C (CCP, p. 731)
21. A (CCP, p. 731)
22. B (CCP, p. 731)
23. D (CCP, p. 732)
24. C (CCP, p. 732)
25. E (CCP, p. 732)
26. C (CCP, p. 733)
27. B (CCP, p. 733)
28. C (CCP, p. 733)
29. E (CCP, p. 733)
30. D (CCP, p. 734)

ANSWER KEY ■ 307

31. D (CCP, pp. 733–734)
32. B (CCP, p. 734)
33. B (CCP, p. 734)
34. D (CCP, p. 735)
35. B (CCP, p. 735)
36. C (CCP, p. 735)
37. A (CCP, p. 735)
38. C (CCP, p. 736)
39. B (CCP, p. 736)
40. A (CCP, p. 736)
41. B (CCP, p. 736)
42. C (CCP, p. 737)
43. B (CCP, p. 737)
44. D (CCP, p. 737)
45. B (CCP, p. 738)
46. A (CCP, p. 738)
47. B (CCP, p. 738)
48. C (CCP, p. 739)
49. D (CCP, p. 739)
50. E (CCP, p. 739)
51. A (CCP, p. 739)
52. C (CCP, p. 740)
53. D (CCP, p. 741)
54. E (CCP, p. 741)
55. C (CCP, p. 742)
56. D (CCP, p. 743)
57. B (CCP, p. 743)
58. A (CCP, p. 743)
59. E (CCP, p. 743)
60. E (CCP, p. 744)
61. C (CCP, p. 745)
62. D (CCP, p. 745)
63. D (CCP, p. 745)
64. E (CCP, p. 746)
65. A (CCP, p. 746)

CHAPTER 25: RENAL AND ACID-BASE EMERGENCIES

1. C (CCP, p. 751)
2. E (CCP, p. 751)
3. C (CCP, p. 753)
4. C (CCP, p. 753)
5. A (CCP, p. 753)
6. D (AP, p. 377)
7. E (AP, p. 673)
8. A (CCP, p. 755)
9. B (AP, p. 666)
10. A (AP, p. 673)
11. D (AP, p. 673)
12. B (AP, p. 673)
13. A (AP, p. 684)
14. C (AP, p. 685)
15. C (AP, p. 675)
16. B (AP, p. 675)
17. E (AP, p. 676)
18. E (CCP, p. 751)
19. D (CCP, p. 755)
20. B (CCP, p. 757)
21. A (CCP, p. 757)
22. C (CCP, p. 759)
23. A (CCP, p. 759)
24. D (CCP, p. 760)
25. E (CCP, p. 761)
26. C (CCP, p. 762)
27. A (CCP, p. 764)
28. C (CCP, p. 764)
29. A (CCP, p. 764)
30. E (CCP, p. 764)
31. B (CCP, p. 765)
32. C (CCP, p. 766)
33. C (CCP, p. 767)
34. E (CCP, p. 762)
35. E (CCP, p. 768)
36. A (PCPP V3, p. 142)
37. C (CCP, pp. 757–759)
38. D (CCP, p. 759)
39. A (PCPP V3, pp. 405–412)
40. E (PCPP V3, pp. 405–412)

CHAPTER 26: INFECTIOUS DISEASE EMERGENCIES

1. C (CCP, p. 774)
2. E (CCP, p. 774)
3. D (CCP, p. 774)
4. B (CCP, p. 774)
5a. G (CCP, pp. 774–775)
 b. H (CCP, pp. 774–775)
 c. F (CCP, pp. 774–775)
 d. E (CCP, pp. 774–775)
 e. D (CCP, pp. 774–775)

f. C (CCP, pp. 774–775)
g. A (CCP, pp. 774–775)
h. B (CCP, pp. 774–775)
6. A (CCP, p. 774)
7. D (CCP, pp. 774–775)
8. B (CCP, p. 775)
9. C (CCP, p. 775)
10. E (CCP, p. 775)
11. E (CCP, p. 775)
12. B (CCP, p. 776)
13. C (CCP, p. 777)
14. B (CCP, pp. 777–778)
15. C (CCP, p. 778)
16. B (CCP, p. 778)
17. E (CCP, p. 778)
18a. E (CCP, p. 779)
  b. C (CCP, p. 779)
  c. B (CCP, p. 779)
  d. D (CCP, p. 779)
  e. A (CCP, p. 779)
19. E (CCP, pp. 778–781)
20. E (CCP, p. 782)
21. E (CCP, p. 782)
22. B (CCP, p. 786)
23. B (CCP, p. 786)
24. C (CCP, p. 787)
25. C (CCP, p. 787)
26. B (CCP, p. 787)
27. C (CCP, p. 789)
28. D (CCP, p. 789)
29. C (CCP, p. 789)
30. D (CCP, p. 789)
31. B (CCP, p. 790)
32. E (CCP, p. 790)
33. C (CCP, p. 790)
34. E (CCP, p. 790)
35. D (CCP, p. 790)
36. A (CCP, p. 791)
37. D (CCP, p. 791)
38. B (CCP, p. 791)
39. A (CCP, p. 792)
40. E (CCP, p. 792)
41. C (CCP, p. 792)
42. B (CCP, p. 793)
43. E (CCP, p. 794)
44. C (CCP, p. 794)

45. A (CCP, p. 795)
46. E (CCP, p. 795)
47. D (CCP, p. 795)
48. A (CCP, p. 796)
49. C (CCP, p. 796)
50. D (CCP, p. 796)
51. A (CCP, p. 796)
52. B (CCP, p. 797)
53. C (CCP, p. 797)
54. B (CCP, p. 797)
55. C (CCP, p. 796)
56. C (CCP, p. 798)
57. B (CCP, p. 798)
58. B (CCP, p. 798)
59. E (CCP, p. 798)
60. C (CCP, p. 800)
61. C (CCP, p. 801)
62. D (CCP, p. 801)
63. D (CCP, p. 801)
64. A (CCP, p. 801)
65. C (CCP, p. 802)
66a. A, B, C, F, H, I, J (CCP, p. 802)
  b. A, B, C, F, H, I, J (CCP, p. 802)
  c. D, E, G, H (CCP, p. 802)
67. B (CCP, p. 802)
68. A (CCP, p. 802)
69. E (CCP, p. 802)
70. D (CCP, p. 803)
71a. 1, A, E (CCP, pp. 803–804)
  b. 1, 2, 3, A, E (CCP, pp. 803–804)
  c. 2, A, B, E (CCP, pp. 803–804)
  d. 4, 5, D, E (CCP, pp. 803–804)
  e. 1, 2, 3, 6, C, D, E (CCP, pp. 803–804)
  f. 1, 2, 3, 4, E (CCP, pp. 803–804)
72. B (CCP, p. 803)
73. A (CCP, p. 803)
74. B (CCP, p. 803)
75. E (CCP, pp. 803–804)
76. D (CCP, p. 804)
77. B (CCP, p. 804)
78. C (CCP, p. 804)
79. E (CCP, p. 804)
80. D (CCP, p. 805)
81. D (CCP, p. 805)
82. B (CCP, p. 805)
83. B (CCP, p. 805)
84. E (CCP, p. 805)

85. C (CCP, p. 805)
86. D (CCP, p. 805)
87. B (CCP, p. 805)
88. C (CCP, pp. 805–806)
89. E (CCP, p. 775)
90. D (CCP, p. 789)

CHAPTER 27: PEDIATRIC MEDICAL EMERGENCIES

1. C (CCP, p. 813)
2. D (CCP, p. 813)
3. D (CCP, pp. 813–816)
4. C (CCP, p. 813)
5. B (CCP, p. 813)
6. C (CCP, p. 814)
7. E (CCP, p. 814)
8. E (CCP, p. 815)
9. D (CCP, p. 816)
10. B (CCP, p. 817)
11. C (CCP, p. 817)
12. C (CCP, p. 817)
13. D (CCP, p. 818)
14. A (CCP, p. 818)
15. D (CCP, p. 819)
16. C (CCP, p. 819)
17. B (CCP, p. 820)
18. A (CCP, p. 820)
19. E (CCP, p. 821)
20. D (CCP, p. 821)
21. A (CCP, p. 822)
22. D (CCP, p. 824)
23. C (CCP, p. 821)
24. A (CCP, p. 824)
25. B (CCP, p. 824)
26. D (CCP, p. 824)
27. D (CCP, p. 825)
28. B (CCP, p. 826)
29. A (CCP, p. 825)
30. B (CCP, p. 827)
31. C (CCP, p. 827)
32. D (CCP, p. 827)
33. C (CCP, p. 828)
34. B (CCP, p. 828)
35. A (CCP, p. 829)
36. D (CCP, p. 830)
37. D (CCP, p. 830)
38. E (CCP, p. 830)
39. A (CCP, p. 830)
40. D (CCP, p. 830)
41. B (CCP, p. 830)
42. A (CCP, p. 830)
43. E (CCP, p. 830)
44. C (CCP, p. 832)
45. A (CCP, p. 832)
46. B (CCP, p. 832)
47. B (CCP, pp. 832–833)
48. C (CCP, p. 833)
49. D (CCP, p. 833)
50. C (CCP, p. 833)
51. C (CCP, p. 833)
52. D (CCP, p. 836)
53. B (CCP, p. 836)
54. D (CCP, p. 836)
55. B (CCP, p. 833)

CHAPTER 28: HIGH-RISK OBSTETRICAL/ GYNECOLOGICAL EMERGENCIES

1. C (CCP, p. 843)
2. A (CCP, p. 843)
3. A (CCP, p. 843)
4. E (CCP, p. 844)
5. B (CCP, p. 843)
6. E (CCP, p. 844)
7. D (AP, p. 583)
8. A (AP, p. 583)
9. A (AP, p. 586)
10. A (AP, p. 590)
11. D (AP, p. 592)
12. E (AP, p. 592)
13. B (AP, p. 594)
14. B (AP, p. 598)
15. A (CCP, p. 849)
16. E (CCP, pp. 850–851)
17. C (AP, p. 583)
18. D (CCP, p. 853)
19. D (CCP, p. 854)
20. A (CCP, p. 855)
21. C (CCP, p. 855)
22. B (CCP, p. 855)
23. D (CCP, pp. 854–855)

24. C (CCP, p. 857)
25. A (CCP, p. 857)
26. A (CCP, p. 858)
27. E (CCP, p. 859)
28. C (CCP, p. 860)
29. B (CCP, p. 861)
30. D (CCP, p. 862)
31. B (CCP, p. 862)
32. A (CCP, p. 862)
33. D (CCP, p. 863)
34. E (CCP, p. 863)
35. D (CCP, p. 865)
36. B (CCP, p. 865)
37. C (CCP, p. 866)
38. E (CCP, p. 867)
39. A (CCP, p. 868)
40. E (CCP, p. 868)
41. D (CCP, p. 869)
42. D (CCP, p. 869)
43. E (CCP, p. 870)
44. E (CCP, p. 870)
45. C (CCP, p. 867)
46. B (PCPP V3, p. 732)
47. D (CCP, p. 867)
48. E (PCPP V3, p. 734)
49. A (PCPP V3, p. 733–734)
50. D (PCPP V3, p. 732)

CHAPTER 29: NEONATAL EMERGENCIES

1. A (CCP, p. 876)
2. E (CCP, p. 876)
3. B (CCP, p. 876)
4. D (CCP, p. 876)
5. A (CCP, p. 876)
6. D (CCP, p. 876)
7. A (CCP, p. 877)
8. C (CCP, p. 877)
9. C (CCP, p. 877)
10. A (CCP, p. 878)
11. E (CCP, pp. 877–878)
12. C (CCP, p. 879)
13. A (CCP, p. 879)
14. C (CCP, p. 879)
15. B (CCP, p. 879)
16. D (CCP, p. 881)
17. A (CCP, p. 881)
18. C (CCP, p. 881)
19. B (CCP, p. 881)
20. D (CCP, p. 882)
21. E (CCP, pp. 879–882)
22. A (CCP, p. 882)
23. A (CCP, p. 883)
24. B (CCP, p. 882)
25. C (CCP, p. 876)
26. C (CCP, p. 882)
27. E (CCP, pp. 882–883)
28. C (CCP, p. 883)
29. A (CCP, p. 883)
30. B (CCP, p. 884)
31. D (CCP, p. 884)
32. C (CCP, p. 884)
33. A (CCP, p. 884)
34. D (CCP, p. 885)
35. B (CCP, p. 885)
36. C (CCP, p. 885)
37. D (CCP, p. 886)
38. A (CCP, p. 886)
39. B (CCP, p. 886)
40. B (CCP, p. 887)
41. D (CCP, p. 887)
42. C (CCP, p. 887)
43. B (CCP, p. 888)
44. D (CCP, p. 888)
45. A (CCP, p. 889)
46. E (CCP, p. 888)
47. E (CCP, p. 889)
48. A (CCP, p. 890)
49. E (CCP, p. 89)
50. B (CCP, p. 89)
51. C (CCP, p. 890)
52. A (CCP, p. 890)
53. B (CCP, p. 890)
54. C (CCP, p. 891)
55. B (CCP, p. 891)
56. D (CCP, p. 892)
57. A (CCP, p. 892)
58. D (CCP, p. 892)
59. B (CCP, p. 893)
60. C (CCP, p. 893)

CHAPTER 30: ENVIRONMENTAL EMERGENCIES

1. B (CCP, p. 897)
2. E (PEP, p. 67)
3. C (PEP, p. 67)
4. E (PEP, p. 67)
5. A (PEP, p. 67)
6. B (PEP, p. 67)
7. C (CCP, p. 897)
8. D (CCP, p. 897)
9. E (CCP, p. 898)
10. D (CCP, p. 898)
11. E (CCP, p. 898)
12. A (CCP, p. 899)
13. C (CCP, p. 899)
14. B (CCP, pp. 898–899)
15. D (CCP, p. 900)
16. D (CCP, p. 900)
17. D (CCP, p. 901; AP pp. 323–325)
18. D (CCP, pp. 902–903)
19. A (CCP, p. 903)
20. A (CCP, p. 903)
21. A (CCP, p. 903)
22. E (CCP, p. 904)
23. B (CCP, p. 904)
24. B (CCP, p. 905)
25. C (CCP, p. 905)
26. E (CCP, p. 905)
27. E (CCP, p. 907)
28. A (CCP, p. 906)
29. E (CCP, p. 906)
30. C (CCP, p. 907)
31. D (CCP, p. 907)
32. B (CCP, p. 907)
33. E (CCP, p. 908)
34. E (CCP, pp. 908–909)
35. C (CCP, p. 909)
36. A (CCP, p. 908)
37. D (CCP, p. 908)
38. E (CCP, p. 910)
39. B (CCP, p. 911)
40. A (CCP, p. 912)
41. C (CCP, p. 912)
42. B (CCP, p. 913)
43. E (CCP, p. 914)
44. D (CCP, p. 899)
45. D (CCP, p. 905)

CHAPTER 31: DIVING EMERGENCIES

1. B (CCP, p. 918)
2. C (CCP, p. 919)
3. E (CCP, p. 919)
4. E (CCP, p. 919)
5. B (CCP, p. 920)
6. D (CCP, p. 920)
7. E (CCP, p. 920)
8. B (CCP, p. 920)
9. A (CCP, p. 920)
10. C (CCP, p. 921)
11. B (CCP, p. 922)
12. A (CCP, p. 918)
13. D (CCP, p. 923)
14. C (CCP, p. 923)
15. E (CCP, p. 923)
16. E (CCP, p. 923)
17. E (CCP, p. 923)
18. C (CCP, p. 923)
19. E (CCP, p. 924)
20. B (CCP, p. 924)
21. B (CCP, p. 924)
22. D (CCP, p. 925)
23. A (CCP, p. 925)
24. E (CCP, p. 925)
25. D (CCP, p. 926)
26. D (CCP, p. 926)
27. E (CCP, p. 926)
28. A (CCP, p. 927)
29. C (CCP, p. 927)
30. E (CCP, p. 927)
31. B (CCP, p. 928)
32. A (CCP, p. 928)
33. B (CCP, p. 928)
34. E (CCP, p. 929)
35. B (CCP, p. 929)
36. D (CCP, p. 930)
37. A (CCP, p. 930)
38. C (CCP, p. 931)
39. D (CCP, p. 931)
40. B (CCP, p. 932)

CHAPTER 32: TOXICOLOGICAL EMERGENCIES

1. B (CCP, p. 938)
2. E (CCP, p. 938)
3. D (CCP, p. 938)
4. C (CCP, p. 938)
5. B (CCP, p. 938)
6. A (CCP, p. 938)
7. E (CCP, p. 938)
8. D (CCP, p. 938)
9. E (CCP, p. 938)
10. A (CCP, p. 939)
11. D (CCP, p. 939)
12. C (CCP, p. 939)
13. D (CCP, p. 939)
14. E (CCP, p. 939)
15. E (CCP, p. 939)
16. D (CCP, p. 939)
17. B (CCP, p. 939)
18. C (CCP, p. 939)
19. E (CCP, p. 939)
20. B (CCP, p. 939)
21. C (CCP, p. 940)
22. D (CCP, p. 940)
23. B (CCP, p. 940)
24. B (CCP, p. 940)
25. A (CCP, p. 941)
26. C (CCP, pp. 940–941)
27. C (CCP, p. 941)
28. B (CCP, p. 941)
29. D (CCP, p. 941)
30. B (CCP, p. 941)
31. D (CCP, p. 941)
32. E (CCP, p. 941)
33. C (CCP, p. 942)
34. B (CCP, p. 942)
35. E (CCP, p. 942)
36. C (CCP, p. 942)
37. D (CCP, p. 942)
38. C (CCP, p. 942)
39. C (CCP, p. 943)
40a. D (CCP, p. 943)
　b. C (CCP, p. 943)
　c. B (CCP, p. 943)
　d. A (CCP, p. 943)
41. C (CCP, p. 943)
42. A (CCP, p. 943)
43. A (CCP, p. 943)
44. C (CCP, p. 943)
45. D (CCP, p. 944)
46. D (CCP, p. 944)
47. E (CCP, p. 944)
48. C (CCP, p. 944)
49. B (CCP, p. 944)
50. C (CCP, p. 944)
51. B (CCP, p. 944)
52. D (CCP, p. 944)
53. A (CCP, p. 944)
54. C (CCP, p. 945)
55. C (CCP, p. 945)
56a. C (CCP, p. 945)
　b. D (CCP, p. 945)
　c. A (CCP, p. 945)
　d. B (CCP, p. 945)
57. E (CCP, p. 946)
58. B (CCP, p. 946)
59. B (CCP, p. 946)
60. C (CCP, p. 947)
61. E (CCP, p. 947)
62. D (CCP, p. 947)
63. E (CCP, pp. 947–948)
64. E (CCP, p. 948)
65. B (CCP, p. 948)
66. C (CCP, p. 949)
67. B (CCP, p. 949)
68. B (CCP, p. 949)
69. A (CCP, p. 949)
70. B (CCP, p. 950)
71. E (CCP, p. 950)
72. D (CCP, p. 951)
73. C (CCP, p. 951)
74. D (CCP, p. 952)
75. C (CCP, p. 952)
76. C (CCP, p. 952)
77. D (CCP, p. 952)
78. C (CCP, p. 953)
79. E (CCP, p. 953)
80. D (CCP, p. 953)
81. B (CCP, p. 953)

CHAPTER 33: WEAPONS OF MASS DESTRUCTION

1. B (CCP, p. 963)
2. C (CCP, p. 962)
3. D (CCP, p. 963)
4. B (CCP, p. 962)
5. E (CCP, p. 963)
6. B (CCP, p. 963)
7. C (CCP, p. 963)
8. D (CCP, p. 963)
9. D (CCP, p. 964)
10. E (CCP, pp. 962–964)
11. D (CCP, p. 965)
12. E (CCP, p. 964)
13. B (CCP, p. 965)
14. E (CCP, p. 965)
15. A (CCP, p. 965)
16. C (CCP, p. 949)
17. D (CCP, p. 966)
18. B (CCP, p. 967)
19. B (CCP, p. 967)
20. D (CCP, p. 967)
21. A (CCP, p. 967)
22. E (CCP, pp. 967–968)
23. D (CCP, p. 968)
24. A (CCP, p. 968)
25. D (CCP, p. 968)
26. B (CCP, p. 969)
27. C (CCP, p. 969)
28. E (CCP, p. 969)
29. E (CCP, p. 970)
30. A (CCP, p. 970)
31. A (CCP, p. 978)
32. C (CCP, p. 979)
33. C (CCP, p. 979)
34. E (CCP, pp. 979–984)
35a. B, D, E (CCP, p. 980)
  b. F (CCP, p. 980)
  c. A, C (CCP, p. 980)
36. A (CCP, p. 981)
37. D (CCP, p. 981)
38. A (CCP, p. 981)
39a. D, F (CCP, pp. 983–984)
  b. A, B (CCP, pp. 983–984)
  c. C, E (CCP, pp. 983–984)
40. D (CCP, p. 984)
41. B (CCP, p. 970)
42. C (CCP, p. 972)
43. B (CCP, p. 972)
44. E (CCP, p. 973)
45. B (CCP, p. 973)
46. C (CCP, p. 973)
47. E (CCP, p. 974)
48. C (CCP, p. 974)
49. B (CCP, p. 974)
50. A (CCP, p. 972)

CHAPTER 34: ORGAN DONATION AND RETRIEVAL

1. B (CCP, p. 990)
2. E (CCP, p. 991)
3. E (CCP, p. 991)
4. C (CCP, p. 991)
5. D (CCP, pp. 991–992)
6. D (CCP, p. 992)
7. B (CCP, p. 992)
8. C (CCP, p. 993)
9. A (CCP, p. 993)
10. E (CCP, p. 994)
11. C (CCP, p. 994)
12. A (CCP, p. 994)
13. D (CCP, p. 994)
14. D (CCP, p. 995)
15. B (CCP, p. 996)
16. B (CCP, p. 997)
17. D (CCP, p. 997)
18. C (CCP, p. 997)
19. E (CCP, pp. 998–999)
20. E (CCP, p. 999)
21. E (CCP, p. 1000)
22. A (CCP, p. 998)
23. D (CCP, p. 998)
24. D (CCP, p. 997)
25. E (CCP, pp. 990–1000)

CHAPTER 35: QUALITY IMPROVEMENT IN CRITICAL CARE TRANSPORT

1. B (CCP, p. 1004)
2. E (CCP, p. 1004)
3. E (CCP, p. 1004)
4. A (CCP, p. 1005)
5. E (CCP, p. 1006)
6. C (CCP, p. 1007)
7. D (CCP, p. 1008)
8. B (CCP, p. 1009)
9. A (CCP, p. 1011)
10. C (CCP, pp. 1011–1012)
11. A (CCP, p. 1015)
12. D (CCP, p. 1017)
13. E (CCP, p. 1015)
14. B (CCP, p. 1016)
15. A (CCP, p. 1005)

CHAPTER 36: COMMUNICATIONS AND DOCUMENTATION

1. C (CCP, p. 1032)
2. D (CCP, pp. 1032–1034)
3. A (CCP, p. 1037)
4. C (CCP, p. 1037)
5. B (CCP, p. 1037)
6. C (CCP, p. 1042)
7. D (CCP, pp. 1042–1043)
8. A (CCP, p. 1043)
9. E (CCP, p. 1044)
10. D (CCP, p. 1047)
11. B (CCP, p. 1047)
12. F (CCP, p. 1047)
13. E (CCP, p. 1047)
14. A (CCP, p. 1047)
15. I (CCP, p. 1047)
16. H (CCP, p. 1047)
17. D (CCP, p. 1048)
18. A (CCP, p. 1048)
19. E (CCP, p. 1018)
20. C (CCP, p. 1048)
21. E (CCP, p. 1047)
22. C (CCP, p. 1046)
23. A (CCP, p. 1044)
24. C (CCP, p. 1041)
25. C (CCP, p. 1040)

CHAPTER 37: THE CRITICAL CARE PARAMEDIC IN THE HOSPITAL ENVIRONMENT

1. E (CCP, p. 1052)
2. D (CCP, p. 1053)
3. C (CCP, p. 1053)
4. D (CCP, p. 1055)
5. A (CCP, p. 1058)
6. D (CCP, p. 1061)
7. C (CCP, p. 1061)
8. A (CCP, p. 1058)
9. B (CCP, p. 1056)
10. E (CCP, pp. 1052–1061)

Final Review
Practice Examination

1. The enzyme carbonic anhydrase is **NOT** found in which of the following tissues?
   A. erythrocytes
   B. brain cells
   C. liver cells
   D. parietal cells of the stomach
   E. none of the above

2. Which of the following formulas is used for calculating minute volume?
   A. $V_T - V_D$
   B. $V_T \times$ respiratory rate
   C. $(V_T - V_D) \times$ respiratory rate
   D. $V_A \times$ respiratory rate
   E. none of the above

3. In patients with which of the following Glasgow Coma Scores (GCS) would endotracheal intubation **NOT** be indicated?
   A. GCS = 9
   B. GCS = 8
   C. GCS < 8
   D. GCS < 9
   E. none of the above

4. The tracing in Figure Final–1 reflects which of the following?
   A. right ventricular pressure
   B. pulmonary artery pressure
   C. pulmonary artery wedge pressure
   D. right atria pressure
   E. radial artery waveform

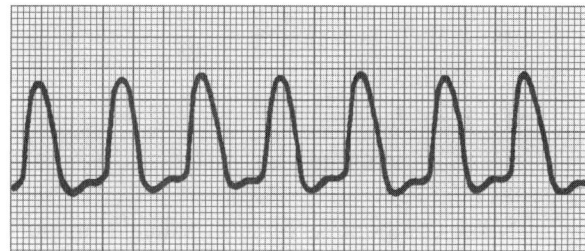

Figure Final–1

5. Which of the following statements regarding the sodium/potassium pump is **FALSE**?
   A. It maintains a high concentration of potassium inside the cell.
   B. Failure can result in cell lysis.
   C. It is the primary user of cellular energy substrates.
   D. It maintains a high concentration of sodium inside the cell.
   E. It uses adenosine triphosphate (ATP) as its energy source.

6. All of the following statements about an intra-aortic balloon pump (IABP) are true EXCEPT:
   A. The balloon is inflated with helium.
   B. It increases coronary artery blood flow.
   C. The ratio of inflations to cardiac contractions can be varied.
   D. It inflates rapidly at the onset of each systole.
   E. none of the above.

7. Which of the following laboratory values is used to measure warfarin (Coumadin) therapy?
   A. partial thromboplastin time (PTT)
   B. prothrombin time (PT)
   C. international normalized ratio (INR)
   D. A and C
   E. B and C

8. Which of the following conditions is NOT a common cause of metabolic acidosis?
   A. shock
   B. diabetic ketoacidosis
   C. steroid usage
   D. renal failure
   E. diuretic usage

9. Some components of aeromedical transport safety might include:
   A. preflight guidelines and equipment checks.
   B. use of safety devices (helmets, clothing, restraint systems).
   C. isolation of the pilot and aircraft controls from the patient compartment.
   D. all of the above.
   E. A and B.

10. The primary tenet of quality in most EMS customer service programs is:
    A. survival to discharge.
    B. unit hour utilization (UHU).
    C. customer satisfaction.
    D. hospital feedback.
    E. none of the above.

11. Helicopters were first used for patient transport during the:
    A. Korean War.
    B. Crimean War.
    C. Vietnam War.
    D. World War II.
    E. Civil War.

12. Which of the following statements about late decelerations in fetal heart rate (FHR) monitoring during labor is TRUE?
    A. They are reassuring.
    B. They reflect fetal head compression.
    C. They are due to umbilical cord compression.
    D. They are due to uteroplacental insufficiency.
    E. none of the above.

13. Which of the following statements regarding spontaneous pneumothorax is FALSE?
    A. Males are more commonly affected.
    B. The patients are often thin.
    C. Smoking is a risk factor.
    D. The left lung is almost always the lung affected.
    E. none of the above

14. Which of the following classification systems is used to describe pediatric fractures?
    A. Salter-Harris
    B. Tscherne
    C. Gustilo
    D. Denis
    E. Neiman-Marcus

15. Which of the following is an absolute CONTRAINDICATION to fibrinolytic therapy?
    A. history of trauma in the past 2 months
    B. prolonged CPR
    C. known cancer

D. active peptic ulcer disease
E. none of the above

16. You are transporting a patient who has received a heparin bolus and a heparin drip. During transport he starts to vomit bright red blood. Which of the following drugs could be administered to reverse the effects of the heparin?
    A. warfarin (Coumadin)
    B. protamine
    C. vitamin K (Aqua-Mephyton)
    D. low-molecular weight heparin
    E. none of the above

17. You have a patient who was involved in a motorcycle crash. He opens his eyes to pain, withdraws by flexion from pain, and utters inappropriate words. What is his Glasgow Coma Scale score?
    A. 4
    B. 6
    C. 7
    D. 8
    E. 9

18. In the choices below, consider cardiac output (CO), intracranial pressure (ICP), and mean arterial pressure (MAP). Which of the following is the formula for cerebral perfusion pressure (CPP)?
    A. CPP = CO × ICP
    B. CPP = CO − ICP
    C. CPP = MAP − ICP
    D. CPP = CO − MAP
    E. none of the above

19. Which of the following is NOT a feature of tetralogy of Fallot?
    A. coarctation of the aorta
    B. subaortic ventricular septal defect
    C. right ventricular infundibular stenosis
    D. aortic valve positioned to override the right ventricle
    E. right ventricular hypertrophy

20. Which of the following describes multiple sclerosis?
    A. degeneration of the upper and lower motor neurons
    B. demyelination of the white matter in the brain and spinal cord
    C. cortical and hippocampal degeneration
    D. results from loss of dopamine-secreting neurons in the substantia nigra
    E. none of the above

21. A blow-out fracture typically affects the:
    A. superior rectus.
    B. superior oblique.
    C. inferior oblique.
    D. inferior rectus.
    E. none of the above.

22. The trigeminal nerve is cranial nerve _____.
    A. II
    B. IV
    C. V
    D. VII
    E. VIII

23. The most commonly seen serious abdominal emergency in neonates that requires surgical intervention is:
    A. necrotizing enterocolitis (NEC).
    B. volvulus.
    C. appendicitis.
    D. diaphragmatic hernia.
    E. none of the above.

24. Of the following, which is NOT an H_2 blocker?
    A. ranitidine (Zantac)
    B. cimetidine (Tagamet)
    C. famotidine (Pepcid)
    D. nizatidine (Axid)
    E. none of the above

25. Which of the following neuromuscular blockers is classified as depolarizing?
    A. vecuronium
    B. pancuronium
    C. mivacurium
    D. atracurium
    E. none of the above

26. Your patient has a blood pressure of 128/80. What is the mean arterial pressure?
    A. 80 mmHg
    B. 90 mmHg
    C. 48 mmHg
    D. 96 mmHg
    E. none of the above

27. The FAA requirement that all nonessential communications be ceased during critical stages of flight is called:
    A. running silent.
    B. muted cockpit.
    C. sterile cockpit.
    D. pilot muting.
    E. none of the above.

28. You are transporting an 18-pound toddler with a third-degree burn. Fluid therapy was started at the transferring hospital. Using the Parkland formula, the patient should receive _____ mL of fluid in the first 8 hours.
    A. 1,500
    B. 1,700
    C. 2,100
    D. 3,400
    E. none of the above

29. Your patient has a history of alcoholism and recently began chemotherapy for colon cancer. After retching clear saliva for the past 24 hours, he begins to vomit bright red blood and has become hypotensive. What is his most likely underlying condition?
    A. peptic ulcer disease
    B. duodenal carcinoma
    C. gastritis
    D. Mallory-Weiss syndrome
    E. none of the above

30. Temperature regulation is primarily controlled in which brain region?
    A. hypothalamus
    B. pons
    C. medulla oblongata
    D. substantia nigra
    E. none of the above

31. Which of the following is NOT a critical finding in neurologic death?
    A. apnea
    B. no motor response to painful stimuli
    C. no brainstem reflexes
    D. explained loss of consciousness
    E. none of the above

32. Which of the following pieces of legislation allows emergency personnel to find out if they were exposed to an infectious disease while rendering patient care?
    A. Centers for Disease Control and Prevention Guidelines
    B. Ryan White Act
    C. Americans with Disabilities Act
    D. Health Insurance Portability and Accountability Act (HIPAA)
    E. none of the above

33. Which of the following diseases is caused by a prion?
    A. Rocky Mountain spotted fever
    B. delta hepatitis
    C. severe acute respiratory syndrome (SARS)
    D. Asian bird influenza (H5N1)
    E. bovine spongiform encephalitis (BSE)

34. You are treating an asthma patient who uses a home nebulizer and has suffered an acute exacerbation. The patient has a peak

expiratory flow rate (PEFR) that is 56% of predicted, an SpO$_2$ of 94%, and both expiratory and inspiratory wheezes. Which of the following statements about this patient is **FALSE**?
   A. The severity of his exacerbation is severe.
   B. Beta agonist therapy should be continued.
   C. The patient should receive corticosteroids.
   D. Supplemental oxygen will be beneficial.
   E. none of the above

35. Ricin is derived from:
    A. uranium.
    B. marine dinoflagellates.
    C. reef fish.
    D. castor beans.
    E. mango fruit.

36. Which of the following drugs would **NOT** be reversed by naloxone (Narcan)?
    A. fentanyl
    B. nalmefene
    C. morphine
    D. codeine
    E. none of the above

37. The sympathetic nervous system is associated with what region(s) of the spinal cord?
    A. thoracic
    B. lumbar
    C. sacral
    D. A and B
    E. A and C

38. A gas has a temperature of 317 K and a volume of 500 cm^3. If the temperature is decreased to 200 K, what would be the volume of the gas?
    A. 553 cm^3
    B. 793 cm^3
    C. 801 cm^3
    D. 253 cm^3
    E. 316 cm^3

39. Which antibody type is most associated with allergic reactions?
    A. IgG
    B. IgE
    C. IgM
    D. IgD
    E. IgA

40. A patient has a pulmonary artery pressure of 26/8 mmHg. What is the mean pulmonary artery pressure?
    A. 18 mmHg
    B. 14 mmHg
    C. 13 mmHg
    D. 10 mmHg
    E. none of the above

41. Which of the following cell types produces cerebrospinal fluid?
    A. astrocytes
    B. microglia
    C. ependymal cells
    D. oligodendrocytes
    E. none of the above

42. What is the normal daily bile production and drainage via a T tube?
    A. 20–30 mL
    B. 700–1,200 mL
    C. 100–120 mL
    D. 2–3 mL
    E. none of the above

43. Ebola is caused by a:
    A. hantavirus.
    B. arenavirus.
    C. filovirus.
    D. coronavirus.
    E. retrovirus.

44. Which gastrourinary organ is most frequently injured in trauma?
    A. kidney
    B. bladder
    C. penis
    D. urethra
    E. none of the above

45. On a lateral radiograph of the neck, epiglottitis can be identified by which of the following signs?
    A. steeple sign
    B. horse's tail sign
    C. Throckmorton's sign
    D. thumb sign
    E. none of the above

46. Which cerebral vessel supplies the medial aspects of the temporal and parietal lobes of the brain?
    A. anterior cerebral artery
    B. middle cerebral artery
    C. posterior cerebral artery
    D. vertebrobasilar artery
    E. none of the above

47. Aqueous humor is found in which area?
    A. posterior cavity
    B. anterior chamber
    C. aqueduct of sylvan
    D. nasolacrimal duct
    E. none of the above

48. Vaccinations are available for all of the following illnesses EXCEPT:
    A. hepatitis A.
    B. hepatitis B.
    C. varicella.
    D. hepatitis C.
    E. variola.

49. What is the most common congenital heart defect?
    A. atrial septal defect
    B. ventricular septal defect
    C. patent *ductus arteriosus*
    D. coarctation of the aorta
    E. tetralogy of Fallot

50. Self-imposed standards or rules of conduct for a group are referred to as:
    A. bylaws.
    B. case law.
    C. ethics.
    D. oaths.
    E. none of the above.

51. Which aspect of the immune defenses attacks and breaks down cell walls, attracts phagocytes, and stimulates inflammation?
    A. complement system
    B. interferons
    C. inflammatory response
    D. immunological surveillance
    E. none of the above

52. What factors are associated with acute respiratory distress syndrome?
    A. near-drowning
    B. pulmonary contusion
    C. multiple trauma
    D. multiple blood transfusions
    E. all of the above

53. Which of the following has the most powerful effect on respiratory activity?
    A. pOH
    B. PO_2
    C. pH
    D. HCO_3^-
    E. none of the above

54. The accessory tract associated with Lown-Ganong-Levine (LGL) syndrome is:
    A. bundle of Kent.
    B. bundle of Purkinje.
    C. James's fibers.
    D. Carson's tract.
    E. none of the above.

55. Which of the following does NOT affect the extent of an electrical injury?
    A. color of skin
    B. type of current
    C. local tissue resistance
    D. duration of contact
    E. pathway of flow

56. The P2 wave seen during intracranial pressure monitoring is due to:
    A. pulse.
    B. cerebral compliance.
    C. closure of the semi-lunar valves.
    D. dural tenting.
    E. none of the above.

57. Your patient has sustained a gunshot to the back. He exhibits motor weakness and the loss of light touch, vibratory and position sense on the right side and loss of pain and temperature sense on the left. Motor loss is greater on the right. This suggests what syndrome?
    A. Brown-Séquard syndrome
    B. anterior cord syndrome
    C. central cord syndrome
    D. cervical cord syndrome
    E. none of the above

58. The most common type of primary brain tumor is:
    A. meningioma.
    B. optic glioma.
    C. medulloblastoma.
    D. astrocytoma.
    E. none of the above.

59. Which of the following conditions increase(s) the risk of hypothermia?
    A. alcoholism
    B. sepsis
    C. shock
    D. chemotherapy
    E. all of the above

60. In regard to hemoglobin-based oxygen-carrying solutions (HBOCs), which of the following statements is FALSE?
    A. They are made of polymerized hemoglobin.
    B. They have a longer shelf-life compared to human blood.
    C. The hemoglobin is in red cells that have been washed to remove infectious agents.
    D. A unit of PolyHeme™ contains the same amount of hemoglobin (50 grams) as whole blood.
    E. Blood typing is not required with HBOCs.

61. Which of the following is NOT a nerve agent?
    A. mustard gas
    B. Tabun (GA)
    C. Sarin (GB)
    D. VX
    E. none of the above

62. Which bacterium has been associated with peptic ulcer disease (PUD)?
    A. *Moraxella cataralis*
    B. *Strep pneumoniae*
    C. *Chlamydia trachomatis*
    D. *Escherechia coli*
    E. none of the above

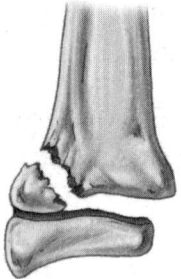

Figure Final–2

63. The fracture type illustrated in Figure Final–2 is classified as:
    A. Salter-Harris Type I.
    B. Salter-Harris Type II.
    C. Salter-Harris Type III.
    D. Salter-Harris Type IV.
    E. Salter-Harris Type V.

64. In terms of intracranial pressure (ICP) monitoring, which of the following statements is TRUE?
    A. The percussion wave (P1) indicates cerebral compliance.
    B. As ICP increases, the amplitude of the pulse pressure wave increases.
    C. The dicrotic wave (P3) reflects closure of the mitral valve.
    D. The tidal wave (P2) reflects the pulse.
    E. none of the above

65. Which of the following is NOT an age-related system change?
    A. increased blood volume and/or RBCs
    B. diminished immune response
    C. reduced sweating
    D. loss of kidney size and function
    E. lower estrogen production in women

66. Which of the following is NOT a finding of compartment syndrome?
    A. pain
    B. pallor
    C. pulselessness
    D. pulsus paradoxus
    E. pressure

Scenario

Questions 67–69 refer to the following scenario:
You are transporting a chest pain patient from a community hospital to a hospital with invasive cardiology capabilities. The patient is a 56-year-old male with a history of smoking, hypertension, and hypercholesterolemia. His vital signs are:

Blood pressure = 110/60 mmHg
Pulse = 102 per minute
Respirations = 18 per minute
SpO_2 = 100% (nasal cannula)

The patient has ST segment elevations in Leads II, III, and AVF and ST segment depression in V2.

67. Which of the following would NOT be of added benefit in evaluating this patient?
    A. 15- or 18-Lead ECG
    B. nitrates
    C. oxygen
    D. aspirin
    E. morphine

68. The patient's blood pressure falls to 90/50 mmHg and his heart rate increases to 122 per minute. Which of the following is indicated?
    A. nitrates
    B. norepinephrine
    C. immediate heparinization
    D. fluid bolus
    E. none of the above

69. Which of the following statements about the patient in the case study is FALSE?
    A. Decreased right ventricular cardiac output (CO) leads to decreased left ventricular CO.
    B. Right ventricular end-diastolic pressure is elevated (RVDP).
    C. Increased RVDP causes a septal shift that causes decreased left ventricular end-diastolic pressure.

D. Increased right ventricular cardiac output (CO) leads to decreased left ventricular CO.
E. none of the above

70. What percentage of carbon dioxide is converted to carbonic acid for transport?
   A. 7%
   B. 70%
   C. 23%
   D. 17%
   E. none of the above

71. Which of the following stimulate(s) uterine contraction?
   A. estrogen
   B. relaxin
   C. fetal growth
   D. oxytocin
   E. all of the above

72. Which of the following is NOT an advantage of patient transport in a fixed-wing aircraft?
   A. rapid departure time
   B. good patient accessibility
   C. lower cost than rotor-wing transport
   D. speed
   E. none of the above

73. Which coronary artery supplies the septum and the anterior wall of the left ventricle?
   A. right coronary artery
   B. left anterior descending coronary artery
   C. left circumflex artery
   D. right circumflex artery
   E. none of the above

74. Which of the following is NOT characteristic of aortic dissection?
   A. arteriosclerosis as the most common cause
   B. usually involves the thoracic aorta
   C. sharp, tearing pain often reported
   D. begins as an intimal tear
   E. none of the above

75. The severity of a subarachnoid hemorrhage can be graded by which of the following scores?
   A. Tscherne
   B. Hunt and Hess
   C. Fisher
   D. B and C
   E. none of the above

76. The typical dose of reteplase (Retavase) is:
   A. 15 milligrams.
   B. 30 milligrams.
   C. 10 units.
   D. 50 milligrams.
   E. 100 units.

77. A Sengstaken-Blakemore tube is used for which of the following conditions?
   A. gastric bypass surgery
   B. short bowel syndrome
   C. high-grade fecal impaction
   D. enteral feeding
   E. none of the above

78. The auditory ossicles are located in what region of the ear?
   A. external ear
   B. middle ear
   C. inner ear
   D. cochlea
   E. none of the above

79. The most common cause of trauma in children is:
   A. motor vehicle collisions.
   B. auto-pedestrian incidents.
   C. child abuse.
   D. bicycling.
   E. falls.

80. Which of the following statements concerning the Allen's test is NOT correct?
    A. It is used to assess perfusion to tissues distal from a site of arterial line placement.
    B. The patient is first asked to clench his fist.
    C. Both the radial and ulnar arteries are compressed and released.
    D. Only the ulnar artery is compressed and released.
    E. none of the above

81. The horizontal and vertical stabilizers are normally affixed to the _____ of a helicopter.
    A. tail boom
    B. main rotor system
    C. tail rotor
    D. undercarriage
    E. all of the above

82. The majority of heat loss from the body occurs via which of the following mechanisms?
    A. radiation
    B. convection
    C. evaporation
    D. conduction
    E. none of the above

83. In terms of organ retrieval and donation, which of the following has the shortest preservation times?
    A. liver
    B. kidney
    C. heart
    D. brain
    E. skin

84. Which of the following statements about diastolic murmurs is FALSE?
    A. They fall after S_2.
    B. They precede S_1.
    C. They occur if the aortic valve is faulty.
    D. They occur if the pulmonic valve is faulty.
    E. none of the above

85. The phenomenon whereby either perfusion or ventilation to an area of the lung decreases is called:
    A. reactive airway disease.
    B. atelectasis.
    C. V/Q mismatch.
    D. VP shunt.
    E. none of the above.

86. The adult normally has _____ teeth.
    A. 22
    B. 28
    C. 30
    D. 32
    E. 36

87. In an inferior wall infarct, you would NOT expect to see ST segment elevation in which of the following ECG leads?
    A. III
    B. AVF
    C. II
    D. V2
    E. none of the above

88. What is the most common isolated valvular lesion?
    A. aortic regurgitation
    B. aortic stenosis
    C. mitral stenosis
    D. mitral regurgitation
    E. pulmonic stenosis

89. For elevations in intracranial pressure (ICP), what is the typical dose of mannitol?
    A. 1.5–2.0 mg/kg
    B. 1.5–2.0 grams
    C. 0.15–0.20 g/kg

D. 25–35 mg

E. 1.5–2.0 g/kg

90. When treating a tar burn, the most important concern is:
    A. removing the tar.
    B. determining the type of tar so a suitable solvent can be selected.
    C. providing an antidote for bitumen.
    D. cooling the tar.
    E. none of the above.

91. The gold standard diagnostic test for abdominal trauma is:
    A. laparotomy.
    B. diagnostic peritoneal lavage (DPL).
    C. computed tomography with contrast.
    D. ultrasound.
    E. none of the above.

92. Which of the following factors is associated with the highest fetal mortality after trauma?
    A. uterine rupture
    B. motorcycle crashes
    C. maternal pelvic fracture
    D. ejection from a motor vehicle
    E. maternal hypotension/hemorrhage

93. Thiamine is indicated for the prevention and/or treatment of which of the following conditions?
    A. Guillain-Barré syndrome
    B. Creutzfeldt-Jacob disease
    C. Wernicke's encephalopathy
    D. myasthenia gravis
    E. none of the above

94. You are transporting a patient who had several seizures and is now postictal. The patient now has a right facial droop, hemiparesis, and lateral eye deviation. The condition most likely is:
    A. astrocytic brain tumor.
    B. acute stroke.
    C. Todd's paralysis.
    D. postictal atresia.
    E. none of the above.

95. What is the pediatric dosage for calcium chloride?
    A. 0.1–0.2 mg/kg
    B. 20 mg/kg
    C. 1 gram
    D. 50 mcg/kg
    E. none of the above

96. Which of the following is NOT one of the four stages of the body's response to burn injury?
    A. fluid-shift phase
    B. rhabdomyolysis phase
    C. emergent phase
    D. resolution phase
    E. hypermetabolic phase

97. The physiological opening between the left and right atria that is functional prior to birth is the:
    A. foramen ovale.
    B. *ductus arterisosus.*
    C. *ductus venosum.*
    D. foramen magnum.
    E. none of the above.

98. The most common causative agent in laryngotracheitis is:
    A. *Haemophilus influenza.*
    B. *Strep. Pneumoniae.*
    C. *Chlamydia trachomitis.*
    D. parainfluenza virus, type I.
    E. variola virus.

99. What is the standard endotracheal tube adapter inside diameter?
    A. 10 cm
    B. 15 cm
    C. 10 mm
    D. 15 mm
    E. none of the above

100. Drooping of the eyelid is termed:
    A. endophthalmos.
    B. diplopia.
    C. ptosis.
    D. exophthalmos.
    E. none of the above.

101. The gas law that states, "The rate at which gases diffuse is inversely proportional to the square root of their densities" is:
    A. Graham's Law.
    B. Gay-Lussac's Law.
    C. Boyle's Law.
    D. Dalton's Law.
    E. Avogadro's Law.

102. You are treating a patient who has sustained a gunshot wound to the abdomen. He is pale and diaphoretic with a systolic pressure of 75 mmHg. His respirations are 24 per minute and pulse is 120 per minute. In regard to this patient, which of the following would NOT be correct?
    A. Cardiac output is increased.
    B. Systemic vascular resistance is increased.
    C. Central venous pressure is increased.
    D. Pulmonary artery occlusion pressure is decreased.
    E. none of the above

103. Which of the following eye injuries is potentially the most threatening to sight?
    A. eyelid laceration
    B. conjunctival hemorrhage
    C. hyphema
    D. A and B
    E. A and C

104. Normal intracranial pressure (ICP) is:
    A. 0–10 mmHg.
    B. 10–20 mmHg.
    C. 20–30 mmHg.
    D. MAP-ICP.
    E. none of the above.

105. Which of the following drugs is classified as a low-molecular-weight heparin?
    A. heparin sodium
    B. warfarin sodium
    C. eptifibatide
    D. abciximab
    E. none of the above

106. You have just delivered an infant during an interfacility transport that was delayed because of bad weather and flooding. At one minute post delivery the infant had the following findings:

    Heart rate: 98 beats per minute
    Respiratory rate: normal rate and effort
    Coughs with nasal stimulation
    Active, spontaneous movement
    Normal color except hands and feet are bluish

    What is this neonate's 1-minute APGAR score?
    A. 6
    B. 7
    C. 8
    D. 9
    E. 10

107. What is the standard induction dose of etomidate for rapid sequence induction (RSI)?
    A. 2 mg
    B. 100 mg
    C. 0.01–0.03 mg/kg
    D. 0.1–0.3 mg/kg
    E. none of the above

108. Which of the following statements about nosocomial pneumonia is NOT correct?
    A. It is acquired in-hospital.
    B. Mortality is higher than in other types of pneumonia.
    C. The use of empiric antibiotics have led to antibiotic-resistant strains.

D. Endotracheal intubation and mechanical ventilation increases risk.
E. none of the above

109. Which of the following is a typical dosage for succinylcholine in prehospital RSI?
    A. 1.0–1.5 mg
    B. 10–15 mg
    C. 1–2 grams
    D. 1.0–1.5 mg/kg
    E. 1.0–1.5 mcg/kg

110. Which of the following drugs can be used to reverse the effects of pancuronium?
    A. succinylcholine
    B. acetylcholine
    C. pyridostigmine
    D. atropine sulfate
    E. none of the above

111. What is the partial pressure of oxygen in the earth's atmosphere at a barometric pressure of 550 mmHg?
    A. 159.6 mmHg
    B. 115.5 mmHg
    C. 33.5 mmHg
    D. 100.2 mmHg
    E. none of the above

112. The first intensive care unit (ICU) was established at which United States hospital?
    A. Mayo Clinic
    B. Parkland Hospital
    C. Johns Hopkins Hospital
    D. Walter Reed Army Medical Center
    E. Cedars-Sinai Medical Center

113. Which if the following is an example of a transabdominal feeding tube?
    A. nasointestinal tube
    B. percutaneous endoscopic gastrostomy (PEG) tube
    C. T-tube
    D. Cantor tube
    E. Miller-Abbott tube

114. Figure Final–3 depicts what Mallampati score?
    A. Class I
    B. Class II
    C. Class III
    D. Class IV
    E. Class V

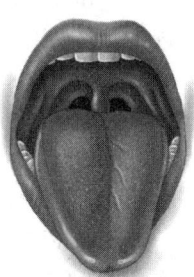

Figure Final–3

115. Which of the following illnesses is NOT typically spread by blood contact?
    A. hepatitis A
    B. hepatitis B
    C. hepatitis C
    D. hepatitis D
    E. none of the above

116. All of the following are ECG findings associated with hypokalemia EXCEPT:
    A. ST segment depression.
    B. peaked T waves.
    C. U waves larger than T waves as potassium falls.
    D. increasing PR interval.
    E. none of the above.

117. Which of the following laboratory tests is/are useful in the diagnosis of acute pancreatitis?
    A. amylase
    B. lipase
    C. creatine kinase
    D. A and B
    E. A and C

118. Which of the following terms is associated with movement of gas molecules?
    A. diffusion
    B. osmosis
    C. Brownian movement
    D. heat
    E. ionization

119. The pressure in an endotracheal tube cuff should never exceed which of the following parameters?
    A. pulmonary capillary wedge pressure
    B. peak-expiratory end-pressure (PEEP)
    C. tracheal capillary pressure
    D. precapillary oncotic pressure
    E. postcapillary oncotic pressure

120. Your patient is 6 feet tall and weighs 176 pounds. What is his body surface area?
    A. 3.9 m^2
    B. 4.1 m^2
    C. 4.8 m^2
    D. 5.6 m^2
    E. none of the above

121. Which of the following findings is/are inconsistent with hypovolemia?
    A. decreased cardiac index
    B. decreased central venous pressure
    C. elevated systemic vascular resistance index
    D. A and B
    E. none of the above

122. Which of the following findings is inconsistent with abruptio placentae?
    A. vaginal bleeding
    B. abdominal pain
    C. recent history of pelvic examination
    D. advanced maternal age (> 35 years)
    E. none of the above

123. Which of the following is NOT a part of brain death determination?
    A. absence of pharyngeal/tracheal reflex
    B. absence of ocular movements
    C. coma
    D. positive Babinski reflex
    E. absence of response to corneal stimulation

124. You are caring for an intubated patient. The endotracheal tube was filled with 4.0 cm^3 of air at sea level. Which of the following will NOT help to minimize tracheal injury when the aircraft ascends to altitude?
    A. using saline instead of air in the ET cuff
    B. using water instead of air in the ET cuff
    C. maintaining cabin pressurization at as low an altitude as possible
    D. adding air to the ET cuff as you ascend to altitude
    E. using a commercial device to regulate ET cuff pressure

125. Which of the following is a contraindication to Foley catheter insertion?
    A. need to measure urinary output
    B. pediatric patient
    C. post prostatectomy
    D. blood at urethral meatus
    E. none of the above

126. The DeBakey classification system is used to classify:
    A. aortic aneurysms.
    B. subarachnoid aneurysms.
    C. aortic dissections.
    D. penetrating cardiac wounds.
    E. none of the above.

127. Which of the following conditions is associated with ingesting reef-dwelling fish?
    A. scombroid
    B. botulism
    C. cnidaria
    D. ciguatera
    E. none of the above

128. The bacteria responsible for plague is:
   A. *Yersinia pestis.*
   B. *Staphylococcus aureus.*
   C. *Treponema pallidum.*
   D. *Mycobacterium leprae.*
   E. none of the above.

129. You are called to treat a patient who complains of 24 hours of nausea, vomiting, and abdominal cramps. He appears very restless and agitated and has prominent piloerection. You note that his nose is constantly dripping and he is constantly yawning. He fails to provide any meaningful history. These findings are most consistent with which of the following conditions?
   A. opiate withdrawal
   B. anticholinergic poisoning
   C. alcohol withdrawal
   D. sympathomimetic ingestion
   E. none of the above

130. Which of the following is NOT a factor in determining buoyancy?
   A. density of the object
   B. relative humidity of the water
   C. specific gravity of the water
   D. A and B
   E. A and C

131. Which of the following ECG findings can be seen with hypothermia?
   A. Nugent wave
   B. Bon Jovi wave
   C. Roth wave
   D. Townshend wave
   E. none of the above

132. Which medication can be used to enhance closure of a patent *ductus arteriosus?*
   A. prostaglandin E_2
   B. indomethacin
   C. cyclosporin
   D. interleukin
   E. none of the above

133. Which of the following findings is NOT indicative of a severe pediatric asthma exacerbation?
   A. increased respiratory rate over 50% of mean
   B. SpO_2 < 90%
   C. 20–40 mmHg pulsus paradoxus
   D. PEFR 70% of predicted
   E. none of the above

134. The virus responsible for SARS is:
   A. myxovirus.
   B. retrovirus.
   C. coronavirus.
   D. paramyxovirus.
   E. none of the above.

135. Which of the following is NOT a single-engine helicopter?
   A. Bell 206
   B. Bell 407
   C. Eurocopter EC 130
   D. Eurocopter AS 355
   E. all of the above

136. Which of the following vasopressors is incompatible with furosemide (Lasix)?
   A. dopamine (Intropin)
   B. amrinone (Inocor)
   C. norepinephrine (Levophed)
   D. metaraminol (Aramine)
   E. dobutamine (Dobutrex)

137. Which of the following statements about the Modified Chest Lead I (MCL-1) is FALSE?
   A. The RA lead is placed on the upper right arm.
   B. The LA lead is placed on the upper left arm.
   C. The LL lead is placed on the left leg.
   D. The LL lead is placed in the right 4th intercostal space.
   E. It is functionally equivalent to Lead V1.

138. Which of the following is NOT an advantage of ground transport over air transport?
    A. larger patient compartment
    B. lower transport costs
    C. safety
    D. relative immunity to weather
    E. none of the above

139. Which of the following ions is most important in muscle contraction?
    A. Ca^{2+}
    B. Na^+
    C. K^+
    D. Mg^{2+}
    E. None of the above

140. The iris is a part of which of the following eye structures/layers?
    A. fibrous tunic
    B. vascular tunic
    C. neural tunic
    D. fovea
    E. none of the above

141. The most common air medical crew configuration in the United States is:
    A. nurse/nurse
    B. paramedic/paramedic
    C. nurse/paramedic
    D. nurse/physician
    E. paramedic/EMT

142. Which of the following is NOT an effect of B-type natriuretic peptide?
    A. relaxes vascular smooth muscle
    B. decreases preload
    C. decreases afterload
    D. promotes fluid retention
    E. none of the above

Scenario

Questions 143–146 refer to the following scenario:
You are transporting a 187-pound 21-year-old male patient who was ejected during a motor vehicle collision. Findings during stabilization were right-sided fractures, an open right-side tibia/fibula fracture, and a contrecoup occipital hematoma found on non-contrast computed tomagrapy (CT). The patient was alert but confused with a reported GCS of 9 to 12 prior to elective intubation at the Level III facility. The patient received etomidate and succinylcholine during the RSI procedure. As you take control of the patient, he is receiving lactated Ringer's at 250 mL/hr and has both a nasogastric tube and Foley catheter in place.

143. The patient begins to move and twitch following the neuromuscular blocker given earlier. Which of the following agents would be the best choice for continued paralysis?
    A. etomidate
    B. succinylcholine
    C. pancuronium
    D. fentanyl
    E. mannitol

144. The patient's urine output for a 30-minute interval is 250 mL. Which of the following statements is TRUE?
    A. Urinary output is 5.9 mL/kg/hour.
    B. Urine output is below normal.
    C. Urine output is normal.
    D. A fluid bolus is indicated.
    E. A and C are correct.

145. The patient begins to develop cardiovascular decompensation. Which of the following interventions would NOT be indicated?
    A. Check ET tube placement.
    B. Check oxygen supply.

C. Check for presence of pneumothorax.

D. Check for secretions or bleeding that might be occluding ET tube.

E. none of the above

146. The tube is in place and the oxygen source is fine. The patient's heart rate begins to slow and he becomes more difficult to ventilate. You notice that the trachea is deviated toward the patient's left. What action should you take?
    A. Administer epinephrine 1:10,000 0.5 mL IVP.
    B. Administer atropine 0.5 mg IVP.
    C. Land and obtain stat chest X-ray.
    D. Needle the left chest.
    E. none of the above

147. You are called to transport a febrile patient from a community hospital to a tertiary care facility. The transferring physician thinks the patient is septic and has ordered various cultures. The patient is a 26-year-old female. She had seen her local MD and was started on promethazine (Phenergan) for vomiting and respiridone (Risperdal) to help with sleep. Her vitals are blood pressure = 160/100 mmHg, pulse 120 beats per minute, respirations 26 per minute, SpO_2 = 99% on nasal cannula, and rectal temperature of 107.9° F. She has a pH of 7.22 and exhibits muscular rigidity. Which of the following statements is TRUE?
    A. The most likely diagnosis is bacterial meningitis.
    B. The most likely diagnosis is neuroleptic malignant syndrome.
    C. Dopamine-2 receptors are blocked.
    D. B and C are correct.
    E. A and C are correct.

148. Which of the following substances is NOT an alkali?
    A. phenol
    B. anhydrous ammonia
    C. wet cement
    D. oven cleaners
    E. none of the above

149. Which of the following is an abnormal vital sign for a neonate?
    A. heart rate of 120 beats per minute
    B. respirations of 26 breaths per minute
    C. blood pressure of 90/60 mmHg
    D. temperature of 37.4° C
    E. none of the above

150. Goblet cells in the respiratory tract secrete:
    A. mucus.
    B. surfactant.
    C. vitamin D.
    D. angiotensin converting enzyme (ACE).
    E. none of the above.

151. Which of the following is typically NOT consistent with a diagnosis of pericarditis?
    A. chest pain
    B. lying down worsens the pain
    C. sitting up or leaning forward worsens the pain
    D. history of malignancy or recent illness or infection
    E. none of the above

152. The pneumotaxic center is located in which of the following structures?
    A. pons
    B. thalamus
    C. hypothalamus
    D. brainstem
    E. medulla oblongata

153. Which of the following statements about frostbite is TRUE?
    A. Cold exposure causes cellular overhydration and cell lysis.
    B. Ice crystals form in the extracellular compartments.
    C. Blood viscosity decreases.
    D. It is classified into three degrees.
    E. none of the above

154. Which of the following infections are caused by the same virus?
    A. herpes and diphtheria
    B. chickenpox and smallpox
    C. shingles and diphtheria
    D. chickenpox and shingles
    E. tetanus and herpes

155. Which of the following statements about AIDS is TRUE?
    A. It is only found in gay cowboys.
    B. HIV-1 is more pathogenic than HIV-2.
    C. The onset of infection is sudden with severe flu-like symptoms.
    D. Opportunistic infections are uncommon.
    E. none of the above

156. Which of the following hormones is NOT produced in the anterior pituitary?
    A. thyroid-stimulating hormone (TSH)
    B. antidiuretic hormone (ADH)
    C. follicle-stimulating hormone (FSH)
    D. growth hormone (GH)
    E. melanocyte-stimulating hormone (MSH)

157. The electrophysiological functional unit in the heart is known as the:
    A. intercalated discs.
    B. bundle of His.
    C. bundle of Kent.
    D. syncytium.
    E. none of the above.

158. Which of the following statements about endotoxins is TRUE?
    A. They are produced by gram-negative bacteria.
    B. They consist of simple sugar molecules.
    C. They come from the cell nucleus.
    D. They are produced by gram-positive bacteria.
    E. C and D

159. Which of the following is usually NOT associated with cephalopelvic disproportion?
    A. primigravida
    B. macrosomia
    C. fetal tumors
    D. postmaturity
    E. patent *ductus arteriosus*

160. All of the following are classified as nucleic-acid base EXCEPT:
    A. adenosine.
    B. guanine.
    C. cytosine.
    D. thymine.
    E. uracil.

161. Which of the following is a dialysis-related complication?
    A. anemia
    B. hypertension
    C. hyperkalemia
    D. infection
    E. all of the above

162. Which of the following may contribute to hypothermia?
    A. exposure time
    B. diabetes

C. beta-blockers

D. age

E. all of the above

163. Which of the following is/are included in a cyanide antidote kit?

   A. sodium nitrite
   B. sodium thiosulfate
   C. pralidoxime
   D. A and B
   E. B and C

164. In regard to the ECG tracing in Figure Final–4, which of the following is TRUE?

   A. The ECG is normal.
   B. The ECG is consistent with pericarditis.
   C. The QRS axis is abnormal.
   D. The ECG is consistent with an inferior STEMI.
   E. none of the above

165. The ECG tracing in Figure Final–4 is most consistent with a diagnosis of:

   A. hypothermia.
   B. hyperkalemia.
   C. hypokalemia.
   D. hypermagnesemia.
   E. none of the above.

166. Decompression sickness is due to an expansion of which of the following gases?

   A. water vapor
   B. oxygen
   C. nitrogen
   D. carbon dioxide
   E. all of the above

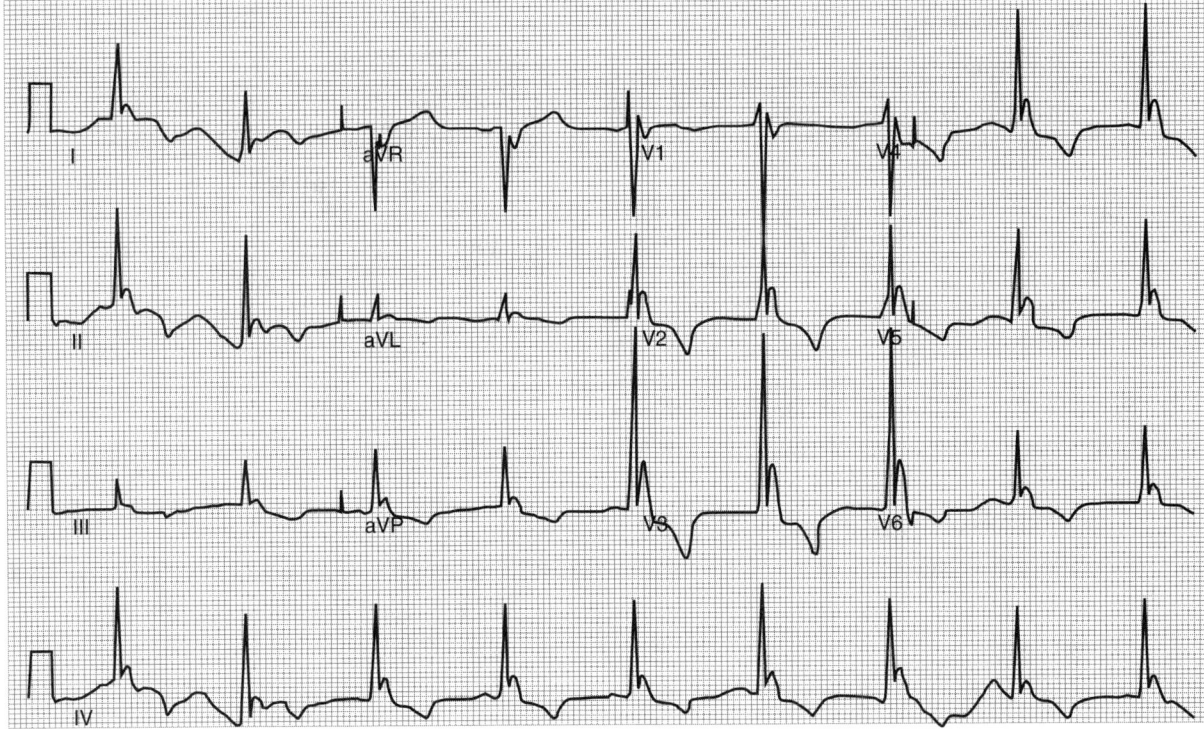

Figure Final–4

167. The quality improvement (QI) charting system that will allow you to readily identify which is the most frequent problem is the:
    A. control chart.
    B. histogram.
    C. Pareto chart.
    D. cause and effect chart.
    E. scatter diagram.

168. Which of the following statements is TRUE?
    A. The atrioventricular valves are closed during ventricular ejection.
    B. The semilunar valves are open during ventricular ejection.
    C. Aortic pressure is highest during ventricular ejection.
    D. all of the above
    E. B and C

169. The capnography waveform in Figure Final–5 is consistent with:
    A. asthma.
    B. congestive heart failure.
    C. pneumothorax.
    D. hypoxemia.
    E. none of the above.

1 sec

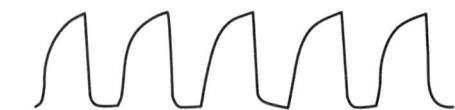

Figure Final–5

170. Which of the following should be a point of concern when transporting a patient at altitude?
    A. endotracheal tube cuff pressure
    B. chest tube drainage
    C. rectal tube cuff pressure
    D. oxygenation
    E. all of the above

171. Which of the following statements about the graphic representation of a murmur in Figure Final–6 is TRUE?
    A. It is a diastolic murmur.
    B. It is a systolic murmur.
    C. It is consistent with mitral stenosis.
    D. It is consistent with aortic regurgitation.
    E. none of the above

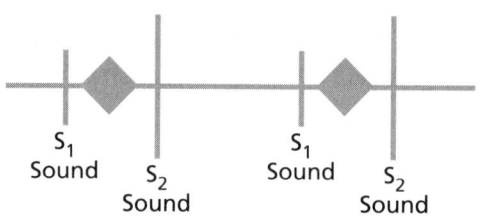

Figure Final–6

172. Which of the following is NOT one of the factors considered in the Monroe-Kellie hypothesis?
    A. jugular venous pressure
    B. brain tissue
    C. blood
    D. cerebrospinal fluid
    E. none of the above

173. Which of the following drugs CANNOT be reversed with flumazenil?
    A. etomidate
    B. midazolam
    C. diazepam
    D. lorazepam
    E. none of the above

174. The creatine kinase isoenzyme that is present in the highest concentration is:
    A. CK-I (BB).
    B. CK-II (MB).

C. CK-III (MM).

D. all are present in equal concentrations.

E. none of the above.

175. Which of the following statements about the pancreas is **FALSE**?

    A. The majority of the pancreas is exocrine.

    B. Lipase levels are elevated in acute pancreatitis.

    C. Amylase levels are elevated in acute pancreatitis.

    D. The pancreas is located in the retroperitoneal space.

    E. all of the above

Scenario

Questions 176–178 refer to the following scenario:

You are transporting a 36-year-old female who took an unknown quantity of desipramine tablets. Her blood pressure is 113/60 mmHg, pulse is 109 beats per minute and irregular, respirations are 12 per minute and regular, SpO_2 on 35% Venturi mask is 100%.

176. In regard to this scenario, which of the following is **NOT** commonly seen with tricyclic antidepressant (TCA) overdose?

    A. coma

    B. convulsions

    C. hypertension

    D. dysrhythmias

    E. acidosis

177. In regard to this scenario, which of the following treatments would **NOT** be indicated?

    A. airway

    B. IV access

    C. fluid administration

    D. glucagon administration

    E. beta-blocker administration

178. In regard to this scenario, it is common to administer sodium bicarbonate to a TCA overdose. What is the purpose of sodium bicarbonate administration in this instance?

    A. to reverse acidosis

    B. to provide adequate sodium for the sodium-ion channels

    C. to prevent dysrhythmias

    D. A and B

    E. A and C

179. Which of the following diseases is no longer naturally occurring?

    A. plague

    B. hemorrhagic fever

    C. smallpox

    D. tularemia

    E. none of the above

180. You have been asked to investigate two accidents in your critical care service and establish a plan to prevent additional similar accidents from occurring. Which of the following tools would be the most helpful?

    A. histogram

    B. Haddon matrix

    C. pie chart

    D. algorithm

    E. none of the above

181. Which of the following is **NOT** an immediate goal of therapy when treating a patient with acute coronary syndrome?

    A. to increase myocardial oxygen supply

    B. to decrease myocardial oxygen demand

    C. to correct disturbances in heart rate and rhythm

    D. to administer prophylactic antidysrhythmics

    E. to reduce pain and relieve stress

182. Which of the following is **NOT** a parameter of the NBG pacemaker code?
    A. I–Chamber(s) Paced
    B. II–Chamber(s) Sensed
    C. III–Response to Setting
    D. IV–Rate Modulation
    E. none of the above

183. The most common causative agent for bronchiolitis in children less than 24 months of age is:
    A. respiratory syncytial virus (RSV).
    B. coronavirus.
    C. paramyxovirus.
    D. bacteria phage.
    E. none of the above.

184. An organ donor has Type B blood (in the ABO system). Which of the following organ types would be compatible from an ABO standpoint?
    A. A
    B. B
    C. AB
    D. O
    E. B and D

185. Which of the following is **NOT** a part of the phonetic alphabet used in aircraft communications?
    A. Alpha
    B. Geronimo
    C. Kilo
    D. Oscar
    E. Whiskey

186. Which of the following snakes is a member of the *Elapidae* family?
    A. rattlesnake
    B. copperhead
    C. coral
    D. water moccasin
    E. none of the above

187. The causative agent in Creutzfeldt-Jakob disease (CJD) is which of the following?
    A. coronavirus
    B. prion
    C. hantavirus
    D. tobacco mosaic virus
    E. none of the above

188. To auscultate the aortic valve, the stethoscope is best placed at the:
    A. second intercostal space (ICS) to the right of the sternum.
    B. second intercostal space (ICS) to the left of the sternum.
    C. fifth intercostal space (ICS) to the left of the sternum.
    D. fifth intercostal space (ICS) at the left mid-clavicular line.
    E. fifth intercostal space (ICS) at the left anterior axillary line.

189. Which of the following is **NOT** a limitation of continuous waveform capnography?
    A. It does not detect endobronchial intubation.
    B. It may be affected by high-levels of oxygen (false low readings).
    C. It may be influenced by excessive water vapor (false high readings).
    D. It may be affected by nitrous oxide administration.
    E. none of the above

190. There are _____ ventricles in the brain.
    A. 2
    B. 3

C. 4
D. 6
E. none of the above

191. Which of the following statements about diagnostic peritoneal lavage is TRUE?
    A. It is indicated for suspected intra-thoracic injury.
    B. It determines the presence of albumin in the abdomen.
    C. It should only be performed by the surgeon who will be making the operative decision.
    D. The catheter is inserted under fluoroscopic guidance.
    E. none of the above

192. Platelets arise from which of the following precursors?
    A. lymphoid stem cells
    B. monoblasts
    C. myeloblasts
    D. megakaryocyte
    E. prooerythroblasts

193. Which of the following is usually NOT a factor in determining whether to initiate and continue cardiac resuscitation while in-flight?
    A. code status of the patient
    B. company policies and procedures for in-flight arrests
    C. availability of resuscitation equipment
    D. endurance of the air medical personnel
    E. none of the above

194. You are transporting a patient with a closed head injury from a Level II trauma center to a Level I trauma center. The patient has multiple contusions on CT—but no skull fractures. His GCS was 5 and he is intubated—but not paralyzed. His ICP as measured via a fiberoptic bolt has been 10–15 mmHg. Suddenly, the patient begins to exhibit decorticate posturing and the ICP increases to 24 mmHg. Which of the following interventions is indicated?
    A. troubleshooting the fiberoptic bolt
    B. elevating the head of the bed
    C. hyperventilation
    D. administration of mannitol
    E. all of the above

195. Which of the following is NOT a part of routine interfacility transfer paperwork?
    A. verification of health care insurance coverage
    B. physician certification that the risks of transport are outweighed by the benefits
    C. signed consent to transport the patient
    D. transport orders for the critical care transport team
    E. copies of all pertinent medical records

196. Which of the following agents is an ACE inhibitor?
    A. esmolol
    B. enalapril
    C. labetalol
    D. clonidine
    E. none of the above

197. Your patient has a transverse maxillary fracture just superior to the apices of the teeth, extending through the maxillary sinus and across the nasal septum. The maxilla moves when the teeth are grabbed and manipulated. This fracture would be classified as:
    A. LeFort I.
    B. LeFort II.
    C. LeFort III.
    D. Salter-Harris Type I.
    E. Salter-Harris Type IV.

198. You are transporting a patient with flash pulmonary edema. The small community hospital administered 20 mg of furosemide and took a chest X-ray. You assess the patient and begin to formulate a treatment plan. Which of the following would NOT be a prudent treatment for the patient?
    A. nitrates
    B. morphine
    C. CPAP/BiPAP
    D. selective administration of beta blockers
    E. none of the above

199. Which of the following is a branch of the Circle of Willis?
    A. anterior cerebral artery
    B. posterior communicating artery
    C. posterior cerebral artery
    D. all of the above
    E. A and C

200. The main purpose of the tail rotor in a helicopter is to:
    A. turn the helicopter
    B. increase the forward speed of the helicopter
    C. counteract torque effects of the main rotor
    D. assist in vertical lift during maximum RPMs
    E. none of the above

Answers for Final Review

Following each answer you will find page numbers indicating where the question topic is discussed in other Brady texts. The texts cited include *Critical Care Paramedic,* ISBN 0-13-119271-X (CCP), the second edition of *Anatomy & Physiology for Emergency Care,* ISBN 0-13-234298-7 (AP), the third edition of *Paramedic Care: Principles & Practice, Volume 1: Introduction to Advanced Prehospital Care,* ISBN 0-13-513704-7 (PCPP V1), the third edition of *Paramedic Care: Principles & Practice, Volume 3: Medical Emergencies,* ISBN 0-13-513702-0 (PCPP V3), and the seventh edition of *Prehospital Emergency Pharmacology,* ISBN 0-13-513822-1 (PEP).

1. E (AP, p. 537)
2. B (PCPP V1, p. 522)
3. A (CCP, p. 142)
4. A (CCP, p. 226)
5. D (CCP, p. 191)
6. D (CCP, p. 241)
7. E (CCP, p. 334)
8. D (CCP, p. 353)
9. D (CCP, p. 14)
10. C (CCP, p. 1004)
11. A (CCP, p. 4)
12. D (CCP, p. 855)
13. D (CCP, p. 614)
14. A (CCP, p. 530)
15. E (PEP, pp. 191–192)
16. B (CCP, pp. 294–295)
17. E (CCP, p. 558)
18. C (CCP, p. 682)
19. A (CCP, p. 888)
20. B (CCP, p. 710)
21. D (CCP, p. 469)
22. C (CCP, p. 462)
23. A (CCP, p. 890)
24. E (CCP, p. 320)
25. E (CCP, p. 146)
26. D (CCP, p. 215)
27. C (CCP, p. 93)
28. B (CCP, p. 504)
29. D (CCP, p. 731)
30. A (CCP, p. 897)
31. E (CCP, p. 991)
32. B (CCP, p. 1063)
33. E (CCP, p. 775)
34. A (CCP, p. 827)
35. D (CCP, p. 804)
36. B (PEP, pp. 340–341)
37. D (CCP, p. 687)
38. D (CCP, p. 56)
39. B (AP, p. 426)
40. B (CCP, p. 232)
41. C (AP, p. 218)
42. C (CCP, p. 743)
43. C (CCP, p. 803)
44. A (CCP, p. 443)
45. D (CCP, p. 822)
46. A (CCP, p. 694)

47. B (CCP, p. 460)
48. D (CCP, pp. 795–801)
49. B (CCP, p. 884)
50. C (CCP, p. 12)
51. A (AP, p. 410)
52. E (CCP, p. 609)
53. E (AP, p. 455)
54. C (CCP, p. 260)
55. A (CCP, p. 510)
56. B (CCP, p. 385)
57. A (CCP, p. 395)
58. D (CCP, p. 703)
59. E (CCP, p. 907)
60. C (CCP, p. 198)
61. A (CCP, p. 964)
62. E (CCP, p. 730)
63. B (CCP, p. 530)
64. B (CCP, p. 386)
65. A (CCP, p. 567)
66. D (CCP, p. 538)
67. B (CCP, p. 266)
68. D (CCP, p. 268)
69. D (CCP, p. 268)
70. B (AP, p. 453)
71. E (CCP, p. 861)
72. E (CCP, p. 19)
73. B (CCP, p. 24)
74. A (CCP, p. 639)
75. D (CCP, pp. 698–699)
76. C (CCP, p. 299)
77. E (CCP, p. 744)
78. B (CCP, p. 458)
79. E (CCP, p. 546)
80. D (CCP, p. 212)
81. A (CCP, p. 19)
82. A (CCP, p. 898)
83. C (CCP, p. 996)
84. E (CCP, p. 629)
85. C (CCP, p. 589)
86. D (CCP, p. 463)
87. D (CCP, p. 633)
88. A (CCP, p. 659)
89. E (CCP, p. 302)
90. D (CCP, p. 515)
91. A (CCP, p. 433)
92. E (CCP, p. 574)
93. C (CCP, p. 706)
94. C (CCP, p. 707)
95. B (CCP, p. 831)
96. B (CCP, pp. 491–492)
97. A (CCP, p. 879)
98. D (CCP, p. 821)
99. D (PCPP V1, p. 548)
100. C (CCP, p. 470)
101. A (CCP, p. 57)
102. A (CCP, p. 199)
103. C (CCP, p. 473)
104. A (CCP, p. 379)
105. E (CCP, pp. 295–296)
106. C (CCP, p. 549)
107. D (CCP, p. 314)
108. E (CCP, p. 612)
109. D (PEP, p. 247)
110. C (CCP, p. 149)
111. B (CCP, p. 53)
112. C (CCP, p. 7)
113. B (CCP, p. 742)
114. B (CCP, p. 168)
115. A (CCP, p. 788)
116. B (CCP, pp. 262–263)
117. D (CCP, p. 345)
118. A (CCP, p. 51)
119. C (CCP, p. 63)
120. B (CCP, p. 231)
121. E (CCP, p. 235)
122. B (CCP, p. 760)
123. D (CCP, p. 991)
124. D (CCP, p. 63)
125. D (CCP, p. 440)
126. C (CCP, pp. 641–642)
127. D (CCP, p. 930)
128. A (CCP, p. 973)
129. A (CCP, p. 939)
130. E (CCP, p. 920)
131. E (CCP, p. 908)
132. B (CCP, p. 886)
133. D (CCP, p. 827)
134. C (CCP, p. 793)
135. D (CCP, p. 81)
136. B (PEP, p. 148)
137. C (CCP, p. 248)
138. E (CCP, p. 19)

139. A (AP, p. 174)
140. B (AP, p. 281)
141. C (CCP, p. 29)
142. D (PEP, pp. 205–206)
143. C (CCP, p. 148)
144. E (CCP, p. 200)
145. E (CCP, p. 590)
146. E (CCP, p. 404)
147. D (CCP, p. 713)
148. A (CCP, p. 513–514)
149. B (CCP, p. 557)
150. A (CCP, p. 581)
151. C (CCP, p. 656)
152. A (CCP, p. 680)
153. B (CCP, p. 909)
154. D (CCP, pp. 786, 796)
155. B (CCP, pp. 786–787)
156. B (AP, p. 315)
157. D (PCPP V3, p. 82)
158. A (PCPP V3, p. 541)
159. E (PCPP V3, p. 681)
160. A (AP, p. 45)
161. E (CCP, pp. 756–757)
162. E (CCP, p. 898)
163. D (CCP, p. 968)
164. E (CCP, p. 252)
165. A (CCP, p. 908)
166. C (CCP, p. 923)
167. C (CCP, p. 1013)
168. D (CCP, p. 625)
169. A (CCP, p. 595)
170. E (CCP, p. 745)
171. B (CCP, p. 629)
172. A (CCP, p. 381)
173. A (CCP, pp. 312–315)
174. C (CCP, p. 343)
175. E (CCP, p. 727)
176. C (CCP, p. 941)
177. E (CCP, p. 941)
178. E (CCP, p. 941)
179. C (CCP, p. 801)
180. B (CCP, p. 363)
181. D (CCP, p. 634)
182. E (CCP, p. 637)
183. A (CCP, p. 827)
184. E (CCP, p. 994)
185. B (CCP, p. 1042)
186. C (CCP, p. 952)
187. B (CCP, p. 714)
188. A (CCP, p. 626)
189. D (CCP, p. 596)
190. C (CCP, p. 680)
191. C (CCP, pp. 433–434)
192. D (CCP, p. 333)
193. E (CCP, p. 675)
194. E (CCP, p. 391)
195. A (CCP, pp. 120–121)
196. B (CCP, p. 280)
197. A (CCP, pp. 469–470)
198. E (CCP, p. 652)
199. D (CCP, p. 684)
200. C (CCP, p. 86)

Index

AAST. *See* American Academy of Surgery for Trauma (AAST)
abdominal and genitourinary trauma, 109–15
  assessment and treatment of, 112–13
  bladder rupture, 113, 114
  bruising, 110
  diagnostic peritoneal lavage, 111
  FAST exam, 111
  kidney injuries, 113, 114, 115
  laparotomy, 110
  liver, 109–10
  Liver Injury Scale, 110
  organs and structures, location of, 109
  renal collecting system, 115
  reproductive system injuries, 113
  Spleen Injury Scale, 110, 113
  ultrasound techniques, 111
Accidental Death and Disability: The Neglected Disease of Modern Society, 87
acetaminophen (APAP) overdose, 260–61
acetylcholine, 37
acid-base emergencies. *See* renal and acid-base emergencies
actinomycetes, 208
acute coronary syndrome, 168
acute pulmonary embolism, 17
acute respiratory distress syndrome (ARDS), 160
acute respiratory failure, 152, 157
ADH. *See* antidiuretic hormone (ADH)
afferent (descending) sensory, 178
AIDS complex, 210

air transport, 9–11
  communications center duties, 10
  coordinator, daily operations, 9
  FAA regulations, 10–11, 24
  fixed wing, 10, 21
  flight crew configuration, 9–10
  helicopter, 10
  medical director duties, 9
  program director responsibilities, 9
  small-airframe rotorcraft, 10, 11, 20–21
airway management and ventilation, 35–41, 235–36
  alveolar minute volume, 35
  Beck Airway Airflow Monitor, 36
  brain and, 35, 36
  carbon dioxide, 35
  Cormack and Lehane grade, 40
  cricothyrotomy, 39
  dissociative agent, 37
  drugs, dosage rates for, 37–38
  Endotracheal Combitubes, 38
  gum elastic bougie, 36
  laryngeal cartilage, 35
  laryngoscope, 36
  lungs, 35, 36
  Mallampati class, 39
  neuromuscular blocking agents, 38
  oxygen, 35
  rescue airways, 38–39, 40
  RSI process, 38
  surfactant, 35
  techniques used, 36
  ventilators, 40–41
altitude physiology, 13–18
  Armstrong's line, 13
  atmospheric zones, 13

barodontalgia, 18
cabin decompression, 17
earth's atmosphere, 13
gas laws, 14
gas pressure and, 13–14, 18
gravitational (G) forces, 16
hypoxia, 14–15
spatial disorientation, 16
alveolar hypoventilation, 152
alveolar minute volume, formula for, 35
Alzheimer's disease, 188
ambulance, types of, 7
American Academy of Surgery for Trauma (AAST), 110
American Board of Medical Specialties, 2
American College of Surgeons, 87
anaerobic metabolism, 44
angiotensin II, 44
anion gap, 82
ANS. *See* autonomic nervous system (ANS)
anthrax, 215, 273
antibiotic-resistant organisms (AROs), 214
antidiuretic hormone (ADH), 201
aortic aneurysm, 168–69
aortic dissection, 168, 169, 172
aortic rupture, 105
APAP overdose, 260–61
APGAR scale, 143
ARDS. *See* acute respiratory distress syndrome (ARDS)
arenaviruses, 216
Armstrong's line, 13
AROs. *See* antibiotic-resistant organisms (AROs)

arteries, cerebral, 178–79, 183
assessment triangle in pediatric trauma, 144
asthma, 158–59
  pediatric, 223
atmospheric zones, 13
atropine sulfate, 37
autonomic nervous system (ANS), 180–81
Avogadro's Law, 14

BAAM. *See* Beck Airway Airflow Monitor (BAAM)
bacterial pneumonia, 17
barodontalgia, 18
Baskett, Peter, 2
Beck Airway Airflow Monitor (BAAM), 36
bilevel continuous positive airway pressure (BiPAP), 17
bilirubin, 83, 241–42
biological agents, 273
BiPAP. *See* bilevel continuous positive airway pressure (BiPAP)
  bites and stings
    marine animal, 252–53
    snake bites, 265–66
    spider bites, 266
bivalent cation, 82
bladder rupture, 113, 114
blood cells, 81–82
blood flow, neonatal, 236–37
blood pressure monitoring, 47
blood urea nitrogen (BUN), 195
botulism, 215
Boyle's Law, 14
bradycardia, 145
brain death and organ donation/retrieval, 276
bronchiolitis, pediatric, 223
BUN. *See* blood urea nitrogen (BUN)
burns and electrical injuries, 125–34
  body's response to, 126
  burn mechanisms of, 125
  carbon monoxide poisoning, 131
  chemical burns, 132–33
  epidermis and dermis layers, 133, 134
  escharotomies, 130–31
  heat defined, 125
  IV fluids, administering, 130
  mechanism of injury, 128
  mortality and, 125
  proteins and cells, 125, 126, 133, 134
  rhabdomyolysis, 132
  rule of nines, 127
  severity of, 131–32
  skin function, 125
  total body surface area, 127–30, 128–29, 130
  zone theory, 125, 126

cabin decompression, 17
Caisson's disease, 17
cannulation, 173
CAP. *See* community acquired pneumonia (CAP)
capnography, end tidal, 156–57
carbonic anhydrase, 17
carbon monoxide poisoning, 131
cardiac and hemodynamic monitoring, 47–51
  blood pressure, 47
  catheters used in
    arterial, 48–49
    Swan-Ganz, 48, 50, 51
  central venous pressure, 48
  intra-aortic balloon pump, 51
  leads and lines used in, 47, 48
  patency of circulation, 47
  phlebostatic axis, 47
  positive-end-expiratory pressure, 49
  subclavian central line, 48
  Swan-Ganz catheter, 48, 50, 51
  tracings, 49, 50
cardiac defects, congenital, 225
cardiac output (CO), 45
cardiac pacemaker, 163
cardiac tamponade, 172
cardiogenic shock, 169–70
cardiovascular emergencies, 163–74
  acute coronary syndrome, 168
  aortic aneurysm, 168–69
  aortic dissection, 168, 169, 172
  cannulation, 173
  cardiac pacemaker, 163
  cardiac tamponade, 172
  cardiogenic shock, 169–70
  congestive heart failure, 171
  dilated cardiomyopathy, 170–71
  heart murmurs, 165
  heart sounds, 164
  hypertensive emergencies, 171–72
  intra-aortic balloon pump, 170, 174
  left ventricle, 163–64
  myocardial infarction, acute, 165, 172
  pericarditis, 172
  peripherally inserted central catheter, 174
  radial arterial line placement, 172–73
  SA node, 163
  stenosis, aortic and mitral, 172
  12-Lead ECG, 166–68
Caroline, Nancy, 2
catheters
  arterial, 6–7, 48–51, 174
  central venous, 6–7
  maintenance of, 6
  peripherally inserted central catheter, 174
  Swan-Ganz, 48, 50, 51
CDC. *See* Centers for Disease Control (CDC)
cell lysis, 44
Centers for Disease Control (CDC), 209
central cord injury, 97
central venous catheter maintenance, 6
central venous pressure (CVP), 45, 48
cerebral arteries, 178–79, 183
cerebrospinal fluid (CSF), 177
CFIT. *See* controlled flight into terrain (CFIT)
Charles' Law, 14
chemical warfare, 268–69
chest contour variations, 154
chest tube insertion, 102–3
chicken pox, 214
cholecystitis, acute, 192
chronic obstructive pulmonary disease (COPD), 160
clostridium tetani, 213
Clostridium tetani, 213
CO. *See* cardiac output (CO)
communications and documentation, 283–85
community acquired pneumonia (CAP), 211
conduction system blocks, 53–54
congenital cardiac defects, pediatric, 225
congenital diaphragmatic herniation, 239
congenital heart defects, neonatal, 239
congestive heart failure, 171
continuous positive airway pressure (CPAP), 159
continuous waveform capnography, 4
controlled flight into terrain (CFIT), 25
COPD. *See* chronic obstructive pulmonary disease (COPD)
Cormack and Lehane grade, 40
corticospinal motor system, 179

INDEX

CPAP. *See* continuous positive airway pressure (CPAP)
cricothyrotomy, 39
critical care paramedic, 7, 287–88
   hospital environment, in the, 287–88
   in-hospital tasks, 287–88
   scope of practice statutes, 287
critical care transport, 2–4
   air, 9–11
   ground, 6–7
   introduction to, 2–4
   quality improvement in, 280–81
croup, pediatric, 222
Croup Scale, 222
CSF. *See* cerebrospinal fluid (CSF)
CVP. *See* central venous pressure (CVP)
cyanide exposure, 270–71

Dalton's Law, 14
DAN. *See* Divers Alert Network (DAN)
decompensated shock, 44
decompression sickness, 251, 252, 254
deliveries, high risk, 231
Deming cycle, 280
Denis system, 140
derangement of function, 44
diabetes insipidus, organ donation/retrieval and, 277
diabetic ketoacidosis (DKA), 204
diagnostic peritoneal lavage (DPL), 111
diagnostic tests. *See* laboratory and diagnostic tests, interpretation of
diaphragmatic herniation, congenital, 239
diaphragmatic rupture, 106
dilated cardiomyopathy, 170–71
dissociative agent, 37
Divers Alert Network (DAN), 252
diverticulitis, 192, 194
diving emergencies, 250–54
   bites and stings by marine animals, 252–53
   deaths, diving, 254
   decompression sickness, 251, 252, 254
   Divers Alert Network, 252
   high-pressure neurologic syndrome, 252
   nitrogen narcosis, 251
DKA. *See* diabetic ketoacidosis (DKA)
DPL. *See* diagnostic peritoneal lavage (DPL)

drownings, 225, 247
drugs
   abuse of, 256
   in critical care, 65–79
   hallucinogens, 257
   over-the-counter, 261, 262
   resuscitation medications, pediatric, 226
   uses and dosage rates of, 66–79

ear trauma. *See* face/ear/ocular/neck trauma
ECG monitoring and critical care, 53–63
   conduction system blocks, 53–54
   hyperkalemia, 56
   Lown-Ganong-Levine syndrome, 56
   Modified Central Leads, 53, 54, 55, 57
   right ventricular infarction, 57
   12-Lead, 166–68
   Wolff-Parkinson-White syndrome, 55
efferent (ascending) sensory, 178
Eisenberg, Mickey, 2
EKG monitoring, 7
electrical injuries. *See* burns and electrical injuries
electroencephalogram, 92–93
ELT. *See* emergency locator transmitter (ELT)
emergency locator transmitter (ELT), 23
encephalopathy, 187
Endotracheal Combitubes (ETCs), 38
endotracheal tubes, 7, 15
environmental emergencies, 244–48
   drownings, 247
   frostbite, 247
   heat exhaustion and stroke, 245–48
   heat loss, 244–45
   hypothermia, 246, 247
   temperature conversions, 244
epidermis and dermis layers, 133, 134
epiglottitis, pediatric, 222–23
equilibrium, inner ear, 16–17
escharotomy, 4, 9, 130–31
ETCs. *See* Endotracheal Combitubes (ETCs)
ethylene glycol poisoning, 204
etomidate, 37
explosive devices, 272–73
external auditory meatus, 94
extraembryonic membrane, 228

extrapyramidal system, 180
extraventricular drain, 94, 95

FAA. *See* Federal Aviation Administration (FAA)
face/ear/ocular/neck trauma, 117–23
   arteries, 117
   assessment of injuries, 122–23
   auditory ossicles, 119
   bones, 118–19
   cardiovascular structures, 120
   cranial nerves, 117, 119
   fascial layers, 120
   glands, 117
   Horner's syndrome, 123
   joints, 117, 121
   laryngopharynx, 120
   neck structures, 120, 121
   nerves, 118, 121
   pinna, 119
   tympanic membrane, 121
   vestibulocochlear complex, 119
FAST exam, 111
Federal Aviation Administration (FAA), 20, 24
fentanyl, 37
fetal terms, 229
fiber-optic bolt, 95
fibrinolytic therapy, 184
Fick's Law, 14
filo-viruses, 216
Fisher scale, 184
fixed wing air transport, 10, 21
flail chest, 104
flight safety and survival, 20–26
   aircraft components, 21–22, 23
   clock method, 24
   controlled flight into terrain, 25
   critical phases of flight, 24
   emergency procedures, 25–26
   Federal Aviation Administration, 20, 24
   fitness standards, 23
   in-flight emergency, 25
   preflight procedures, 24
   protective equipment, 20, 23
   safety committee tasks, 20
   weight considerations, 22
fracture classification, 137–38, 140
frostbite, 247

gases, 263–64
gas exchange, 151–52
gas laws, 14
gas pressure, 13–14, 18
gastritis, 193
gastroenteritis, 213
gastrointestinal emergencies, 192–99

blood urea nitrogen, 195
cholecystitis, acute, 192
diagnostic imaging studies, 196
diverticulitis, 192, 194
gastritis, 193
GI bleeds, 193, 194, 195
Grey Turner's sign, 196
intestinal components, 192–93
Levine tube, single-lumen, 197
liver cirrhosis, 193, 195
liver disease and failure, 197
Mallory-Weiss tear, 194
pancreatitis, acute, 192, 196
peptic ulcers, 192, 193
Salem sump nasogastric tube, 197
Stress-related erosive syndrome, 193
treatments of, 195–96
tubes for, 198–99
gastrostomy tube replacement, 4
Gay-Lussac's Law, 14, 16
GCS. See Glasgow Coma Score/Scale (GCS)
genitourinary trauma. See abdominal and genitourinary trauma
geriatric trauma, 147–48
GI bleeds, 193, 194, 195
Glasgow Coma Score/Scale (GCS), 88, 92, 145–46
Global Initiative for Chronic Obstructive Lung Disease (GOLD), 160
global positioning satellite (GPS), 11
glycolysis, 43
GOLD. See Global Initiative for Chronic Obstructive Lung Disease (GOLD)
GPS. See global positioning satellite (GPS)
Graham's Law, 14
gravitational (G) forces, 16
Grey Turner's sign, 196
ground transport, 6–7
gum elastic bougie, 36
gynecological emergencies. See obstetrical and gynecological emergencies, high risk

HACE. See high-altitude cerebral edema (HACE)
hallucinogens, 257
hantaviruses, 216
HAPE. See high-altitude pulmonary edema (HAPE)
HBOCs. See hemoglobin-based oxygen carrying solutions (HBOCs)
heart, donation and retrieval of, 277
heart failure, 165, 171, 172

heart murmurs, 165
heart rate, fetal, 229–30
heart sounds, 164
heat, defined, 125
heat exhaustion and stroke, 245–48
heat loss, 244–45
Heimlich valve, 154
helicopter transport, 10
HELLP syndrome, 231
hemicraniectomy, 95
hemodynamic monitoring. See cardiac and hemodynamic monitoring
hemoglobin-based oxygen carrying solutions (HBOCs), 44, 45
hemorrhagic shock, 89
hemothorax, 101–2
Henry's Law, 14
hepatic portal hypertension, 193
high-altitude cerebral edema (HACE), 17
high-altitude pulmonary edema (HAPE), 17
high-pressure neurologic syndrome (HPNS), 252
hip fractures, types of, 139
HIV, 210
Horner's syndrome, 123
hospital environment, paramedic in, 287–88
HPNS. See high-pressure neurologic syndrome (HPNS)
Hunt and Hess scale, 184
Hymenoptera, 265
hyperkalemia, 56
hypertensive emergencies, 171–72
hypoglycemia, pediatric, 225
hypoperfusion, 224
hypothalamic compression, 96, 97
hypothalamus, 180
hypothermia, 246, 247
hypoxia, 14–15

IAPB. See intra-aortic balloon pumps (IAPB)
ICP. See intracranial pressure (ICP)
Ideal Gas Law, 14
IFR. See instrument flight rules (IFR)
ILS. See instrument landing system (ILS)
infectious disease emergencies, 207–18
actinomycetes, 208
AIDS complex, 210
anthrax, 215
antibiotic-resistant organisms, 214
arenaviruses, 216
botulism, 215
Centers for Disease Control, 209
chicken pox, 214

clostridium tetani, 213
community acquired pneumonia, 211
elements of, basic, 208
gastroenteritis, 213
hantaviruses, 216
HIV, 210
influenza, 211
microorganisms, 207, 208
mumps virus, 213
mycotoxins, 218
organisms, 207
OSHA documents, 208–9
severe acute respiratory syndrome, 212
smallpox, 215
toxic shock syndrome, 214
treatments, 217
tuberculosis, 211–12
United States Standards, 209
vaccines, 218
viruses, 207
Yersinia pestis (plague), 214, 215
in-flight emergency, 25
influenza, 211
initial assessment for patient transport, 29
instrument flight rules (IFR), 11
instrument landing system (ILS), 11
Intensive Care Unit, first, 2
intestinal components, 192–93
intra-aortic balloon pumps (IAPB), 6, 51, 170, 174
intracranial compartment, 96
intracranial pressure (ICP), 93, 94, 97, 98–99
intraosseous needle placement, 4
invasive hemodynamic monitoring, 6, 7
ischemia, 182–83
isoenzyme sources, 83

kidneys, 201, 202
injuries to, 113, 114, 115
renal and acid-base emergencies, 201–5, 202
renal collecting system, 115
renal failure, 204–5
stones, 202

labor, in high risk delivery, 230–31
laboratory and diagnostic tests, interpretation of, 81–85
anion gap, 82
bilirubin, 83
bivalent cation, 82
blood cells and, 81–82
isoenzyme sources, 83

laparotomy, 110
laryngeal cartilage, 35
laryngopharynx, 120
laryngoscope, 7, 36
left ventricle, 163–64
Levine tube, single-lumen, 197
Lindegaard ratio, 185
liver cirrhosis, 193, 195
liver disease and failure, 109–10, 197
Liver Injury Scale, 110
Lown-Ganong-Levine syndrome, 56
lungs, 35, 36
lung sounds, 155–56

Mallampati class, 39
Mallory-Weiss tear, 194
MAOIs. See monoamine oxidase inhibitors (MAOIs)
MASH, 3
material safety data sheet (MSDS), 263
mechanism of injury (MOI), 128
mechanism of injury/nature of illness (MOI/NOI), 29, 128
mediastinitis, 17
Medicare, 3, 6
meningococcal meningitis, 185–86
metals, 265
methanol poisoning, 203
microorganisms, 207, 208
microwave landing system (MLS), 11
midline shift, 94
MLS. See microwave landing system (MLS)
Modified Central Leads, 53, 54, 55, 57
MOI. See mechanism of injury (MOI)
MOI/NOI. See mechanism of injury/nature of illness (MOI/NOI)
monoamine oxidase inhibitors (MAOIs), 259
Monroe-Kellie hypothesis, 96
MSDS. See material safety data sheet (MSDS)
mumps virus, 213
mustard gas, 271
mycotoxins, 218
myocardial contusion, 107
myocardial infarction, acute, 165, 172

Nagel, Eugene, 2
NEC. See necrotizing enterocolitis (NEC)
neck trauma. See face/ear/ocular/neck trauma

necrotizing enterocolitis (NEC), 241
Neisseria gonorrhea, 84
neonatal emergencies, 235–42
  airway, managing the, 235–36
  assessment and treatment of, 242
  bilirubin, 241–42
  blood flow, 236–37
  diaphragmatic herniation, congenital, 239
  heart defect, congenital, 239
  hypoglycemia, 235
  necrotizing enterocolitis, 241
  patent *ductus arteriosus,* 240
  persistent pulmonary hypertension of the newborn, 237
  respiratory failure, 237, 238
  tetralogy of Fallot, 240–41
  thermoregulation, inability to maintain, 235
neurohumoral agents, 44
neurologic emergencies, 176–90
  afferent (descending) sensory, 178
  Alzheimer's disease, 188
  arteries, cerebral, 178–79, 183
  assessing and transporting patients, 182–89
  autonomic nervous system, 180–81
  brain structure, 176–77, 181
  cerebrospinal fluid, 177
  corticospinal motor system, 179
  diagnostic imaging equipment, 182
  efferent (ascending) sensory, 178
  encephalopathy, 187
  extrapyramidal system, 180
  fibrinolytic therapy, 184
  Fisher scale, 184
  Hunt and Hess scale, 184
  hypothalamus, 180
  ischemia, 182–83
  meningococcal meningitis, 185–86
  motor control and, 179–80
  nerve tracts, proprioreceptive, 180
  spina bifida, 189–90
  spinal cord, 177–78
  stroke deficit assessments, 184
  vasospasm, 185
  vestibulocochlear nerve, 180
neurologic trauma, 92–99
  brain functions and, 93, 94
  central cord injury, 97
  electroencephalogram, 92–93
  evaluation tests, 92
  external auditory meatus, 94
  extraventricular drain, 94, 95
  fiber-optic bolt, 95
  Glasgow Coma Scale, 92

hemicraniectomy, 95
hypothalamic compression, 96, 97
intracranial compartment, 96
intracranial pressure, 93, 94, 97, 98–99
management of, 96
midline shift, 94
Monroe-Kellie hypothesis, 96
spinal cord injury, 98
tentorial herniation, 93
traumatic brain injury, 98
neuromuscular blocking agents, 38
Newton's First Law, 16
Newton's Second Law, 16
nitrogen narcosis, 251
nonsteroidal anti-inflammatory drugs (NSAIDs), 140, 194
NSAIDs. See nonsteroidal anti-inflammatory drugs (NSAIDs)

obstetrical and gynecological emergencies, high risk, 228–33
  assessment and treatment of, 232–33
  deliveries, 231
  extraembryonic membrane, 228
  fetal terms, 229
  heart rate, fetal, 229–30
  HELLP syndrome, 231
  labor, 230–31
  placenta previa, 230
obstetrical trauma, 148–49
ocular trauma. See face/ear/ocular/neck trauma
open pneumothorax, 103
organ donation and retrieval, 276–78
  brain death and, 276
  diabetes insipidus and, 277
  heart, 277
organisms, 207
orthopedic care, principles of, 136–40
  fracture classification, 137–38, 140
  hip fracture types, 139
  skeletal system, 136–37
OSHA documents, 208–9
oxygenation failure syndromes, 152

pancreatitis, acute, 192, 196
Pantridge, J. Frank, 2
patent *ductus arteriosus,* 240
patient care report (PCR), 284
patient transport, 28–33. See also air transport; flight safety and survival
  by air
  airway intervention, 30

burn patients, 29
critical care, 6–7, 9–11, 280–81
detailed physical examinations, 31–32
EMTALA/COBRA guidelines, 32
family members and, dealing with, 32–33
by ground, 6–7
high-priority patients, 30
information gathering, 28
initial assessment, 29
mechanism of injury/nature of illness and, 29
in neurologic emergencies, 182–89
pediatric, 143–45, 146
rapid physical examination, 30–31
rapid trauma assessment, 29
stabilizing for, 29
PCR. See patient care report (PCR)
pediatric medical emergencies, 220–26
anatomical characteristics, pediatric patients, 220–21
asthma, 223
bronchiolitis, 223
congenital cardiac defects, 225
croup, 222
Croup Scale, 222
drownings, 225
epiglottitis, 222–23
hypoglycemia, 225
hypoperfusion, 224
respiratory emergencies, 221–22, 225
resuscitation medications, administering, 226
shock, 224–25
pediatric trauma, 142–47
APGAR scale, 143
assessment triangle, 144
bradycardia, 145
fear and anxiety, minimizing, 142–43
Glasgow Coma Score/Scale, 145–46
shock, treatment for, 146–47
transporting, 143–45, 146
transporting, examining for, 143–45, 146
Pediatric Trauma Score, 88–89
PEEP. See positive-end-expiratory pressure (PEEP)
peptic ulcers, 192, 193
percussive sounds, 155
pericardial tamponade, 104, 105
pericardiocentesis, 105
pericarditis, 172

peripherally inserted central catheter (PICC), 174
persistent pulmonary hypertension of the newborn (PPHN), 237
pharmacology. See drugs
physical examination, detailed, 31–32
PICC. See peripherally inserted central catheter (PICC)
placenta previa, 230
plague, 273
pneumonia
 bacterial, 17
 community acquired, 211
poison control centers, 256
PolyHeme™, 45
positive-end-expiratory pressure (PEEP), 17, 49
PPHN. See persistent pulmonary hypertension of the newborn (PPHN)
proprioceptive nerve tracts, 180
pulmonary emergencies. See respiratory emergencies
pulse oximeter, 156
pulsus paradoxus, 104–5
pyogenic granuloma, 17

quality improvement (QI) programs, 281

radial arterial line placement, 172–73
radiation, 271–72
rapid physical examination, 30–31
rapid sequence induction (RSI), 38
renal and acid-base emergencies, 201–5
 antidiuretic hormone, 201
 buffer systems, 202, 203
 diabetic ketoacidosis, 204
 ethylene glycol poisoning, 204
 kidneys, 201, 202
 kidney stones, 202
 methanol poisoning, 203
 renal failure, 204–5
 salicylate poisoning, 204
renal collecting system, 115
renal failure, 204–5
reproductive system injuries, 113
rescue airways, 38–39, 40
respiratory emergencies, 151–61
 acute respiratory distress syndrome, 160
 alveolar hypoventilation, 152
 asthma, 158–59
 capnography, end tidal, 156–57
 chest contour variations, 154
 chronic obstructive pulmonary disease, 160

continuous positive airway pressure, 159
gas exchange, 151–52
Global Initiative for Chronic Obstructive Lung Disease, 160
Heimlich valve, 154
lung sounds and, 155–56
oxygenation failure syndromes, 152
pediatric, 221–22, 225
percussive sounds, 155
pulmonary agents and, 270
pulmonary contusion, 106
rescue airways, 38–39, 40
respiratory epithelium, 151–52
respiratory failure
 acute, 152, 157
 neonatal, 237, 238
severe acute respiratory syndrome, 212
ventilation and perfusion mismatch, 153, 154
respiratory epithelium, 151–52
resuscitation medications, pediatric, 226
Revised Trauma Score, 88
rhabdomyolysis, 132
right ventricular infarction, 57
RSI. See rapid sequence induction (RSI)

Sagan's First Law, 16
Salem sump nasogastric tube, 197
salicylate overdose and poisoning, 204, 261
SA node, 163
SARS. See severe acute respiratory syndrome (SARS)
severe acute respiratory syndrome (SARS), 212
shock, 43–45
 anaerobic metabolism, 44
 assessment and management of patient, 43–45
 cell lysis, 44
 decompensated shock, 44
 derangement of function, 44
 glycolysis, 43
 hemoglobin-based oxygen carrying solutions, 44, 45
 neurohumoral agents, 44
 pediatric, 146–47, 224–25
 PolyHeme™, 45
 types of, 45
Six-sigma programs, 280
skeletal system, 136–37
small-airframe rotorcraft air transport, 10, 11, 20–21

smallpox, 215
snake bites, 265–66
spatial disorientation, 16
spider bites, 266
spina bifida, 189–90
spinal cord, 177–78
spinal cord injury, 98
Spleen Injury Scale, 110, 113
SRES. *See* Stress-related erosive syndrome (SRES)
stenosis, aortic and mitral, 172
Stress-related erosive syndrome (SRES), 193
stroke deficit assessments, 184
subclavian central line, 48
succinylcholine, 37
SVR. *See* systemic vascular resistance (SVR)
Swan-Ganz catheter, 48, 50, 51
systemic vascular resistance (SVR), 45

TBSA. *See* total body surface area (TBSA)
TCA. *See* tricarboxylic acid (TCA)
temperature conversions, 244
tentorial herniation, 93
tetralogy of Fallot, 240–41
thermoregulation, inability to maintain, 235
Third Law of Thermodynamics, 16
thoracic trauma, 101–7
  aortic rupture, 105
  assessment of, 101
  chest tube insertion, 102–3
  diaphragmatic rupture, 106
  emergency management of, 101
  flail chest, 104
  hemothorax, 101–2
  myocardial contusion, 107
  open pneumothorax, 103
  pericardial tamponade, 104, 105
  pericardiocentesis, 105
  pulmonary contusion, 106
  pulsus paradoxus, 104–5
  tracheobronchial disruption, 106
total body surface area (TBSA), 127–30, 128–29, 130
toxicological emergencies, 256–66
  acetaminophen overdose, 260–61
  drug abuse, 256
  gases, 263–64
  hallucinogens, 257
  Hymenoptera, 265
  MAOIs, 259
  material safety data sheet, 263
  metals, 265
  over-the-counter drugs, 261, 262
  poison control centers, 256
  salicylate overdose, 261
  signs and symptoms, 262–63
  snake bites, 265–66
  spider bites, 266
  toxidrome, 257, 258, 259
  warfare agents, 264
toxic shock syndrome (TSS), 214
toxidrome, 257, 258, 259
tracheobronchial disruption, 106
Transcranial Doppler, 185
transport. *See* patient transport
transvenous pacing, 6
trauma, introduction to, 87–90
  Glasgow Coma Score, 88
  hemorrhagic shock, 89
  Pediatric Trauma Score, 88–89
  Revised Trauma Score, 88
  TRISS scoring system, 88
traumatic brain injury, 98
tricarboxylic acid (TCA), 43
TRISS scoring system, 88
TSS. *See* toxic shock syndrome (TSS)
tuberculosis, 211–12
12-Lead ECG, 166–68

ultrasound techniques, 111
United States Standards, 209

vaccines, 218
vasospasm, 185
vecuronium, 37
ventilation. *See* airway management and ventilation
ventilation and perfusion (V/Q) ratio, 153, 154
ventilators, 40–41
vertigo, 17
vestibulocochlear complex, 119
vestibulocochlear nerve, 180
VFR. *See* visual flight rules (VFR)
viruses, 207
visual flight rules (VFR), 10–11
V/Q ratio. *See* ventilation and perfusion (V/Q) ratio

warfare agents, 264
WASS. *See* wide area augmentation system (WAAS)
weapons of mass destruction, 268–74
  anthrax, 273
  biological agents, 273
  chemicals, 268–69
  cyanide exposure, 270–71
  explosive devices, 272–73
  mustard gas, 271
  plague, 273
  pulmonary agents, 270
  radiation, 271–72
wide area augmentation system (WAAS), 11
Wolff-Parkinson-White syndrome, 55

Yersinia pestis (plague), 214, 215